Harty's endodontics in clinical practice

Commissioning Editor: *Alison Taylor*
Development Editor: *Fiona Conn*
Project Manager: *Mahalakshmi Nithyanand*
Designer/Design Direction: *Charles Gray*
Illustration Manager: *Bruce Hogarth*
Illustrator: *Antbits*

Harty's endodontics in clinical practice

Sixth edition

Edited by

Bun San Chong BDS (Lond), MSc. (Lond), PhD (Lond), LDS RCS (Eng), FDS RCS (Eng), MFGDP (UK), MRD

Specialist in Endodontics
London, UK

Illustrations by

Antbits

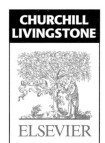

Edinburgh London New York Oxford Philadelphia St Louis Sydney Toronto 2010

CHURCHILL LIVINGSTONE
ELSEVIER

First Edition published 1976
Second Edition published 1982
Third edition published 1990
Fourth edition published 1997
Fifth edition © 2004, Elsevier Science Limited
Sixth edition © 2010, Elsevier Limited. All rights reserved.

ISBN 978 0 7020 3156 4

British Library Cataloguing in Publication Data
A catalogue record for this book is available from the British Library

Library of Congress Cataloging in Publication Data
A catalog record for this book is available from the Library of Congress

Notice

Knowledge and best practice in this field are constantly changing. As new research and experience broaden our knowledge, changes in practice, treatment and drug therapy may become necessary or appropriate. Readers are advised to check the most current information provided (i) on procedures featured or (ii) by the manufacturer of each product to be administered, to verify the recommended dose or formula, the method and duration of administration, and contraindications. It is the responsibility of the practitioner, relying on their own experience and knowledge of the patient, to make diagnoses, to determine dosages and the best treatment for each individual patient, and to take all appropriate safety precautions. To the fullest extent of the law, neither the Publisher nor the Editor assumes any liability for any injury and/or damage to persons or property arising out of or related to any use of the material contained in this book.

The Publisher

ELSEVIER your source for books, journals and multimedia in the health sciences

www.elsevierhealth.com

Working together to grow libraries in developing countries

www.elsevier.com | www.bookaid.org | www.sabre.org

ELSEVIER   BOOK AID International   Sabre Foundation

The publisher's policy is to use **paper manufactured from sustainable forests**

Printed in China

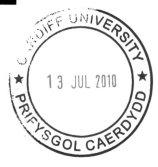

Preface

The new edition of this long-established book has come full circle, back to where it began. Fred Harty, after whom this book is named, was responsible for the first three editions and I have been a specialist in endodontics for over 20 years in the practice founded by Fred.

Tom Pitt Ford was responsible for the fourth and fifth editions of this book. We had other plans for further collaboration but, unfortunately, Tom passed away in the early stages of this project and so this edition is dedicated to him as a fitting tribute.

Tom was the Professor of Endodontology, Vice-Dean of King's College London Dental Institute at Guy's, King's College and St Thomas' Hospitals, and previously Director of Education. He was also Director of Institutional and Academic Audit at King's College, London. A man of extraordinary talent, Tom's death is an irreplaceable loss to dentistry and in particular the specialty of endodontics. Clinician, teacher, researcher, author and administrator, Tom's roles were numerous and his contributions to advancing endodontics immeasurable. Those privileged to have trained or worked with him, including many of the contributors to this edition, will forever remember and admire his example of diligence, perseverance and attention to detail.

The aim of this book is for it to be an authoritative guide to proven, current clinical endodontic practice. It is primarily intended as an essential undergraduate text for dental students in the United Kingdom. Since it is imperative that practitioners keep up to date, continuing education is now a mandatory requirement, so the book is also intended for dental practitioners seeking to update their knowledge, to help and support especially those who have chosen to embark on continuing education courses.

Despite the recognition and the establishment of a specialist list in endodontics in the United Kingdom, endodontic treatment will continue to be carried out mostly in general dental practice. Students and new graduates should not only be competent in treating the majority of endodontic cases but also be able to recognize, where appropriate, the need for referral to a specialist. A growing number of patients can now benefit from management of challenging or complex endodontic treatment by specially trained practitioners and can expect to receive a predictable outcome.

Diagnosis is the first step in the care and management of any patient so a new chapter on this topic is included in this edition. The style of referencing has also been replaced with the Vancouver system so that it is unobtrusive and easy to read. Illustrations, including line artwork, are now in full colour.

It is inevitable that there will be some duplication of material in this book and this should be viewed as reinforcement of relevant information. Different contributors will also have different writing styles and preferred terminology but, hopefully, not at the expense of clarity and cohesion.

I am grateful to all the contributors for providing their perspective on the topics covered in this new edition. I would also like to thank the publishers. I acknowledge the patience and understanding of my family, Grace, James and Louisa.

B.S. Chong
2009

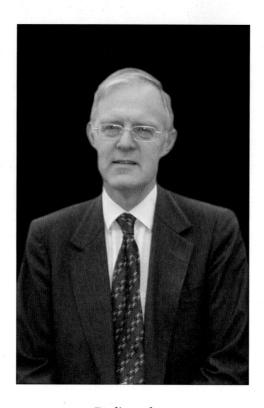

Dedicated to
Professor Thomas Russell Pitt Ford
BDS (Lond), LDS RCS (Eng), PhD (Lond),
FDS RCPS (Glas), FDS RCS (Eng), FDS RCS (Edin)
1949–2008

Contributors

Nicholas P. Chandler BDS, MSc., PhD, LDS RCS (Eng),
FDS RCPS (Glas) FDS RCS (Edin), FFD RCSI
Associate Professor of Endodontics,
School of Dentistry, University of Otago, Dunedin,
New Zealand

Bun San Chong BDS, MSc., PhD, LDS RCS (Eng),
FDS RCS (Eng), MFGDP (UK), MRD
Specialist in Endodontics,
London, UK

Henry F. Duncan BDS, MClinDent, MRD RCS (Edin),
FDS RCS (Edin)
Lecturer/Consultant in Endodontics,
Dublin Dental School & Hospital, Trinity College Dublin,
Dublin, Ireland

Michael P. Escudier MBBS, BDS, FDS RCS, FDS (OM)
RCS (Eng), FFGDP (UK)
Senior Lecturer/Honorary Consultant in Oral Medicine,
Dental Institute, King's College London, UK

Massimo Giovarruscio DDS
Specialist in Endodontics, Rome, Italy

James L. Gutmann DDS, Cert Endo, PhD, FICD,
FACD, FADI
Professor Emeritus, Baylor College of Dentistry, Texas A & M
University System, Dallas, Texas, USA

Francesco Mannocci MD, DDS, PhD
Senior Lecturer/Honorary Consultant in Endodontology,
Dental Institute, King's College London, UK

Philip J.C. Mitchell BDS, LDS RCS (Eng), MSc.,
MRD RCS (Edin)
Senior Specialist Clinical Teacher/Specialist in Endodontics,
Dental Institute, King's College London, UK

Amanda L. O'Donnell BDS, MFDS (Eng), MClin Dent,
MPaedDent, FDS RCS (Eng)
Consultant in Paediatric Dentistry,
UCL Eastman Dental Institute, London, UK

Dag Ørstavik Cand Odont, Dr Odont.
Professor of Endodontics,
Institute of Clinical Dentistry, University of Oslo, Oslo,
Norway

Shanon Patel BDS, MSc., MClinDent, MFDS RCS (Eng),
MRD RCS (Edin)
Specialist in Endodontics,
Dental Institute, King's College London, London, UK

Heather E. Pitt Ford LDS RCS (Eng), FDS RCS (Eng)
Associate Specialist in Paediatric Dentistry,
Dental Institute, King's College London, UK

John D. Regan BDentSc., MSc., MS
Honorary Associate Professor,
Baylor College of Dentistry, Texas A & M University System,
Dallas, Texas, USA

John S. Rhodes BDS, MSc., MFGDP (UK),
MRD RCS (Edin)
Specialist in Endodontics,
Poole, Dorset, UK

Ilan Rotstein DDS
Professor of Endodontics,
Chair, Surgical Therapeutic and Bioengineering Sciences,
Associate Dean, Continuing Oral Health
Professional Education,
University of Southern California School of Dentistry
Los Angeles, California, USA

James H.S. Simon BA, DDS
Professor of Endodontics, Director, Advanced
Endodontic Program,
University of Southern California School of Dentistry
Los Angeles, California, USA

Andrew D.M. Watson BDS, MSc., DGDP (UK), MRD
Specialist in Endodontics, Cheshire, UK

Contents

Contents

Contents

Contents

Chapter | 1 |

Introduction and overview

B.S. Chong

SUMMARY

The science and art of endodontics has come a long way since the early days. A brief review of the history of endodontics is helpful in understanding its influence on current practice. The scope of modern endodontics is now wider and encompasses a variety of procedures. Patients are no longer willing to accept tooth loss and have higher treatment and care expectations. Microorganisms have an essential role in the pathogenesis of pulpal and periapical diseases. The host defence response against root canal infection includes numerous inflammatory mediators and a range of cells. Continuing research is increasing our knowledge of the root canal microbiota, which will hopefully result in dedicated strategies to manage the different types of root canal infection. Advances in endodontics are continuing and many recent developments have been successfully translated into everyday clinical practice.

INTRODUCTION

Endodontology is the branch of dental sciences concerned with the form, function, health of, injuries to and the diseases of the dental pulp and periradicular region, and their relationship with systemic well-being and health. Endodontic treatment can be defined as the prevention or treatment of apical periodontitis, the principal disease. The concept of treating the pulp of the tooth to preserve the tooth itself is a relatively modern development in the history of dentistry and it may be useful to review, very briefly, the history of pulp treatment in order to appreciate better modern views on endodontic treatment. Toothache has been a scourge of mankind from the earliest times. Both the Chinese and the Egyptians left records describing caries and alveolar abscesses. The Chinese believed that these abscesses were caused by a white worm with a black head which lived within the tooth. The 'worm theory' was current until the middle of the eighteenth century when doubts were raised,[1] but they could not be expressed forcibly because those in authority still believed in the worm theory.[2] The Chinese treatment for an abscessed tooth was aimed at killing the worm with a preparation that contained arsenic. The use of this drug was taught in most dental schools as recently as the 1950s in spite of the realization that it was self-limiting and that extensive tissue destruction occurred if even minute amounts of the drug leaked into the soft tissues. Pulp treatment during Greek and Roman times was aimed at destroying the pulp by cauterization with a hot needle or boiling oil, or with a preparation containing opium and hyoscyamus. About the end of the first century AD, it was realized that pain could be relieved by drilling into the pulp chamber to obtain drainage. In spite of modern antibiotics, there is

© 2009 Elsevier Ltd, Inc, BV
DOI: 10.1016/B978-0-7020-3156-4.00004-8

still no better method of relieving the pain of an abscessed tooth than drainage.

Endodontic knowledge remained static until the sixteenth century when pulpal anatomy was described. Until the latter part of the nineteenth century, root canal therapy consisted of alleviating pulpal pain and the main function of the opened root canal was to provide retention for a dowel crown.[3,4] At the same time, bridgework became popular and many dental schools taught that no tooth should be used as an abutment unless it was first devitalized.[5] Root canal therapy became commonplace partly for these reasons and also because the discovery of cocaine led to painless pulp extirpation. The injection of 4% cocaine as a mandibular nerve block was first reported in 1884;[4] and 20 years later, the first synthetic local anaesthetic, procaine was produced. Around this time, reports of endodontic surgery appeared.[6] The first radiograph of teeth was taken in 1896,[3,7] shortly after the discovery of X-rays by Roentgen in 1895. This further popularized root canal therapy and gave it some respectability. About the same time dental manufacturers began to produce special instruments, which were used primarily to remove pulp tissue or clean debris from the canal. There was no concept of filling the root canals since the object of the procedure was to provide retention for a post crown.

By 1910 'root canal therapy' had reached its zenith and no self-respecting dentist would extract a tooth. Every root stump was retained and a crown constructed. Sinus tracts often appeared and were treated by various ineffective methods for many years. The connection between the sinus tract and the pulpless tooth was known but not acted upon. In 1911, William Hunter[8,9] attacked 'American dentistry' and blamed bridgework for several diseases of unknown aetiology. He reported recovery from these conditions in a few patients following extraction of their teeth. It is interesting to note that he did not condemn root canal therapy itself but rather the ill-fitting bridgework and the sepsis that surrounded it. About this time microbiology became established and the findings of microbiologists added fuel to the fire of Hunter's condemnations. Radiography, which at first helped the dentist, now provided irrefutable evidence of apical periodontitis surrounding the roots of pulpless teeth.

Whilst the theory of 'focal infection' was not enunciated by Billings[10] until 1918, Hunter's condemnations started a reaction to root canal therapy, and there began the wholesale removal of both non-vital and perfectly healthy teeth. The blame for obscure diseases was placed on the dentition, and as dentists could not refute this theory, countless mouths were mutilated. Naturally, not all dentists accepted this wholesale dental destruction. Some, particularly in continental Europe, continued to save teeth in spite of the focal sepsis theory. It is difficult to know why dentists in continental Europe disregarded this theory and one explanation may be that their patients equated the loss of teeth with a loss of virility, and therefore, did not allow their dentists to mutilate their dentitions. Alternatively, it could be that these practitioners were not so readily swayed by fashion as were their British colleagues.

MODERN ENDODONTICS

The re-emergence of endodontics as a respectable branch of dental science began in the 1930s.[11,12] The occurrence and degree of bacteraemia during tooth extraction was shown to depend on the severity of periodontal disease and the amount of tissue damage at operation. The incongruity between microbiological findings in the treatment of chronic oral infection and the histological picture was demonstrated. When the gingival sulcus was disinfected by cauterization before extraction, microorganisms could not be demonstrated in the bloodstream immediately postoperatively.

Gradually, the concept that a 'dead' tooth, one without a pulp, was not necessarily infected began to be accepted. Further, it was realized that the function and usefulness of the tooth depended on the integrity of the periodontal tissues and not on the vitality of the pulp.[13] Another important advance was clarification of the 'hollow tube' theory[14] by research using sterile polyethylene tube implants in rats.[15,16] The tissue surrounding the lumina of clean, disinfected tubes, which were closed at one end, was relatively free of inflammation and displayed a normal capacity for repair. When such tubes were filled with muscle, the inflammatory reaction was only severe around the openings of the tubes containing tissue contaminated with Gram-negative cocci. These findings place stress on the microbial contents of the tube; if the tube contains microorganisms then the potential for repair is far less favourable than when the lumen of the tube is clean and sterile.[17] This infected situation is likely to be found in most root canals requiring treatment. The concept that 'apical seal' was important led to the search for filling and sealing materials that were stable, non-irritant and provided a perfect seal at the apical foramen. With the more recent realization of the importance of coronal leakage[18,19] and the biodegradation of root canal fillings, total filling of the root canal space, including lateral and accessory canals, has assumed much greater importance.

Until relatively recently, practitioners were preoccupied with a mechanistic approach to root canal treatment and to the perceived effects of various potent drugs on the microorganisms within the root canal rather than a total antimicrobial approach of effective cleaning, adequate shaping and complete filling of the root canal space.[20] This preoccupation diverted attention from the effects of such drugs on the periapical tissues. Medicaments that kill microbes may also be toxic to living tissue.[21] The consequences of such materials passing out of the tooth into the surrounding vital tissues can be localized tissue necrosis. These avoidable problems cause distress to patients and can lead to litigation. Effective elimination of microorganisms from root canal system is best achieved by instrumentation combined with irrigation.

SCOPE OF ENDODONTICS

The extent of the subject has altered considerably in the last 50 years. Formerly, endodontic treatment confined itself to root canal filling techniques by conventional methods; even endodontic surgery, which is an extension of these methods, was considered to be in the field of oral surgery. Modern endodontics has a much wider field[22,23] and includes the following:

- the differential diagnosis and treatment of orofacial pain of pulpal and periradicular origin
- prevention of pulpal disease and vital pulp therapy
- root canal treatment
- management of post-treatment endodontic disease
- surgical endodontics
- bleaching of endodontically treated teeth
- treatment procedures related to coronal restorations using a core and/or a post involving the root canal space
- endodontically related measures in connection with crown-lengthening and forced eruption procedures
- treatment of traumatized teeth.

ROLE OF MICROORGANISMS

The Chinese belief that dental abscesses were caused by small organisms, worms, persisted until the eighteenth century. At the end of the nineteenth century Miller[24] demonstrated the role of bacteria in root canal infection, and noted that different microorganisms were found in the root canal compared with the open pulp chamber. Shortly afterwards, systematic culturing of root canals was undertaken.[25] Unfortunately, these methods, which were potentially so valuable for improving the outcome of root canal treatment, were used to condemn much of the dentistry carried out at the time.[9] During the 1930s, microbiological techniques were used to re-establish the scientific basis of root canal treatment. However, techniques at that time only readily identified aerobic bacteria, and led to confusing results in later clinical studies.[26,27] This resulted in clinicians being complacent about the role of microorganisms, and performing treatment simply as a technical exercise.

The development of anaerobic culturing allowed the identification of many previously unknown microorgan-

isms present in root canals.[28] This led rapidly to the demonstration that the majority of these microorganisms were anaerobes,[29,30] and the realization that canals previously considered sterile contained anaerobes alone. Furthermore, when traumatized teeth were examined, there was a close correlation between the presence of anaerobic bacteria in the root canal and a periapical radiolucency;[30] in the absence of infection, the necrotic pulp and stagnant tissue fluids cannot induce or perpetuate a periapical lesion. This was later demonstrated experimentally in teeth where the pulp tissue had been removed; only in those where the pulp was infected did periapical inflammation occur.[31] Although anaerobic culturing of root canals is not a technique applicable to everyday clinical practice, the results of research have provided rational explanations for pulp and periapical diseases and its treatment.[32] Microorganisms, which previously could not be cultured, and so were mistakenly considered absent, can now be identified. Over 50% of the oral microbiota is still uncultivable.[33,34] However, the use of molecular biology techniques has enabled the identification of microbes that would be undetectable by conventional culturing techniques.[33,35,36] As knowledge in this area expands, our understanding of the root canal microbiota is changing. The presence of specific or combination of microorganisms and their implications are yet to be fully appreciated.[37]

Most root canal infections contain a mixture of microorganisms with bacteria being the main candidate pathogen.[30,38,39] It has also been shown that the relative proportions of different microorganism are determined by the local environmental conditions.[39] Endodontic pathogens do not occur at random but are found in specific combinations.[40] If a selection of microorganisms is inoculated into root canals in fixed proportions, their relative numbers will change over time, with a decline in aerobes and an increase in anaerobes.[39] It has also been established that combinations of microorganisms are more likely to survive than inocula of single species.[38] It is clear that one species can produce substances that others can metabolize in order to survive, forming complex ecological and nutritional relationships.[32]

Microorganisms are normally confined to the root canal system in pulpless teeth and exist in two forms:

- planktonic – loose collections or suspensions within the root canal lumen
- biofilm – dense aggregate, forming plaques on and within the root canal wall.

The intraradicular infection may be divided into three categories:

- Primary – caused by microorganisms that initially invaded and colonized the necrotic pulp.
- Secondary – caused by microorganisms that were not present in the primary infection but were introduced into the root canal system following dental intervention.

- Persistent infection – caused by microorganisms associated with the primary or secondary infection that managed to survive treatment procedures and nutritional deprivation.

It is unusual for microorganisms to be present in periapical lesions; the host defences prevent them from invading the periapical tissues.[41] However, in certain circumstances and with some species, microorganisms may establish an extraradicular infection, which can be dependent or independent of the intraradicular infection; thankfully, the incidence of independent extraradicular infection in untreated teeth is low.[42]

TISSUE RESPONSE TO ROOT CANAL INFECTION

The role of infection in the demise of damaged pulps was demonstrated in a classic study by Kakehashi and co-workers in the 1960s,[43] and eventually led to a biological approach to operative dentistry.[44] The presence of microorganisms, their byproducts or damaged tissue in the root canal can cause apical periodontitis, typically at the apical foramen but also around the foramina of any lateral or accessory canals or at a fracture. The periapical inflammation prevents the spread of infection from the tooth into the alveolar bone, otherwise osteomyelitis would occur. The inflammatory lesion contains inflammatory mediators and numerous inflammatory cells, e.g. polymorphonuclear leucocytes, macrophages, B- and T-lymphocytes and plasma cells.[45] The interaction between these cells and the antigenic substances from the root canal results in the release of a large number of inflammatory mediators. The inflammatory mediators include neuropeptides, the complement system, lysozymes and metabolites of arachidonic acid.[46] Prostaglandins, leucotrienes and cytokines play an important role in the development of periapical lesions.[45,46]

As long as antigens emerge from the canal foramina, there will be a continuing inflammatory response, mediated in a number of different ways. This is a very dynamic response to rapidly multiplying microorganisms in the root canal, and may not be readily apparent to the clinician observing a radiograph or a histologist examining a slide of fixed cells. Endodontic treatment is primarily directed at effective elimination of the microorganisms, allowing inflammation to subside and healing to occur.

QUALITY ASSURANCE

The general public across the world now expect professional people to deliver a high standard of service; dentistry, and endodontic treatment in particular, is no exception. In the UK, guidance has been published by the regulatory body on the standards expected of,[47] and the scope of practice for,[48] the whole dental team. The European Society of Endodontology has issued quality guidelines for endodontic treatment.[49] It is essential that dental practices have a quality control system to ensure that each step in history, diagnosis and treatment is carried out in a logical and consistent manner. This is to ensure a high standard of care and treatment, known as clinical governance. Patients are increasingly well informed and will not tolerate poor standards, e.g. in sterilization procedures or out-of-date views. In the UK and in line with many other countries, one of the largest source of dental negligence claims relate to endodontics.[50] The dramatic rise in litigation is a reflection that patients are increasingly prepared to seek redress for any failures regarding their care or treatment.

In a recent survey in England of newly qualified dentists in vocational training to join the National Health Service, most expressed a lack of preparedness with regards to complex/molar endodontics, with 66% rating their preparedness as 'poor' and 3% 'very poor'.[51] Those dentists who have undertaken further training to become specialists are expected to achieve consistently high standards in diagnosis and treatment. However, general practitioners cannot continue to practise in the way that they were taught at dental school many years ago; they must keep up to date and offer referral to an appropriate specialist when the treatment required is beyond their skill. This change has already occurred in the USA and is spreading to other countries. In the UK, continuing professional development is now mandatory for recertification with the regulatory body and practitioners are also required to refer patients for further advice or treatment when it is necessary, or if requested by the patient.[47]

Almost all endodontic procedures can be carried out with a predictable outcome. Root canal treatment has a reported success rate of over 90%,[52,53] even though closer analysis reveals that retreatment of teeth with apical periodontitis is less successful than initial treatment in teeth without apical periodontitis.[52,54] It is essential that individual practitioners monitor their outcomes against accepted criteria,[55] and that their treatment protocols conform to published guidelines.[49] Success of treatment can be measured in different ways[56] and should encompass not only clinical but also radiological evidence.

RECENT DEVELOPMENTS

The dental pulp may be damaged as a result of caries or infection consequent to trauma or operative dentistry. With a reduced incidence of dental caries, a greater emphasis on preventing sports injuries, and the preparation of smaller cavities combined with better restorative materials in operative dentistry, the expectation is a decline in the number of teeth with damaged pulps. However, the trend and popularity of 'cosmetic' dentistry potentially risks irreversibly compromising the pulp. The degree to which adhesive restorative materials will be successful in preventing pulp damage in clinical practice is another unquantifiable variable.

Recent progress in the understanding of the cellular and molecular processes involved in the dentine/pulp complex has heralded a new era of regenerative dentistry.[57] The media trumpeted research in this field with the assertion that one day everyone will be able to grow a completely new set of teeth. The identification of stem cells in the dental pulp, the bioactive molecules within the dentine matrix and specific processes promoting tissue regeneration will, hopefully, translate into biologically-based therapies in everyday clinical practice. The ability to control tissue injury, microbial infection, and inflammation will tip the balance so that instead of necrosis there will be regeneration and maintenance of pulpal vitality. Case reports have appeared on the revascularization of necrotic pulps in immature permanent teeth.[58,59] In the new and allied field of regenerative endodontics, the ultimate goal is to replace diseased, damaged or missing pulp tissues with healthy tissues to revitalize teeth.[60,61]

The management of persistent infection in previously endodontically treated teeth is challenging.[62,63,64] Endodontic pathogens have the capability to adapt, including the formation of biofilms, in response to changes in the root canal environment.[65,66] As the breadth of microbial diversity in the oral cavity has been revealed by molecular techniques,[33] several newly identified species/phylotypes have emerged as potential pathogens.[67] Findings have revealed new candidate endodontic pathogens, including as-yet-uncultivated bacteria and taxa, which may participate in the mixed infections associated with apical periodontitis in previously treated teeth.[61,68] Improved knowledge of the microbiota should, eventually, lead to dedicated strategies for managing different types of root canal infection, including those that are recalcitrant.

Images captured on X-ray films or via digital sensors are two-dimensional 'shadowgraphs' with inherent problems of geometric distortions and anatomical noise.[69] Cone Beam Computed Tomography (CBCT) is a relatively new imaging technique.[70] It is designed to overcome some of the deficiencies of conventional radiography.[71] CBCT produces undistorted and accurate images of the area under investigation enhancing diagnosis and in the process aiding, for example, the planning of endodontic surgery and the management of resorption lesions. Since CBCT is able to detect lesions that are not discernible on conventional radiographs, it should also enable more objective assessment of healing after endodontic treatment.

Since its introduction, the use of the operating microscope in endodontics has increased[72] and it has become an invaluable tool.[73] From diagnosis to canal location, through to canal preparation and filling, the improved vision and illumination afforded by the operating microscope is immensely beneficial.

Techniques, and in particular instruments, for preparation of root canals has altered substantially in recent years.[74,75] A crown-down concept is now the major approach to shaping and cleaning the root canals.[76] Manufacturers are always introducing, onto the market, newer instruments for preparation of root canals. The development of nickel-titanium rotary systems continues unabated, coupled with the promise of speed, ease and efficiency. However, not all claims can be substantiated and any instrument or technique is only as good as the operator. Endodontic treatment should always be guided by biological and evidence-based principles. Speed, expediency and technical wizardry does not guarantee a favourable treatment outcome.

There has been a quiet revolution in endodontic surgery. This treatment modality is no longer a substitute for failure to manage properly the root canal system non-surgically. The indications for endodontic surgery are reduced and non-surgical retreatment should first be considered. Newer root-end filling materials, among other advances, including developments in surgical armamentarium, the implementation of microsurgical techniques, enhanced illumination and magnification have helped improve the predictability and outcome of endodontic surgery.[77] The use of amalgam as a root-end filling material is confined to history with zinc oxide-eugenol materials and Mineral Trioxide Aggregate (MTA) now being widely used.[77] In the first prospective clinical study on the use of MTA as a root-end filling material, a high rate of success (92%) was achieved.[78] Further development of this novel material, with the unique ability to encourage hard tissue deposition, has helped promote the use of MTA not only as a root-end filling, but also a perforation sealant and pulp capping agent. Other similar tissue regenerative materials are being investigated.

The advent of implants has led to clinicians being confronted with the decision to either extract a tooth and place an implant or preserve the natural tooth by root canal treatment. There are debates about the advantages of implants versus endodontics[79,80,81] fuelled by the myopic perception within both camps that one discipline is a threat to the other. This has led to the movement to incorporate implant placement into endodontic surgery. In reality, both disciplines are complementary to each other.[82] Endodontic treatment of a tooth represents a feasible, practical and economical way to preserve function in a vast array of cases and in selected situations in which prognosis is poor, a dental implant is a suitable alternative.[83]

The importance of good coronal restoration of root-filled teeth has been highlighted.[18,19] This is facilitated by the use of adhesive materials where appropriate, and the placement of suitable bases, and well-fitting restorations.

Despite conflicting arguments about the relative importance between the quality of the root filling and the coronal restoration on treatment outcome, there can be no disagreement that both should be performed well[84,85,86] and are mutually beneficial to the long-term prognosis of the root treated tooth.[52,87]

A majority of endodontic treatment is within the capability of general practitioners but there will, inevitably, be cases that are best managed by specialists. Endodontic referral practice is undertaking more root canal retreatment because of technical deficiencies in the original treatment. In many cases, this is difficult and challenging but success can be very rewarding, particularly when in the past, the alternative would have been extraction. It is encouraging that many more patients are refusing to allow a tooth with an exposed or infected pulp to be extracted, but instead ask for it to be saved by root canal treatment.

High quality endodontic treatment will make a significant contribution to good oral health.

LEARNING OUTCOMES

At the end of this chapter, readers will be able to understand and discuss the:

- history of endodontics and its influence on current practice;
- scope of modern endodontics;
- essential role of microorganisms in the pathogenesis of pulpal and periapical diseases;
- tissue response to root canal infection;
- high standard of endodontic care and treatment expected by patients;
- recent developments in endodontics.

REFERENCES

1. Gutmann JL. History of Endodontics. In: Ingle JI, Bakland LK, Baumgartner JC, editors. Ingle's Endodontics. 6th ed. Hamilton, Ontario, Canada: BC Decker; 2008. p. 36–85.

2. Curson I. History and endodontics. Dental Practitioner and Dental Record 1965;15:435–439.

3. Cruse WP, Bellizzi R. A historic review of endodontics, 1689–1963, Part 1. Journal of Endodontics 1980;6:495–499.

4. Cruse WP, Bellizzi R. A historic review of endodontics, 1689–1963, Part 2. Journal of Endodontics 1980;6:532–535.

5. Prinz H. Dental Chronology. A Record of the More Important Historic Events in the Evolution of Dentistry. London, UK: Kimpton; 1945.

6. Gutmann JL, Harrison JW. Surgical Endodontics. Boston, MA, USA: Ishiyaku EuroAmerica; 1994.

7. Grossman LI. Endodontics 1776–1976: a bicentennial history against the background of general dentistry. Journal of the American Dental Association 1976;93:78–87.

8. Cruse WP, Bellizzi R. A historic review of endodontics, 1689–1963, Part 3. Journal of Endodontics 1980;6:576–580.

9. Hunter W. The role of sepsis and antisepsis in medicine. Lancet 1911;1:79–86.

10. Billings F. Focal Infection. New York, NY, USA: Appleton; 1918.

11. Fish EW, MacLean I. The distribution of oral streptococci in the tissues. British Dental Journal 1936;61:336–362.

12. Okell CC, Elliott SD. Bacteraemia and oral sepsis with special reference to the aetiology of subacute endocarditis. Lancet 1935;2:869–872.

13. Marshall JA. The relation to pulp-canal therapy of certain anatomical characteristics of dentin and cementum. Dental Cosmos 1928;70:253–263.

14. Rickert UG, Dixon CM. The controlling of root surgery. Paris, France: Eighth International Dental Congress. IIIa; 1931. p. 15–22.

15. Torneck CD. Reaction of rat connective tissue to polyethylene tube implants. Part I. Oral Surgery, Oral Medicine, Oral Pathology 1966;21:379–387.

16. Torneck CD. Reaction of rat connective tissue to polyethylene tube implants. Part II. Oral Surgery, Oral Medicine, Oral Pathology 1967;24:674–683.

17. Wu MK, Moorer WR, Wesselink PR. Capacity of anaerobic bacteria enclosed in a simulated root canal to induce inflammation. International Endodontic Journal 1989;22:269–277.

18. Chong BS. Coronal leakage and treatment failure. Journal of Endodontics 1995;21:159–160.

19. Saunders WP, Saunders EM. Coronal leakage as a cause of failure in root-canal therapy: a review. Endodontics and Dental Traumatology 1994;10:105–108.

20. Kawashima N, Wadachi R, Suda H, et al. Root canal medicaments. International Dental Journal 2009;59:5–11.

21. Chong BS, Pitt Ford TR. The role of intracanal medication in root canal treatment. International Endodontic Journal 1992;25:97–106.

22. American Association of Endodontists. Glossary of Endodontic Terms. 7th ed. Chicago, IL, USA: American Association of Endodontists; 2003.

23. European Society of Endodontology. Undergraduate curriculum guidelines for endodontology. International Endodontic Journal 2001;34:574–580.

24. Miller WD. An introduction to the study of the bacterio-pathology of the dental pulp. Dental Cosmos 1894;36:505–528.

25. Onderdonk TW. Treatment of unfilled root canals. International Dental Journal 1901;22:20–22.

26. Bender IB, Seltzer S, Turkenkopf S. To culture or not to culture? Oral Surgery, Oral Medicine, Oral Pathology 1964;18:527–540.

27. Seltzer S, Turkenkopf S, Vito A, Green D, Bender IB. A histologic evaluation of periapical repair following positive and negative root canal cultures. Oral Surgery, Oral Medicine, Oral Pathology 1964;17:507–532.

28. Möller AJR. Microbiological examination of root canals and periapical tissues of human teeth. Thesis, Akademiforlaget, Gothenberg, Sweden, 1966 p 1–380.

29. Kantz WE, Henry CA. Isolation and classification of anaerobic bacteria from intact chambers of non-vital teeth in man. Archives of Oral Biology 1974;19:91–96.

30. Sundqvist G. Bacteriological studies of necrotic dental pulps. Thesis. University of Umea, Umea, Sweden; 1976. p. 1–94.

31. Möller AJR, Fabricius L, Dahlén G, et al. Influence on periapical tissues of indigenous oral bacteria and necrotic pulp tissue in monkeys. Scandinavian Journal of Dental Research 1981;89:475–484.

32. Sundqvist G. Taxonomy, ecology, and pathogenicity of the root canal flora. Oral Surgery, Oral Medicine, Oral Pathology 1994;78:522–530.

33. Munson MA, Pitt-Ford T, Chong B, et al. Molecular and cultural analysis of the microflora associated with endodontic infections. Journal of Dental Research 2002;81:761–766.

34. Siqueira JF Jr, Rôças IN. Uncultivated phylotypes and newly named species associated with primary and persistent endodontic infections. Journal of Clinical Microbiology 2004;43:3314–3319.

35. Siqueira JF Jr, Rôças IN. Exploiting molecular methods to explore endodontic infections: Part 1 – Current molecular technologies for microbiological diagnosis. Journal of Endodontics 2005;31:411–423.

36. Siqueira JF Jr, Rôças IN. Exploiting molecular methods to explore endodontic infections: Part 2 -Redefining the endodontic microbiota. Journal of Endodontics 2005;31:488–498.

37. Nair PNR. Abusing technology? Culture-difficult microbes and microbial remnants. Oral Surgery, Oral Medicine, Oral Pathology, Oral Radiology and Endodontology 2007;104:569–570.

38. Fabricius L, Dahlén G, Holm SE, Möller AJR. Influence of combinations of oral bacteria on periapical tissues of monkeys. Scandinavian Journal of Dental Research 1982;90:200–206.

39. Fabricius L, Dahlén G, Öhman AE, Möller AJR. Predominant indigenous oral bacteria isolated from infected root canals after varied times of closure. Scandinavian Journal of Dental Research 1982;90:134–144.

40. Peters LB, Wesselink PR, van Winkelhoff AJ. Combinations of bacterial species in endodontic infections. International Endodontic Journal 2002;35:698–702.

41. Pitt Ford TR. The effects on the periapical tissues of bacterial contamination of the filled root canal. International Endodontic Journal 1982;15:16–22.

42. Siqueira JF Jr, Rôças IN. Update on endodontic microbiology: candidate pathogens and patterns of colonisation. ENDO (London England) 2008;2. p. 7–20.

43. Kakehashi S, Stanley HR, Fitzgerald RJ. The effects of surgical exposures of dental pulps in germ-free and conventional laboratory rats. Oral Surgery, Oral Medicine, Oral Pathology 1965;20:340–349.

44. Bergenholtz G, Cox CF, Loesche WJ, Syed SA. Bacterial leakage around dental restorations: its effect on the pulp. Journal of Oral Pathology 1982;11:439–450.

45. Kiss C. Cell-to-cell interactions. Endodontic Topics 2004;8:88–103.

46. Takahashi K. Microbiological, pathological, inflammatory, immunological and molecular biological aspects of periradicular disease. International Endodontic Journal 1998;31:311–325.

47. General Dental Council. Standards for dental professionals. London, UK: General Dental Council; 2005.

48. General Dental Council. Scope of practice. London, UK: General Dental Council; 2009.

49. European Society of Endodontology. Quality guidelines for endodontic treatment: consensus report of the European Society of Endodontology. International Endodontic Journal 2006;31:921–930.

50. Nehammer CF, Chong BS, Rattan R. Endodontics. Clinical Risk 2004;10:45–48.

51. Patel J, Fox K, Grieveson B, Youngson CC. Undergraduate training as preparation for vocational training in England: a survey of vocational dental practitioners' and their trainers' views. British Dental Journal 2006;201(Suppl):9–15.

52. Friedman S. Expected outcomes in the prevention and treatment of apical periodontitis. In: Ørstavik D, Pitt Ford TR, editors. Essential Endodontology. 2nd ed. Oxford, UK: Blackwell Munksgaard; 2008. p. 408–471.

53. Ng Y-L, Mann V, Rahbaran S, Lewsey J, Gulabivala K. Outcome of primary root canal treatment: systematic review of the literature – Part 2. Influence of clinical factors. International Endodontic Journal 2008;41:6–31.

54. Sjögren U, Hägglund B, Sundqvist G, Wing K. Factors affecting the long-term results of endodontic treatment. Journal of Endodontics 1990;16:498–504.

55. Chong BS. Highlighting deficiencies. British Dental Journal 2008;204:596–597.

56. Chong BS. Managing Endodontic Failure in Practice. London, UK: Quintessence Publishing Co. Ltd; 2004. p. 1–10.

57. Smith AJ, Lumley PJ, Tomson PL, Cooper PR. Dental regeneration and materials: a partnership. Clinical Oral Investigations 2008;12:103–108.

58. Reynolds K, Johnson JD, Cohenca N. Pulp revascularization of necrotic bilateral bicuspids using a modified novel technique to eliminate potential coronal

discolouration: a case report. International Endodontic Journal 2009;42:84–92.

59. Thibodeau B, Trope M. Pulp revascularization of a necrotic infected immature permanent tooth: case report and review of the literature. Pediatric Dentistry 2007;29:47–50.

60. Hargreaves KM, Giesler T, Henry M, Wang Y. Regeneration potential of the young permanent tooth: what does the future hold? Journal of Endodontics 2009;34(Suppl):S51–S56.

61. Murray PE, Garcia-Godoy F, Hargreaves KM. Regenerative endodontics: a review of current status and a call for action. Journal of Endodontics 2007;33:377–390.

62. Nair PNR. On the causes of persistent apical periodontitis: a review. International Endodontic Journal 2006;39:249–281.

63. Siqueira JF Jr, Rôças IN. Clinical implications and microbiology of bacterial persistence after treatment procedures. Journal of Endodontics 2008;34:1291–1301.

64. Wu M-K, Dummer PMH, Wesselink PR. Consequences of and strategies to deal with residual post-treatment root canal infection. International Endodontic Journal 2006;39:343–356.

65. Chávez de Paz LE. Redefining the persistent infection in root canals: Possible role of biofilm communities. Journal of Endodontics 2004;33:652–662.

66. Svensäter G, Bergenholtz G. Biofilms in endodontic infections. Endodontic Topics 2004;9:27–36.

67. Siqueira JF Jr, Rôças IN. The microbiota of acute apical abscesses. Journal of Dental Research 2009;88:61–65.

68. Sakamoto M, Siqueira JF Jr, Rôças IN, Benno Y. Molecular analysis of the root canal microbiota associated with endodontic treatment failures. Oral Microbiology Immunology 2008;23:275–281.

69. Patel S, Dawood A, Whaites E, Pitt Ford T. New dimensions in endodontic imaging: Part 1. Conventional and alternative radiographic systems. International Endodontic Journal 2009;42: 447–462.

70. Patel S, Dawood A, Pitt Ford T, Whaites E. The potential applications of cone beam computed tomography in the management of endodontic problems. International Endodontic Journal 2007;40: 818–830.

71. Patel S. New dimensions in endodontic imaging: Part 2. Cone Beam Computed Tomography. International Endodontic Journal 2009;42:463–475.

72. Kersten DD, Mines P, Sweet M. Use of the microscope in endodontics: results of a questionnaire. Journal of Endodontics 2008;34:804–807.

73. Kim S, Baek S. The microscope and endodontics. Dental Clinics of North America 2004;48:11–18.

74. Hülsmann M, Peters OA, Dummer PMH. Mechanical preparation of root canals: shaping goals, techniques and means. Endodontic Topics 2005;10:30–76.

75. Young GR, Parashos P, Messer HH. The principles of techniques for cleaning root canals. Australian Dental Journal 2007;52(Suppl): S52–S63.

76. Peters OA. Current challenges and concepts in the preparation of root canal systems: a review. Journal of Endodontics 2004;30:559–567.

77. Chong BS, Pitt Ford TR. Root-end filling materials: rationale & tissue response. Endodontic Topics 2005;11:114–130.

78. Chong BS, Pitt Ford TR, Hudson MB. A prospective clinical study of Mineral Trioxide Aggregate and IRM when used as root-end filling materials in endodontic surgery. International Endodontic Journal 2003;36:520–526.

79. Blicher B, Baker D, Lin J. Endosseous implants versus nonsurgical root canal therapy: a systematic review of the literature. General Dentistry 2008;56: 576–580.

80. Dawson AS, Cardaci SC. Endodontics versus implantology: to extirpate or integrate? Australian Endodontic Journal 2008;32: 57–63.

81. Torabinejad M, Anderson P, Bader J, et al. Outcomes of root canal treatment and restoration, implant-supported single crowns, fixed partial dentures, and extraction without replacement: a systematic review. Journal of Prosthetic Dentistry 2007;98: 285–311.

82. Wolcott J, Meyers J. Endodontic re-treatment or implants: a contemporary conundrum. Compendium of Continuing Education in Dentistry 2006;27: 104–110.

83. Iqbal MK, Kim S. A review of factors influencing treatment planning decisions of single-tooth implants versus preserving natural teeth with nonsurgical endodontic therapy. Journal of Endodontics 2008;34:519–529.

84. Chugal NM, Clive JM, Spångberg LS. Endodontic infection: some biologic and treatment factors associated with outcome. Oral Surgery, Oral Medicine, Oral Pathology, Oral Radiology and Endodontics 2003;96:81–90.

85. Chugal NM, Clive JM, Spångberg LS. Endodontic treatment outcome: effect of the permanent restoration. Oral Surgery, Oral Medicine, Oral Pathology, Oral Radiology and Endodontology 2007;104: 576–582.

86. Kirkevang L-L, Væth M, Hörsted-Bindslev P, et al. Risk factors for developing apical periodontitis in a general population. International Endodontic Journal 2007;40: 290–299.

87. Ng Y-L, Mann V, Rahbaran S, et al. Outcome of primary root canal treatment: systematic review of the literature – Part 1. Effects of study characteristics on probability of success. International Endodontic Journal 2007;40:921–939.

Chapter | 2 |

General and systemic aspects of endodontics

M.P. Escudier

SUMMARY

A patient's general health may have an impact on endodontic treatment. In addition, pain is the predominant complaint associated with endodontic disease. This chapter will cover the diagnosis of orofacial pain of both odontogenic and non-odontogenic origin. The potential influence of a number of systemic conditions and disorders, as well as medication, on treatment planning and management of endodontic patients will be discussed. Sections on the use of antibiotics and analgesics in endodontic cases have also been included.

INTRODUCTION

The treatment of periapical infection using modern endodontic techniques is safe and effective, provided it is appropriately applied and undertaken by competent clinicians. In line with this, a full assessment of both the medical history and the clinical situation should be undertaken prior to commencing treatment. Comprehensive and sensible treatment planning based on a careful analysis of the information gathered will help to protect the patient from harm and the dental practitioner from criticism, legal or otherwise.

The dental practitioner is largely dependent on the medical history to identify systemic disease or therapy that may affect patient management. It is, therefore, vital that this is comprehensive and regularly updated. In addition, any areas of uncertainty or concern should be discussed with the patient's physician prior to commencing treatment. Many patients have systemic disorders, which are well-controlled by therapy and, therefore, unlikely to influence the outcome of dental treatment. However, the therapy itself may influence their management, for example patients taking prednisolone or warfarin.

The assessment will initially consist of the history and a clinical examination, which will provide a differential diagnosis. It should be remembered that the history is the single most important factor in arriving at a diagnosis.[1] However, the clinical examination and subsequent investigations will increase the clinician's confidence in the diagnosis, even though they may contribute relatively few new facts.[2] The fear of transmission of HIV (human immunodeficiency virus) or hepatitis viruses as well as prions has highlighted the importance of applying current guidelines for cross-infection control in endodontics as in any other aspect of clinical dentistry.[3]

DIFFERENTIAL DIAGNOSIS OF DENTAL PAIN

The commonest cause of pain in the orofacial region is dental disease leading to pulpal pain (see Chapter 3). As such, dental surgeons are experienced and competent in the diagnosis and management of this complaint. However, the differential diagnosis of pain in the teeth, jaws and face is far wider than is sometimes appreciated. Pain may be:

- referred from a distant origin, e.g. cardiac
- have an unusual local cause, e.g. osteomyelitis
- psychogenic in origin, e.g. atypical facial pain
- neurological, e.g. trigeminal neuralgia
- modified by apparently unrelated factors, e.g. previous cerebrovascular accident.

This broader diagnostic sieve should be remembered, particularly if the pattern of presentation is unusual, the examination findings are sparse or conflicting, or if pain persists or develops in spite of, apparently, successful treatment. The essence of good clinical practice is a methodical and disciplined approach (history, followed by examination, followed by special investigations – usually radiographic, followed by analysis and conclusion). In the case of orofacial pain this is extremely well dealt with in other texts.[4]

Pain history

A thorough, structured pain history will provide a diagnosis in the majority of cases and will help identify those areas in need of further investigation. This should commence with the patient being asked to describe the pain in their own words, before asking direct questions. Certain, core information (Table 2.1) should be elicited in all cases.[4]

Examination

The assessment of a patient starts with their entry into the clinical setting. This will enable observation of the general demeanour as well as any locomotor problems, walking aids or possible neurological deficits. It may enable identification of a facial swelling, and particular attention should be paid to facial symmetry, notably that of the cheeks, the mandibular angle region and the nasolabial

Table 2.1 Pain history

Duration	When did your pain start? Have you ever had a pain like this before?
Character	What type of pain is it?
Periodicity	When do you get the pain? Does it come and go? Is there any particular pattern to the pain?
Severity	How severe is your pain?
Site	Where is your pain?
Radiation	Does your pain spread to other areas?
Provoking factors	Does anything make your pain worse?
Relieving factors	Does anything make your pain better?
Associated factors	Have you noticed anything else about your pain?

folds. Observation of the patient's face during the history taking may reveal a subtle neurological feature requiring formal assessment of cranial nerve function. An assessment of the level of pain can be made using the facial expression,[5] although it is important to remember that facial expressions can be manipulated. Hence avoidance of, or flinching from, examination may be a more accurate indication of a trigger spot or tenderness than response to questioning during examination. The observation of mandibular movements is the essential preliminary to examination of temporomandibular joint function.

The features of a comprehensive examination of the teeth and jaws are described in Chapter 3. The soft tissues of the cheeks, palate, tongue and floor of the mouth may also yield vital, relevant information. The necessity of a detailed occlusal examination depends on the history and clinical setting. Similarly, the history will determine the necessity or desirability of formal assessment of the temporomandibular apparatus. The maxillary sinus as a cause of pain is considered below. Thermal or electrical stimulation of suspect teeth, differential local anaesthetic injections, and removal of restorations all have their place in diagnosis. In addition, radiography is essential, but all these techniques must supplement the history and clinical examination, and never replace them.

Persistent orofacial pain

The orofacial region (including the teeth) is a common site for the expression of pain or discomfort as a manifestation of underlying psychosocial disharmony. It may represent anything from a plea for help to a symptom of frank psychosis. The dental surgeon should avoid being manipulated by the patient, or their relatives, into undertaking treatment when the diagnosis is uncertain or the evidence conflicting. In such circumstances, it is better to defer active treatment until a definitive diagnosis can be obtained. In many such cases, the pain will either resolve spontaneously or provide further evidence to assist in the diagnosis, e.g. development of a hemifacial rash of herpes zoster. A review appointment should be arranged with the caveat that the patient may return sooner should the need arise. The dental practitioner also has the opportunity to refer the patient for a second opinion at any time, particularly where the diagnosis continues to remain unclear.

Certain features in the history often help in the diagnosis of idiopathic facial pain. The pain is often unremitting and may have been present for months or even years. The stated severity may be out of proportion to the observed level of distress, disturbance of life or self-therapy. The pain may not follow anatomical boundaries and may be described as throbbing, nagging, aching, miserable or cruel in nature. It does not usually disturb sleep, although there may be a coincident disturbance of sleep pattern. In addition, other chronic pain conditions such as headache, low back pain and abdominal or pelvic pain are often present. There may also be obvious secondary gain (family or social) for the sufferer. In such cases it is important to seek further information in relation to the patient's social history and family circumstances. There is often a history of long-term or recent distressing life events, e.g. bereavement, divorce or job loss.[4]

Depression is common in chronic pain patients and may be effectively detected by two simple questions:[6] 'during the last month have you often been bothered by feeling down, depressed or hopeless?' and 'during the past month have you been bothered by having little interest or pleasure in doing things?' Psychiatric treatment or psychotherapy is often beneficial and may be curative. Such cases are often best referred to an oral physician as direct referral to a psychiatrist may meet with difficulties.

MAXILLARY SINUS

The close proximity of the maxillary sinuses to the maxillary teeth can make the diagnosis of pain in these segments difficult. The distinction between pain of dental origin and sinusitis may be helped by the presence of obvious dental disease, or a typical acute or recurrent sinusitis with nasal discharge. Acute sinusitis rarely occurs without preceding symptoms of 'a cold', and tenderness to pressure of a whole quadrant of teeth is characteristic. In such cases, the use of broad-spectrum antibiotics, e.g. amoxicillin 500 mg, three times a day for 7–14 days, may

be of benefit.[7] However, the clinician will need to weigh the small benefits of the antibiotic treatment against the potential for adverse effects at both the individual and general population levels.[7] Periapical infection of premolar or molar teeth may lead to purulent discharge into the sinus with associated pain. A further consideration is the risk of penetration of the sinus wall or even the sinus lining by endodontic instruments, or during apical surgery. This may result in acute sinusitis from bacterial contamination. The condition may resolve spontaneously but the prescription of a broad-spectrum antibiotic and nasal decongestant (see below) is usual practice.

Small oroantral communications usually heal spontaneously, and in the case of apical surgery, the replacement of the surgical flap is sufficient to seal the opening. The identity of microorganisms involved in sinus infection is often unclear and broad-spectrum antibiotics may be required, e.g. amoxicillin 500 mg, three times a day. It is usual to continue therapy for 5 days although a one-off 3g dose of amoxicillin is equally effective. If there is poor drainage of the sinus, e.g. a history of chronic sinusitis, nasal drops (0.5% ephedrine) should be prescribed. In addition, inhalations, such as menthol and eucalyptus, have a soothing effect and may be of benefit.

A connection between sinus disease and root canal treatment was reported. They relate to aspergillosis of the maxillary antrum following root canal treatment with zinc-oxide based cements that are known to promote cultures of the fungus *Aspergillus*.[8,9,10]

SYSTEMIC DISEASE AND ENDODONTICS

Disabled or debilitated patients cannot be expected to readily tolerate complex and lengthy treatment procedures. However, even in severe ill-health, some patients have a strong desire to retain their natural teeth, and the dentist's duty is to try to respond. Even in terminal illness, simple treatment can be a great aid to comfort, masticatory function and morale. Good decision-making is dependent on frank and thoughtful discussion with the patient and his medical advisers. In some conditions, e.g. cardiac abnormalities, endodontic treatment should only be carried out if a high standard of treatment can be achieved, which may involve referral to a specialist.

Both the patient's general prognosis and the prognosis for the tooth being treated must be considered; this may lead to the decision to extract the tooth rather than undertake root canal treatment. In chronic diseases, subject to cyclical remission, either spontaneously or with treatment, it is sensible to defer dental intervention until the optimum physical health is achieved. This is particularly true of haematological disorders, e.g. leukaemia, especially if the patient receives periodic transfusion or cycles of chemotherapy. Sufferers from haemorrhagic diatheses will not require factor replacement or antifibrinolytic therapy for root canal treatment alone, but may do if a local anaesthetic is to be given or endodontic surgery undertaken. In all such cases, the patient's haematologist should be consulted to discuss any necessary preoperative or perioperative measures. There is insufficient evidence to show that the presence of systemic disease has a major influence on the healing of periapical lesions. Hence, a positive approach should be taken to treatment even in immunocompromised patients.[11]

Progressive narrowing of pulp chambers and root canals (due to excessive dentine formation) in patients receiving substantial doses of corticosteroids following renal transplantation has been observed.[12] There is no need for antibiotic prophylaxis when undertaking dental treatment in these patients, although some renal transplant units still advise the need for prophylaxis. In such circumstances, it would be advisable to discuss the individual case with the unit concerned.

Endodontics and infective endocarditis

Infective endocarditis (IE) is an uncommon but life-threatening condition with an overall mortality of 20%. Since 1955 antibiotic prophylaxis has been recommended for at risk individuals on the basis that endocarditis usually follows bacteraemia as a result of certain dental procedures and the bacteria responsible are usually sensitive to antibiotics.[13] However, the evidence for the use of antibiotic prophylaxis relied heavily on extrapolation from animal models[14] and their application to humans has been questioned. Similarly, the assumption that antibiotic prophylaxis is effective for the prevention of IE has not really been proven.[15]

Recent guidelines by the British Society for Antimicrobial Chemotherapy[16] and the American Heart Association[17] have challenged existing dogma by highlighting the prevalence of bacteraemias that arise from everyday activities such as toothbrushing, the lack of association between episodes of IE and prior interventional procedures, and the questionable efficacy of antibiotic prophylaxis regimens. Against this background, the Department of Health (England) asked the National Institute for Health and Clinical Excellence (NICE), the body responsible for recommending what treatment and medication should be available on the National Health Service, to look at conflicting advice in relation to antibiotic prophylaxis against IE. After an independent review of the available scientific evidence, NICE has recommended that for people at risk of developing IE undergoing dental procedures:[18]

- antibiotic prophylaxis is not recommended;
- chlorhexidine mouthwash should not be offered;

- any episodes of infection should be investigated and treated promptly to reduce the risk of endocarditis developing.

NICE also recommended that healthcare professionals should offer people at risk of infective endocarditis clear and consistent information about prevention; these include:

- the benefits and risks of antibiotic prophylaxis, and an explanation as to why antibiotic prophylaxis is no longer routinely recommended;
- the importance of maintaining good oral health;
- symptoms that may indicate infective endocarditis and when to seek expert advice;
- the risks of undergoing invasive procedures, including non-medical procedures such as body piercing or tattooing.

Endodontics in patients with prosthetic hip joints

There is no special risk to patients with hip or knee prostheses from any form of dental treatment, and certainly not from endodontic procedures.[19] However, some orthopaedic patients are still advised of the need for antibiotic prophylaxis and in such cases, it would be advisable to discuss the individual situation with the surgeon concerned.

Endodontics in patients taking warfarin or corticosteroids

Increasing numbers of patients are taking regular medication for a variety of conditions. Amongst those of particular relevance to the management of dental patients are warfarin and corticosteroids. Warfarin is a commonly used oral anticoagulant in the management of several medical conditions. Its action is monitored by means of the International Normalised Ratio (INR); the desired therapeutic range (deep vein thrombosis INR 2.0–3.0, prosthetic heart valve INR 3.0–4.0) and the duration of treatment is dependent on the medical condition. In such cases, the first question is whether the warfarin therapy is to be discontinued at any time? If it is, then a decision can be made as to whether the proposed treatment can be deferred until that time. However, if treatment is required, or the warfarin therapy is ongoing, the INR will need to be reconsidered. Warfarin therapy should not be stopped or altered prior to dental treatment without the agreement of the anticoagulant team.

Endodontic treatment, with or without local anaesthesia (except inferior alveolar nerve blocks), can safely be undertaken with an INR of 4.0 or less[20] and provided the INR is stable. Apical surgery, involving raising a mucoperiosteal flap and bone removal, is best avoided above an

INR of 2.5, as are inferior alveolar nerve blocks. In all cases the INR should be formally checked within 24 hours, prior to the procedure and ideally on the day of treatment.[20] Patients presenting with an INR much higher than their normal value, even if it is less than 4.0, should have their procedure postponed and should be referred back to the clinician maintaining their anticoagulant therapy.[20] The use of low-dose aspirin as an anti-platelet drug is also unlikely to pose significant problems provided appropriate local measures are employed.[21]

Corticosteroids may be administered topically, via an inhaler or systemically. Systemic corticosteroids taken above a dose of 7.5 mg (10 mg in some guidelines) daily for over a month, or in high doses (>40 mg per day) for periods as short as a week may cause adrenocortical suppression. In the case of high doses for short periods ('pulsed') the effects are not clinically significant after a month off treatment and deferral of treatment until this time would be prudent. In the case of long-term corticosteroid therapy, prophylaxis is required and is best administered either orally or intravenously. Two regimes may be employed depending on the preference of the patient and clinician. The first requires that the patient doubling the normal daily dose the day before, the day of and the day after treatment. The second is a one-off dose of 100 mg hydrocortisone administered orally 1 hour prior to treatment, or intravenously a few minutes before treatment.

It should also be noted that some inhaled corticosteroids, e.g. fluticasone, may cause adrenal suppression. Similarly, potent topical corticosteroids prescribed by dermatologists, e.g. Eumovate (clobetasone butyrate), applied to large areas, particularly if ulcerated, may also produce suppression and require corticosteroid prophylaxis prior to dental treatment.

Endodontics in patients taking bisphosphonates

Bisphosphonates are increasingly prescribed to reduce the morbidity of osteoclast-mediated bone diseases such as osteopenia, osteoporosis, fibrous dysplasia, Paget's disease, multiple myeloma and metastatic bone cancer. The relevance of these drugs to the dental surgeon is their association with osteonecrosis of the jaws following dental intervention. The condition has a predilection for the molar region and, in particular, in the mandible.

The risk of bisphosphonate-associated osteonecrosis (BON) is related to the type, dose and duration of bisphosphonate therapy as well as the nature of the dental intervention. Intravenous bisphosphonate therapy (pamidronate, zoledronate) confers a much higher risk of BON (up to 20%) than oral therapy (alendronate, residronate and ibandronate) where the risk is 0–0.04%.[22] The risk of BON increases with the duration of therapy, most cases developing after a mean of around 9 months of treatment for intravenous bisphosphonates. All cases of BON in patients taking oral therapy developed after at least 3 years of therapy with the incidence and severity increasing linearly thereafter.[22] The risk is also increased by concomitant corticosteroid therapy.

Endodontic treatment is preferable to extraction if a tooth is restorable. Routine endodontic technique should be used although manipulation beyond the apex is to be avoided.[23] If extractions or bone surgery are necessary, the patient should be informed of the risk of BON and alternative treatment options considered. In some situations, depending on risk, removal of the clinical crown and endodontic treatment, to allow passive exfoliation of the remaining root may be appropriate. In all cases a conservative surgical technique should be adopted with primary closure, if possible.[23] In addition, immediately before and after any surgical procedures involving bone, the patient should be instructed to rinse gently with a chlorhexidine-containing mouthwash until the wound has healed. The regimen may be extended depending on the progress of healing. The use of prophylactic antibiotics after a surgical procedure should be based on the risk of developing an infection and not on the patient's bisphosphonate therapy. There is no evidence that the use of antibiotics is effective in preventing BON.[23]

USE OF ANTIBIOTICS IN ENDODONTICS

Antibiotics or other antimicrobial drugs are either bacteriocidal (kill susceptible bacteria) or bacteriostatic (arrest their multiplication), and so allow the natural defence processes to combat infection, and healing to progress (Table 2.2). They do not relieve pain or reduce swelling and should not be used to treat pulpitis,[24] but reserved to control a spreading cellulitis or a periapical abscess together with drainage. Overuse should be avoided to prevent further increase in resistant strains of

Table 2.2 Useful antibacterial drugs
Treatment of infections
Phenoxymethylpenicillin capsules, 250 mg one or two 6-hourly, at least 30 minutes before food, for 4–7 days
Amoxicillin capsules, 250 mg one or two 8-hourly for 4–7 days
Augmentin capsules, 375 mg one or two 8-hourly for 4–7 days
Metronidazole tablets, 200 mg one or two 8-hourly for 3–5 days

microorganisms[25] and adherence to clinical guidelines is recommended.[26]

Ideally, the choice of an antibiotic should be based on the results of identification and sensitivity testing of the microorganisms responsible for the infection. This is seldom feasible in clinical practice and requires culture techniques in a laboratory setting, as simple Gram staining and microscopy is of little help. However, most of the bacteria associated from dentoalveolar infection are still sensitive to penicillins and hence, if not allergic, phenoxymethylpenicillin 250 mg or 500 mg, four times a day for 5 days, depending on the severity of the infection, is appropriate.[26] Amoxicillin 250 mg, three times a day for 5 days may be preferred because of its efficient absorption. Metronidazole 200 mg or 400 mg, three times a day for 3 to 5 days will assist in the elimination of anaerobes and may be used alone or in combination with penicillin. The newer penicillinase-resistant antibiotic Augmentin (amoxicillin 250 mg and clavulanic acid 125 mg) may be preferred for ease of use and patient compliance. A potential unwanted side-effect of the use of broad-spectrum antibiotics is interference with absorption of the oestrogen component of combined oral contraceptives, with consequent loss of effect. Women taking such preparations concurrently should be advised not to rely on this method of contraception alone for one month after the end of the antibiotic course. In addition, antibiotics are known to potentiate the action of warfarin, which may upset the therapeutic control.[27] Erythromycin and other macrolide antibiotics interact with warfarin unpredictably and only in certain individuals. Metronidazole also interacts with warfarin and should be avoided if possible. If necessary, the patient should, therefore, be advised to contact their anticoagulant centre for appropriate follow-up.

CONTROL OF PAIN AND ANXIETY

Pain and anxiety control are central to successful endodontic treatment. The drugs available for local analgesia and for sedation are both safe and effective, but, as with any potent therapeutic agent, need to be employed with skill and discretion, particularly in patients who are taking other medication regularly. A whole spectrum of techniques of control of pain and anxiety are applicable in endodontics as in other dental treatment. These range from simple persuasion and a comforting and sympathetic manner, through to sedation. Local anaesthetic techniques are well established, and 2–4 ml of lidocaine (lignocaine) 2% with 1:80,000 adrenaline (epinephrine) is a safe and effective preparation for all patients. An aspirating syringe system should be used to help avoid inadvertent intravascular injection. Only in very rare cases where true allergy to lidocaine is proven, need an alternative solution, e.g. prilocaine with felypressin, be used.

Table 2.3 Useful analgesics

Mild to moderate pain
Aspirin tablets, 300 mg (or aspirin tablets dispersible, 300 mg) one to three every 4–6 hours as necessary, maximum 4 g/day
Paracetamol tablets, 500 mg one to two every 6 hours as necessary, maximum 4 g/day
Ibuprofen tablets, 200 mg one to two every 4–6 hours, as necessary, preferably after food, maximum 2.4 g/day

Moderate to severe pain
Dihydrocodeine tablets, 30 mg one every 4–6 hours, as necessary after food, maximum 1.8 g/day

Severe pain
Pethidine tablets, 50 mg one to two every 4 hours, maximum 6 g/day

Conscious sedation using either an inhaled mixture of nitrous oxide and oxygen, or intravenous administration of midazolam, is a safe and effective way of overcoming anxiety. Such techniques are only rarely required for root canal treatment, however, sedation may more often be required for apical surgery.

Analgesics

Analgesics may be used to treat existing pain, or to reduce postoperative pain (Table 2.3). Analgesics administered preoperatively, as a pre-emptive measure, are useful in reducing postoperative pain. Aspirin and paracetamol (acetaminophen) remain the most effective and widely used remedies for local pain of mild to moderate severity. Aspirin is contraindicated in patients with peptic ulceration, bleeding diatheses, or who are taking systemic corticosteroids. It is also not advised in children because of the risk of causing Reye's syndrome. When paracetamol is used, it is essential to warn patients not to exceed the daily maximum dose of 4 g, because of the risk of severe and sometimes fatal liver damage. Other non-steroidal anti-inflammatory drugs (NSAIDs) such as ibuprofen may be used if preferred and may be used in combination with paracetamol if required. For patients who are taking warfarin, analgesics such as ibuprofen, aspirin and diclofenac should not be used.[27]

Dihydrocodeine tartrate is used to relieve more severe pain, but frequently causes unpleasant side-effects, including dizziness and nausea, and may prove ineffective. On the rare occasions that severe pain persists, then pethidine 50 mg, one or two tablets 4-hourly, can be given and the patient's condition reviewed the next day. Local treatment, e.g. drainage and irrigation of a root canal, making a tooth free of occlusal contact, replacement of a failed temporary filling following root canal cleaning, or irrigation of a surgical wound, are far more effective ways of dealing with pain than the indiscriminate use of analgesics.

BRITISH NATIONAL FORMULARY

This formulary,[19] which includes the Dental Practitioner's Formulary, published jointly by the British Medical Association and the Royal Pharmaceutical Society of Great Britain is a succinct and authoritative guide to prescribing for the dentist and is regularly updated. It is an invaluable source of advice and information and should be available in every dental surgery. The sections on antibiotics

and analgesics as well as information on potential drug interactions, prescribing during pregnancy and medical emergencies in dental practice are particularly useful. A dentist's guide to using this formulary and advice on rational prescribing was recently published as a two-part series of articles.[28,29] Further information on medical aspects of dentistry, is available in 'Medical Problems in Dentistry'.[30]

LEARNING OUTCOMES

After reading this chapter, the reader should:

- be aware of the differential diagnosis of orofacial pain
- understand the relevance of concurrent, systemic disease as well as medication to treatment planning and management of endodontic patients
- be familiar with the use of analgesics and antibiotics in endodontic cases.

REFERENCES

1. Hampton JR, Harrison MJ, Mitchell JR, et al. Relative contributions of history-taking, physical examination and laboratory investigations to diagnosis and management of medical outpatients. British Medical Journal 1975;2:486–489.

2. Roshan M, Rao AP. A study on relative contributions of the history, physical examination and investigations in making medical diagnosis. Journal of the Association of Physicians of India 2000;48:771–775.

3. Department of Health. Health Technical Memorandum 01-05: Decontamination in primary care dental practices. London: Department of Health; 2008.

4. Zakrzewska J, Harrison SD. Pain Research and Clinical Management: Volume 14, Assessment and management of orofacial pain. Amsterdam: Elsevier; 2002.

5. Solomon PE, Prkahin KM, Farewell V. Enhancing sensitivity to facial expression of pain. Pain 1997;71: 279–284.

6. Whooley MA, Avins AL, Miranda J, Browner WS. Case–finding instruments for depression. Two questions are as good as many. Journal of General Internal Medicine 1997;12:439–445.

7. Ahovuo-Saloranta A, Borisenko OV, Kovanen N, et al. Antibiotics for acute maxillary sinusitis. Cochrane Database Systemic Reviews 2008;Art. No. (2):CD000243.

8. Beck-Mannagetta J, Necek D. Radiologic findings in aspergillosis of the maxillary sinus. Oral Surgery, Oral Medicine, Oral Pathology 1986;62:345–349.

9. Giardino L, Pontieri F, Savoldi E, Tallarigo F. Aspergillus mycetoma of the maxillary sinus secondary to overfilling of a root canal. Journal of Endodontics 2006;32: 692–694.

10. Khongkhunthian P, Reichart PA. Aspergillosis of the maxillary sinus as a complication of overfilling root canal material into the sinus: report of two cases. Journal of Endodontics 2001;27:476–478.

11. DePaola LG, Peterson DE, Overholser Jr CD, et al. Dental care for patients receiving chemotherapy. Journal of the American Dental Association 1986;112:198–203.

12. Näsström K, Forsberg B, Petersson A, Westesson PL. Narrowing of the dental pulp chamber in patients with renal diseases. Oral Surgery, Oral Medicine, Oral Pathology 1985;59:242–246.

13. Durack DT. Prevention of infective endocarditis. New England Journal of Medicine 1995;332:38–44.

14. Pallasch TJ. Antibiotic prophylaxis: problems in paradise. Dental Clinics of North America 2003;47: 665–679.

15. Prendergast BD. The changing face of infective endocarditis. Heart 2006;92:879–885.

16. Gould FK, Elliott TSJ, Foweraker J et al. Guidelines for the prevention of endocarditis: report of the Working Party of the British Society for Antimicrobial Chemotherapy. The Journal of Antimicrobial Chemotherapy 2006;57:1035–1042.

17. Wilson W, Taubert K, Gewitz M et al. Prevention of infective endocarditis. Guidelines from the American Heart Association: A Guideline from the American Heart Association Rheumatic Fever, Endocarditis and Kawasaki Disease Committee, Council on Cardiovascular Disease in the Young and the Council on Clinical Cardiology, Council on Cardiovascular Surgery and Anaesthesia and the Quality of Care and Outcomes Research Interdisciplinary Working Group. Circulation 2007;116:1736–1754.

18. Prophylaxis against infective endocarditis: NICE guidelines. National Institute for Health and Clinical Excellence. Online. Available: <http://www.nice.org.uk/nicemedia/pdf/CG64NICEguidance.pdf>; 2008.

19. British National Formulary. London: British Medical Association & Royal Pharmaceutical Society of Great Britain; September 2008.

20. Surgical management of the primary care dental patient on warfarin. North West Medicines Information Centre, Liverpool, UK. Online. Available: <http://www.nelm.nhs.uk/en/NeLM-Area/Evidence/Medicines-Q--A/Surgical-management-of-the-primary-care-dental-patient-on-warfarin/?query=warfarin+++surgical+management&rank=5>; 2007.

21. Ardekian L, Gaspar R, Peled M, et al. Does low-dose aspirin therapy complicate oral surgical procedures? Journal of the American Dental Association 2000;131:331–335.

22. Marx RE, Cillo JE, Ulloa JJ. Oral bisphosphonate-induced osteonecrosis: Risk factors, predilection of risk using serum CTX testing, prevention and treatment. Journal of Oral and Maxillofacial Surgery 2007;65:2397–2410.

23. Edwards BJ, Hellstein JW, Jacobsen PL et al. Updated recommendations for managing the care of patients receiving oral bisphosphonate therapy: An advisory statement from the American Dental Association Council on Scientific Affairs. Journal of the American Dental Association 2008;139:1674–1677.

24. Nagle D, Reader A, Beck M, Weaver J. Effect of systemic penicillin on pain in untreated irreversible pulpitis. Oral Surgery, Oral Medicine, Oral Pathology, Oral Radiology & Endodontics 2000;90:636–640.

25. World Health Organisation. Antibiotic resistance: synthesis of recommendations by expert policy groups. Online. Available: <http://www.who.int/drugresistance/Antimicrobial_resistance_recommendations_of_expert_polic.pdf>; 2001.

26. Adult antimicrobial prescribing in primary dental care for general dental practitioners. London, UK: Faculty of General Dental Practice UK, Royal College of Surgeons of England; 2006.

27. Managing patients who are taking warfarin and undergoing dental treatment. National Patient Safety Agency, London, UK. Online. Available: <http://www.npsa.nhs.uk/nrls/alerts-and-directives/alerts/anticoagulant/>; 2009.

28. Wray D, Wagle SMS. A dentist's guide to using the BNF: part I. British Dental Journal 2008;204:437–439.

29. Wray D, Wagle SMS. A dentist's guide to using the BNF: part II. British Dental Journal 2008;204:487–491.

30. Scully C, Cawson RA. Medical problems in dentistry. 5th ed. Amsterdam: Churchill Livingstone/Elsevier; 2005.

Chapter | 3 |

Diagnosis

S. Patel, B.S. Chong

SUMMARY

Diagnosis is the first step in the care and management of any patient. A systematic and organized approach is important in order to avoid misdiagnosis. Special test and additional investigations may be necessary to help confirm a provisional diagnosis. Until and unless a clear diagnosis is possible, invasive and irreversible treatment may have to be delayed. However, once a confirmed diagnosis has emerged, in conjunction with the patient, the various treatment options can then be considered. Depending on patient's preference, a treatment plan is formulated and then carried out to resolve the patient's complaint. Referral to a specialist may, sometimes, be necessary to help establish a diagnosis or if complex endodontic treatment is required.

INTRODUCTION

Diagnosis is the process of identifying a disease or an abnormal condition by collecting and evaluating the patient's presenting signs and symptoms, and the results of further investigations. A clear diagnosis can only be reached when information is collected systematically and interpreted accurately. Without a correct diagnosis, the clinician will not be able to manage and provide appropriate treatment to resolve the patient's complaint.

© 2009 Elsevier Ltd, Inc, BV
DOI: 10.1016/B978-0-7020-3156-4.00006-1

If a diagnosis cannot be reached, irreversible treatment may have to be delayed. The maxim 'first do no harm' is a reminder it may be better to do nothing than something that risks causing more harm than good. If a diagnosis cannot be established, a referral to an appropriate specialist should be considered.

HISTORY

Taking an accurate history from the patient is the first step in diagnosis. The clinician can then decide the direction the diagnostic process should take, for example, the additional investigations or special tests required. Subject to confirmation, a tentative diagnosis may be possible at this stage.

As well as helping to establish the reasons for the patient's attendance, the history may also reveal the patient's attitude and motivation towards dental treatment. The clinician may be alerted to potential patient management problems, for example, if the patient mentioned previous difficulties in achieving adequate anaesthesia or an intolerance to having dental instruments in the mouth.

Presenting complaint

Patients should be questioned sympathetically and asked to describe their complaint in their own words; this should then be documented. Their cooperation and ability to describe their complaint accurately will greatly aid diagnosis. The questions asked should be open ended and not leading, for example, 'What brings you to see me today?' With endodontic problems, pain and/or swelling are usually the predominant complaints. Typically with pain, a series of follow-up questions is necessary to help establish the character, duration, severity and other features of the pain or discomfort (see Chapter 2, Table 2.1).

History of presenting complaint

Often, the presenting complaint is not new but previous symptoms may have been mild or they may have temporarily abated. The patient may be unaware that treatment is required or may have even chosen to ignore the problem, especially if no longer causing symptoms. However, a historical perspective and the chronology of the presenting complaint are still necessary as it will provide relevant information for arriving at a diagnosis.

Dental history

It is helpful to gain an insight into the patient's past and present dental history including pattern of attendance. Some patients may only attend when they are in pain, whilst others may see their dentist on a more regular basis. It is also important to determine if the patient has recently had dental treatment in the region of interest because unless it is purely coincidental, it may be related to the presenting complaint. Other relevant snippets of information gleaned from the dental history may provide clues to possible factors contributory to the patient's complaint. For example, a history of dental trauma may explain symptoms of irreversible pulpitis associated with an otherwise clinically unremarkable tooth.

Medical history

An up-to-date medical history is required. Unless already documented, normally the patient is requested to complete a medical history form beforehand, which the clinician will then go through with the patient. It is imperative to ascertain if there are any medical conditions or medications that the patient may be taking, which may alter their dental management. In addition, patients should be asked if they are allergic to latex (rubber dam and rubber gloves), household bleach (sodium hypochlorite) and iodine; materials they will be in contact with during endodontic treatment. The subject of the patient's general health and potential impact on endodontic treatment is covered in Chapter 2.

EXAMINATION

Extraoral

The patient's general well-being and demeanour will be noticeable during consultation. Signs of facial asymmetry, swelling and/or trismus may also be apparent (Fig. 3.1). However, less obvious signs may only be revealed follow-

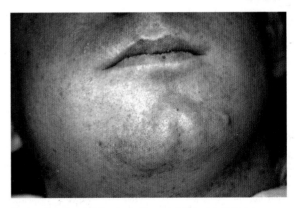

Figure 3.1 An extraoral swelling and associated facial asymmetry that will be obvious upon meeting the patient.

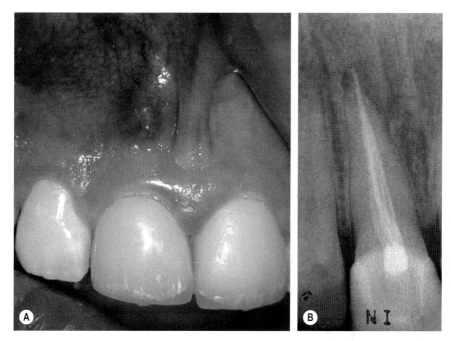

Figure 3.2 (A) Clinical view of the buccal sinus tract associated with a maxillary central incisor. (B) Periapical radiograph of tooth showing an overextended and sub-optimal root canal filling.

ing closer examination. The lymph glands, temporomandibular joint and muscles of mastication are assessed. The degree of mouth opening possible should also be noted because if limited, access for endodontic treatment may be hindered.

Intraoral

Soft tissues

The general state of the soft tissues should be assessed. Scalloping of the lateral borders of the tongue and/or frictional keratosis of the buccal mucosa may indicate a parafunctional habit. The area of interest requires more detailed assessment (see later). Signs, such as a swelling or the presence of a sinus tract should be noted (Fig. 3.2).

Hard tissues

The dentition, including the state and quality of existing restorations is assessed; this will provide an overall clinical view of the patient's dental history (Fig. 3.3). Combined with the oral hygiene status, general periodontal probing profile and caries experience, these are relevant when devising a treatment plan.

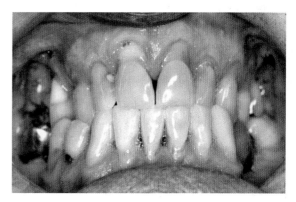

Figure 3.3 The state of the dentition will provide an overall clinical view of the patient's past dental history.

If evident, the severity and distribution of tooth surface loss should be recorded. Localized wear facets and fracture lines may indicate an occlusal component to the patient's symptoms (Fig. 3.4). If a cracked tooth is suspected it may be necessary to assess individual cusps by occlusal loading (see later). Transillumination, using a light source placed on the side of the tooth may help reveal otherwise hard

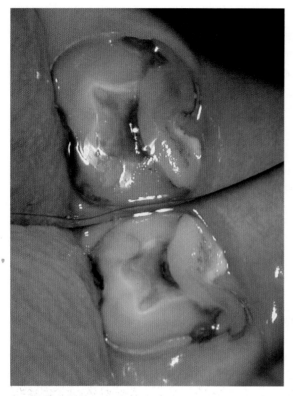

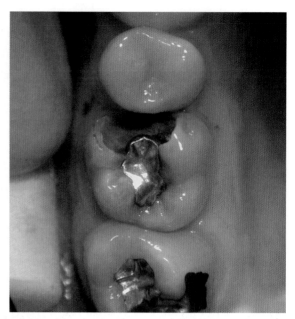

Figure 3.6 A large carious cavity in a maxillary right first molar. The clinical picture suggested possible pulpal involvement and the need for endodontic treatment.

Figure 3.4 Excessive generalised tooth surface loss in this mandibular left second molar has resulted in pulpal symptoms.

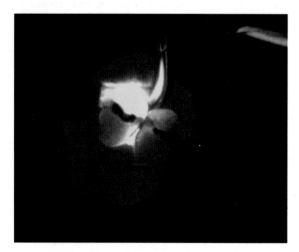

Figure 3.5 Transillumination using a fibreoptic light.

to detect fracture lines (Fig. 3.5). Special dyes, such as methylene blue (Vista-Blue, Vista Dental Products, Racine, WI, USA) may also be used to highlight a fracture line once its approximate position is known. In general, the use of magnification and enhanced illumination greatly aid visualisation allowing a detailed examination (see Chapter 6).

Specific tooth/teeth

The area of interest and specific tooth/teeth are assessed in more detail. The occlusion and the strategic nature of the tooth are considered, for example, if a tooth is unopposed or non-functional. The colour of the tooth, should be compared with adjacent teeth; any darkening of the clinical crown may be related to a history of trauma.[1] The possible causes of pulpal or periapical diseases are noted, for example, the presence of primary or secondary caries (Fig. 3.6), fracture lines (Fig. 3.7) and extensive dentine exposure due to tooth surface loss. The restorability of the tooth must be assessed. The extent of any caries, the size of existing restorations and the amount of original tooth substance left will provide an indication about restorability; there is further discussion on this subject later.

Palpation

The buccal/labial and palatal/lingual mucosa are palpated. Light finger pressure is applied in a rolling motion on the soft tissues using, normally, an index finger (Fig. 3.8). Signs of tenderness usually indicate inflammation of the underlying tissue.

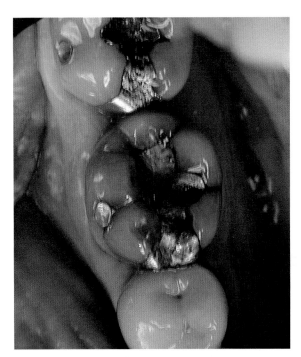

Figure 3.7 A mandibular right first molar with stained crack lines and an old amalgam restoration that is leaking, with evidence of secondary caries underneath.

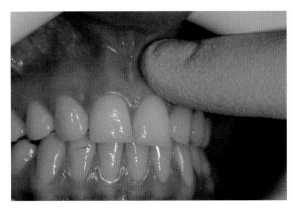

Figure 3.8 Light finger pressure is applied in a rolling motion to palpate the soft tissues.

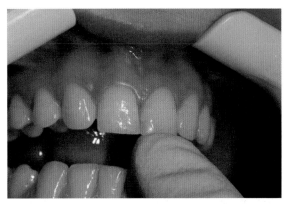

Figure 3.9 Tooth percussion performed using a forefinger.

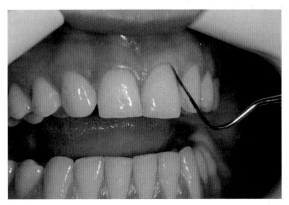

Figure 3.10 The periodontal probe must be walked around the tooth to ensure that any isolated narrow periodontal defects are not missed.

Percussion

Teeth are percussed in an axial and buccal direction using a forefinger (Fig. 3.9) or the end of a mirror handle. Tenderness to gentle percussion indicates inflammation of the periodontal ligament surrounding the tooth; this may be of pulpal or periodontal in origin.

Mobility

With fingers or combined with a mirror handle, any abnormal tooth mobility should be noted. Common causes of increased mobility include periodontal disease, root fracture and acute apical periodontitis.

Periodontal probing

Probing depths should be assessed by 'walking' the periodontal probe around the entire circumference of the tooth (Fig. 3.10). The probing profile for root fractures and iatrogenic perforations is, characteristically, an isolated localised loss of attachment. Whereas loss of attachment due to periodontal disease is usually more generalised and not associated with a singular defect. Furcation involvement may indicate advanced periodontal disease (Fig. 3.11) or an iatrogenic root perforation.

INVESTIGATIONS

Pulp sensitivity tests

Currently available sensitivity tests assess the neural response, and not the vascular supply of the pulp, the

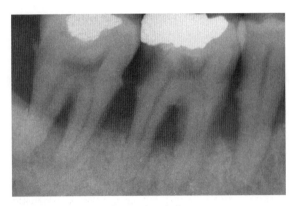

Figure 3.11 Advanced periodontal disease.

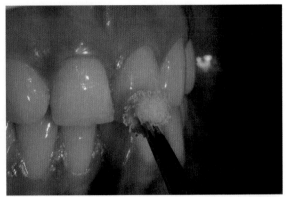

Figure 3.12 Cold thermal test; a refrigerant is sprayed on a small cotton pellet and applied to the tooth.

assumption with these tests is that the neural status reflects the blood supply status of the tooth.[2,3] With any sensitivity test, an explanation should be given to the patient about the rationale for the test. Otherwise, particularly with an anxious patient, false positive responses will result. An adjacent tooth, considered healthy, should be tested first; this will act as the control and allow the patient to experience the likely response.

Thermal tests

Cold test

Cold thermal tests work by causing contraction of the dentinal fluid within the dentine tubules; this rapid outward flow of movement results in 'hydrodynamic forces' acting on the Aδ nerve fibres.[4,5] There is a sharp sensation, lasting for up to a few seconds after the cold stimulus has been removed from the tooth.[6] Several types of cold tests are available; the main difference between them is the operating temperature.

Ice sticks (0°C) are made by filling discarded, sterilized local anaesthetic needle covers with water and placing them in the freezer. They have the advantage of being inexpensive and easy to prepare. However, false negative responses can occur as a result of water droplets contacting adjacent teeth and gingivae, as the ice melts. Commercially available refrigerant spray containing tetrafluoroethane (−50°C) is convenient and easy to use. It is sprayed onto a small cotton pellet and then applied to the tooth (Fig. 3.12). Carbon dioxide snow (−78.5°C) is also very effective. Carbon dioxide is expressed into a plunger mechanism from a pressurised gas cylinder, and then compressed into a stick of carbon dioxide snow. This is then placed on the tooth to be tested using a special applicator. Being the coldest, carbon dioxide snow is particularly useful for assessing teeth restored with full coverage restorations.

Teeth may also be isolated individually with rubber dam, and then bathed with cold water. This test is a par-

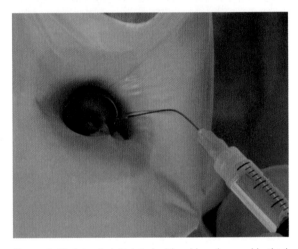

Figure 3.13 A tooth is isolated with rubber dam and bathed with cold water; this is repeated for each tooth in the quadrant to try to reproduce the patient's symptoms.

ticularly useful test when a patient is complaining of a poorly localized pain provoked by cold (Fig. 3.13). The colder the applied stimulus the more reliable the test as there is a greater temperature reduction within the dentine-pulp complex.[7,8] This is important in posterior teeth as the thickness of both dentine and enamel is greater than that in anterior teeth. A negative response may be because the applied stimulus is not cold enough. A prolonged and lingering response usually indicates irreversible pulpitis. Cold tests appear to be more effective in assessing nerve status than heat tests.[9,10]

Heat test

Heat may be applied to a tooth using a heat-softened gutta-percha stick. A thin layer of petroleum jelly should first be applied to the test surface to prevent the gutta-percha sticking to the tooth. Another way of applying heat to a tooth is by running a rubber prophylaxis cup dry, in a slow handpiece, to generate frictional heat on the crown of the tooth[11] but this method is seldom used; a false positive response may be obtained because of the vibrations, and particularly if the patient is anxious.

Individual teeth may also be isolated with rubber dam and warm water applied. Again, this test is particularly useful when the patient complained of poorly localized heat sensitivity. Prolonged application of heat to a tooth can result in stimulation of C-fibres, resulting in lingering pain.[12] For testing purposes and for this reason, heat should only be applied to a tooth for a maximum of 5 seconds.[3]

Electric pulp test

Electric pulp testers (EPTs) are battery operated units (Fig. 3.14). They produce negative pulses of electricity, with a maximum current of a few milliamperes. The current can be adjusted; it is either controlled by the operator or it increases automatically when the unit is activated.[13] The

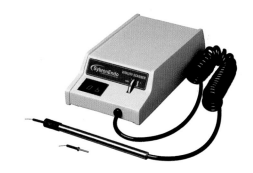

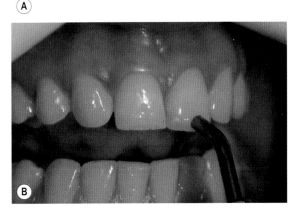

Figure 3.14 (A) A typical electric pulp tester. (B) The probe is placed on the incisal third of the crown of the tooth; toothpaste is used to help improve conduction.

tooth to be assessed is isolated with cotton wool and dried. Depending on the EPT, the patient is asked to hold the handle of the probe, or a lip hook is placed, to form one loop of the circuit. The tip of the probe is usually coated with a conducting medium (e.g. toothpaste) to improve electrical transmission to the tooth. When the probe is placed onto the tooth (Fig. 3.14), the circuit is complete. If desired, strips of rubber dam or cellulose strips may be used interproximally to reduce the likelihood of electrical conduction to adjacent teeth.[3]

As the test proceeds, the strength of the electrical stimulus will increase and when sensation is elicited, the patient is advised to either let go of the handle of the probe which breaks the circuit, or signal to the clinician so the probe may be removed. The reading on the EPT, either numerical or arbitrary is then recorded. If numerical, the digital readout is relative rather than an accurate quantitative measurement of the health status of the pulp. Apart from a total lack of response suggesting a lack of vitality, EPT readings are merely an indication, a comparative measurement as healthy teeth will respond over a range of values. The threshold for obtaining a positive response depends on the position of the probe on the tooth and the thickness of the enamel and dentine. The probe of the EPT should be placed adjacent to the pulp horn as this is where there is the highest density of nerves. In the case of anterior and posterior teeth this is at the incisal and mid-third region of the tooth respectively[14,15,16] (Fig. 3.14). The thicker the enamel and dentine, the higher the excitation threshold; for this reason, the probe should be placed where the enamel is thinnest.[17] This explains why for a given test, the excitation threshold increase from incisor to premolar to molar teeth as the thickness of the overlying enamel and dentine increases.[12,18]

A tingling or warm sensation indicates a healthy 'positive' response. This is a result of Aδ nerve fibres being stimulated, resulting in an ionic shift in the dentinal fluid causing a localized depolarisation and the generation of an action potential from the healthy nerve.[19] A lingering, dull ache following the removal of the EPT probe is a result of stimulation of the C-fibres, which is indicative of irreversible pulpal inflammation. No response from electric pulp testing indicates that the tooth is non-vital, i.e. the pulp is necrotic. Saliva conduction through the periodontal ligament may result in a false positive reading; a negative response may also be due to the failure to complete the electrical circuit. A review on electric pulp testing was published recently;[20] included is the important reminder that electric pulp tests can be unreliable, especially in the case of immature and concussed teeth.

A study to evaluate the ability of thermal and electrical tests to register pulp vitality[2] reported that the probability of a non-sensitive reaction representing a necrotic pulp was 89% with the cold test, 88% with the electrical test and 48% with the heat test. It also indicated that the probability of a sensitive reaction representing a vital pulp was

90% with the cold test, 84% with the electrical test and 83% with the heat test. The results of this study would suggest that, in descending order of accuracy: the cold test followed by the electrical test and then the heat test.

Test cavity preparation

Historically, test cavity preparation has been suggested as a technique to assess the pulp status when all other tests are inconclusive. Local anaesthetic is not administered and a small bur is used with copious irrigation to prepare a small cavity down the centre of the tooth into dentine.[21] If the patient feels sensitivity, this may indicate that the tooth is vital; alternatively, it may indicate that the tooth is unhealthy as Aδ fibres may still be viable in necrotic pulp tissue. No response indicates a lack of pulpal vitality. However, if the pulp tissue has receded away from the centre of the tooth and an excessive amount of tertiary dentine has been deposited within the root canal system, the dentinal tubules being transected may not communicate with the vital odontoblastic processes, hence a negative response.

The patient's response to all sensitivity testing is subjective.[22,23] There is a poor correlation between signs and symptoms, and pulpal and periapical histopathology.[10,24,25,26] When the results of five studies were analysed in an attempt to correlate clinical findings with the histopathological status of teeth, it was concluded that the results of these tests were more likely to be correct when teeth are healthy than diseased.[27] Sensitivity tests by itself are of limited value; they should be used when indicated as an adjunct, as part of the diagnostic process.[24,28]

Bite/cusp loading tests

Tenderness to bite is indicative of inflammation of the periodontium and a common presenting symptom. The more specific cusp loading bite test using some form of wedging device is indicated for patients with a suspected cusp, tooth or root fracture presenting with poorly localized pain on biting.[29] The patient is instructed to bite firmly on a cotton roll (Fig. 3.15A) or a commercially available 'Tooth Slooth' (Professional Results, Inc., Laguna Niguel, CA, USA) (Fig. 3.15B). The biting pressure results in the temporary separation of the fractured segments, thus reproducing the patient's symptoms. Neighbouring teeth are used as controls.

Selective local anaesthesia

If symptoms, particularly pain, are poorly localized or referred, it will be difficult to identify the source. Often, patients may be able to indicate that the pain is from the left or right side of their mouth but they may be unsure if it is from the mandible or maxilla. If pulp sensitivity

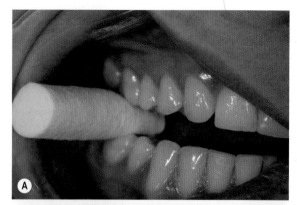

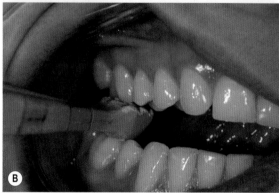

Figure 3.15 Bite/cusp loading test. (A) The patient is asked to bite on a cotton roll to try and reproduce symptoms of localized tenderness to chewing. (B) A wedging device may be used to apply more specific pressure to individual cusps.

testing is equivocal, then selective local anaesthesia may be helpful. Using the intraligamental local anaesthetic injection technique, the clinician should first selectively anaesthetize teeth in the maxillary quadrant starting from the distal sulcus of the most posterior tooth. The local anaesthetic is then administered more forward, one tooth at a time, until the pain disappears. If, after an appropriate interval, the pain persists, selective local anaesthesia should, similarly, be performed in the mandibular quadrant. Selective local anaesthesia is usually better at pinpointing the arch or quadrant rather than a specific tooth.

Blood flow assessment

Various 'physiometric' tests have been investigated to evaluate the actual blood supply within the tooth. They include Laser Doppler Flowmetry (LDF), pulse oximetry[30,31] and the measurement of tooth temperature using thermocouples, thermistors, infrared thermography and cholesteric liquid crystals;[32] most of these methods are experimental.

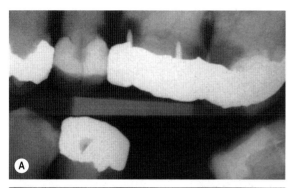

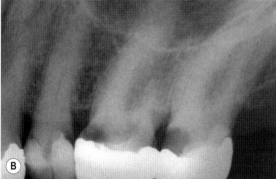

Figure 3.16 (A) A bitewing and (B) a periapical radiograph of the maxillary left quadrant combined to provide information about the quality of existing restorations, extent of caries, crestal bone levels, pulpal calcifications, root morphology and apical health.

LDF, which is a non-invasive technique, appears to be the most promising.[3,33] A probe which emits a low energy laser beam is placed against the surface of the tooth. This laser beam travels along the enamel prisms and dentinal tubules to reach the pulp tissue. On reaching the pulp tissue, some of the light from the laser beam is absorbed and scattered by red blood cells within the capillary plexus resulting in a Doppler shift in the frequency of the light reflected back to the probe.[34,35] The LDF amplifies this reflected light and detects its pulsatility and signal strength. Fourier analysis, a mathematical technique, can be used to improve the diagnostic accuracy of LDF.[33] As well as assessing the blood supply of the tooth, the other major advantages of LDF include more objective and reliable results compared with sensitivity tests.[32,36] LDF is particularly helpful when the results of other investigations are inconclusive;[37] it has also been used to detect the pulpal status of traumatized teeth.[38,39] Unfortunately, LDF does have its disadvantages, these include being more time-consuming to perform, technique sensitive and it cannot be used on extensively restored or decayed teeth.[3]

Radiographs

Radiographs are an essential component of the diagnostic process.[40] Images from conventional radiography are captured on X-ray films or digital sensors. With the latter, the sensors are either charged-coupled devices (CCDs) or storage phosphor plates (SPPs). CCD sensors are relatively bulky and are available as wired or wireless versions; captured images allow immediate viewing. SPP sensors are almost equivalent in thickness to conventional X-ray films and there is no wire connection but irradiated sensors have to be scanned in a processing unit before images can be viewed.

Periapical radiographs may be supplemented with bitewing radiographs; this view may reveal additional information regarding the quality of any restoration present, extent of caries in relation to the pulp, calcifications in the pulp chamber and crestal bone levels[41] (Fig. 3.16). Radiographs should be taken using the paralleling technique, aided by a beam-aiming device, rather than the bisecting angle technique to reduce geometric distortions thus resulting in more accurate images of the apical anatomy.[42] In addition, the use of a beam-aiming device allows similar positioning to be reproduced when radiographs are taken at a later date[43,44] for review or comparative purposes. All radiographs condense the complex three-dimensional anatomy of the tooth and its surrounding alveolar anatomy into a two-dimensional image. The parallax technique may be used to detect, for example, additional root canals and improve perception of the spatial relationship of the root apices to their relevant surrounding structures (Fig. 3.17).

Cone Beam Computed Tomography (CBCT) is a relatively new imaging technique that has been exclusively designed for scanning the maxillofacial skeleton.[45,46] CBCT overcomes some of the deficiencies of conventional radiography.[47,48] A series of exposures is taken in a single rotation of a cone shaped X-ray source and the reciprocal detector around the patient's head.[49] The patient radiation dose is of the same order of magnitude as conventional radiography.[50,51,52] Reconstruction algorithms convert these two-dimensional images into a three-dimensional volume of data and using sophisticated software, processed into a format which closely resembles that produced by conventional CT scanners. Selecting and moving the cursor on one image automatically alters the reconstructed slices in three orthogonal planes: axial, sagittal and coronal, thus allowing images to be scrolled through in real time.[53,54,55,56] CBCT produces undistorted and accurate images of the area under investigation. Studies have concluded that CBCT detects endodontic lesions before they become visible on conventional radiographs[57,58,59,60,61] (Fig. 3.18). This should help improve diagnosis, and may also result in a more objective assessment of healing of root treated teeth.[54] The compact size of the CBCT scanner and ease of use has resulted in a relatively rapid uptake in

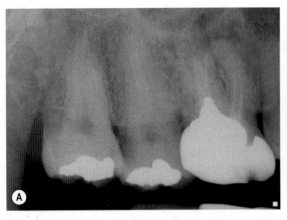 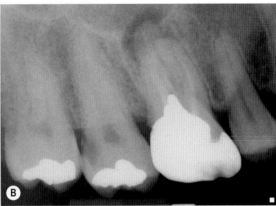

Figure 3.17 Additional radiographs may be helpful. The first periapical radiograph (A) reveals an inadequately root treated maxillary right first molar and distal caries in the adjacent second molar; the second, parallax radiograph (B) reveals more details.

dentistry.[54,62] However, the cost of the equipment is not inconsiderable and limitations include scatter caused by metallic restorations; the resolution (2–3 lines/mm) is also inferior to conventional radiography (15–20 lines/mm). At present, CBCT is not yet universally available in dental practices.

DIFFERENTIAL DIAGNOSIS

Differential diagnosis is the process of distinguishing between diseases or conditions of similar characteristics by comparing their presenting signs and symptoms. The differential diagnosis of dental pain in general is covered in Chapter 2; pulpal and periapical conditions are covered in this chapter.

There is no universally agreed diagnostic terminology, classification scheme or system for pulpal and periapical diseases. The terms symptomatic/asymptomatic have been suggested to replace acute/chronic; the changes to reflect the nature of the patient's presenting complaint instead of the histological description. The terms apical, periapical and periradicular are often used interchangeably. The choice of terminology is a matter of personal preference and invariably some latitude is necessary. In this chapter, the more conservative terms have been retained.

Pulpal conditions

Normal pulp

A tooth with a normal pulp will be symptom-free. The results of clinical examination will be unremarkable, and the tooth will respond normally to sensitivity testing.

Reversible pulpitis

There is mild or transient pulpal inflammation. This may result in the tooth causing sharp pain lasting for up to 5–10 seconds, which does not linger, after the applied stimulus has been removed. Common causes of reversible pulpitis include caries and coronal leakage. Radiological examination may confirm the presence of caries or a defective restoration; the periapical tissues will appear normal. Removal of the causal factor/s will, usually, result in alleviation of pulpal inflammation and the patient's symptoms.

Irreversible pulpitis

The pulp has suffered a more severe insult and is irreversibly inflamed; therefore, the tooth cannot be treated conservatively. Symptoms of irreversible pulpitis may range from a throbbing pain, initiated by hot or cold stimuli and lasting minutes to hours, to spontaneous intermittent bouts of aching pain lasting for hours. Symptoms may be exacerbated when the patient lies down or bends over; this is due to increased intra-pulpal pressure. As mentioned earlier, the results of clinical examination do not, necessarily, correlate with the true histopathological status of the pulp.[10,24,25,63] This is especially true with irreversible pulpitis, which may progress relatively symptom-free to pulp necrosis and subsequent apical periodontitis.[64]

Clinical examination may reveal caries or a defective restoration; this may be confirmed by radiological examination but the periapical tissues may appear normal. An attempt to reproduce the patient's symptoms is prudent, to confirm the diagnosis. With the application of thermal stimulus there is usually an initial sharp shooting Aδ fibre type pain lasting for a few seconds, then after a few seconds

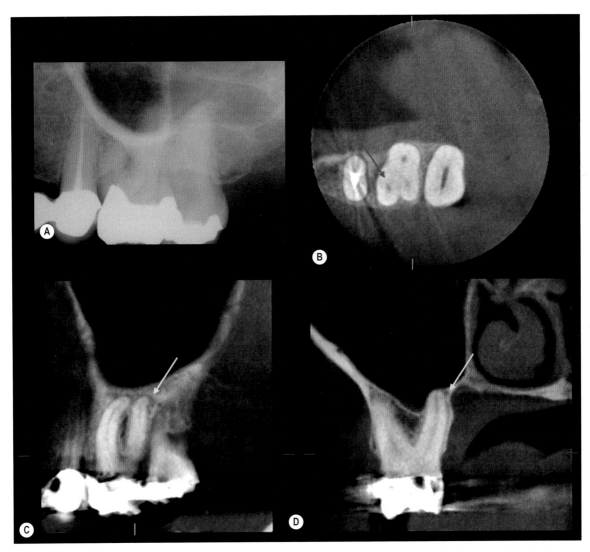

Figure 3.18 (A) A periapical radiograph of the maxillary left first molar showing, apparently, normal periapical health. (B) Axial, (C) sagittal and (D) coronal reconstructed views from Cone Beam Computed Tomography showing the presence of a periapical radiolucency associated with the distobuccal and palatal roots (yellow arrow) and the presence of only one mesiobuccal canal (red arrow).

of quiescence, a dull throbbing C-fibre ache develops which may take minutes to hours to subside even after the stimulus has been removed.[65,66] Once the offending tooth has been identified and irreversible pulpitis confirmed, preservation of the pulp is not possible and pulp removal is necessary.

Pulp necrosis

This term describes the partial or complete necrosis of the pulp caused by a loss of, or inadequate blood supply.

If the necrotic tissue has not become infected, then the periapical tissues will appear normal radiologically. Until the periodontium is involved, the tooth is usually symptom-free. Single-rooted teeth usually do not respond to sensitivity testing. However, in multi-rooted teeth, the pulp may still be partially vital; as a result, sensitivity testing may produce a negative or positive response, depending on the status of the neural supply adjacent to the tooth surface being tested. Root canal treatment is indicated if the diagnosis of pulp necrosis is confirmed.

Periapical conditions

Normal periapical tissues

The tooth is symptom-free and there is no tenderness to palpation or percussion. Radiological examination will reveal a normal periodontal ligament space and no evidence of periapical pathosis.

Acute apical periodontitis

The tooth in question will be exquisitely tender to touch, biting or percussion. Radiological examination may reveal a slight widening of the periodontal ligament space. A negative response to sensitivity testing indicates an endodontic cause.

Acute periapical abscess

Patients suffering from acute periapical abscess will usually present complaining of an intense throbbing pain. The tooth in question will be very tender to touch, percussion and palpation. There may be discernible mobility as the tooth is elevated from its bony socket. The tooth will not respond to sensitivity tests. An intra or extraoral swelling may be present (Fig. 3.19). In severe cases, there may be lymphadenopathy, malaise and the patient may have an elevated temperature. Radiologically, the periapical tissues may appear normal, or there may be a periapical radiolucency. The abscess will have to be drained via the root canal by instituting root canal treatment and incision and drainage is also required for any fluctuant swelling (Fig. 3.19).

Chronic apical periodontitis

Patients may be symptom-free, alternatively, they may report that the tooth feels different or it may be slightly tender to chewing. Clinically, the tooth may be tender to percussion or palpation and does not respond to sensitivity testing. Radiologically, there may be a widening of the periodontal ligament space or more usually, a periapical radiolucency may be present (Fig. 3.20). A 'phoenix' abscess is an acute exacerbation of chronic apical periodontitis and arises in a tooth with a pre-existing periapical radiolucency.

Chronic periapical abscess

The tooth is usually symptom-free, not sensitive to biting pressure but may 'feel different' to the patient upon percussion. It is not responsive to pulp sensitivity tests and radiologically, there will be a periapical radiolucency. Chronic periapical abscess may be distinguished from chronic apical periodontitis because the former will usually be associated with a draining sinus tract. If the sinus tract is sited at the gingival margin, there will be a localized, narrow periodontal pocket. A gutta-percha point may be gently inserted into the sinus tract and a radiograph taken to track the source and confirm the causative tooth (Fig. 3.21).

RESTORABILITY

If a tooth is to be retained as a functional unit in the dental arch after endodontic treatment, it has to be restored to both form and function. Therefore, the restorability of the tooth has to be considered before providing treatment. If there are any doubts about restorability, it may be necessary to remove the entire existing restoration to check.[67] Only after it has been established that there is sufficient sound coronal tooth structure remaining should endodontic treatment proceed. This approach has the added benefit of allowing the clinician to visualize and consider the eventual post-endodontic restoration required.

Recently, a 'Tooth Restorability Index' (TRI) was devised to assist the clinician in deciding how to restore root treated tooth.[68] Prior to restoration, the tooth is divided into sextants. The amount of remaining sound coronal tooth structure in each sextant is given a grade ranging from 0–3 depending on its quantity, height and width. The scores from each sextant are then combined, the resulting score will help guide the clinician in planning

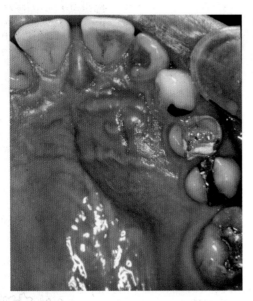

Figure 3.19 An acute periapical abscess related to the maxillary left first premolar. The palatal swelling will have to be incised and drained, and root canal treatment instituted if the tooth is to be retained.

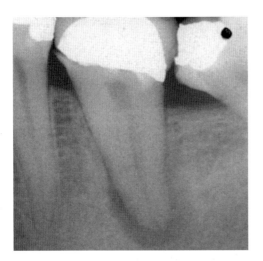

Figure 3.20 A mandibular left first molar with chronic apical periodontitis. The tooth is restored with a crown and is symptom-free but the radiograph reveals a periapical radiolucency.

which type of post-endodontic restoration is suitable for the tooth. The restoration of endodontically treated teeth is covered in Chapter 15.

TREATMENT OPTIONS

Upon reaching a diagnosis, the patient should be advised of the different endodontic treatment options available. As part of the decision-making process, the advantages, disadvantages and the prognosis for each treatment option should be discussed with the patient. The treatment plan should be tailored to the patient's specific problem, taking into account the patient's preference. In addition, the clinician should be competent and confident in carrying out the treatment plan. If not, the case may be best referred to a specialist for management (Fig. 3.22). Endodontic case assessment forms[69,70] have been devised to help the clinicians evaluate the potential complexity of endodontic treatment. Similar forms have been found to be useful for assessing the potential complexity of endodontic treatment, therefore helping the general practitioner decide whether to refer the patient to a specialist.[71]

Watch and review

If there is no clear diagnosis or the patient is undecided on treatment, then a more cautious approach may be adopted. The tooth is monitored until a definitive diagnosis or decision on treatment has been reached. If appropriate and necessary, for the time being, only symptomatic treatment is provided, for example, analgesics for pain.

Save tooth

If a tooth is potentially saveable and the patient preference is for its retention, then treatment should be provided in the effort to keep the tooth.

Lose tooth

If the prognosis is likely to be poor despite intervention, or the patient does not want to retain a potentially salvageable tooth, then extraction may be necessary

SPECIFIC ENDODONTIC TREATMENT OPTIONS

Pulp monitoring

If there is insufficient and inconclusive evidence that endodontic intervention is required, periodic reviews may be necessary to monitor pulpal status. A common example is cases of trauma, where teeth have to be reassessed and special tests may have to be repeated to evaluate pulpal vitality. The rationale for such an approach should be explained to the patient and if there are any new developments, the need for treatment should be reconsidered.

Pulp preservation

The aim of this treatment option is to maintain pulpal vitality by removing irritants that may provoke pulpal inflammation. The treatments commonly used to preserve pulp vitality include indirect pulp capping, direct pulp capping and pulpotomy. This subject is covered in Chapter 5.

Pulp extirpation

When the vital pulp is irreversibly damaged, its removal is inevitable. Pulp extirpation is often the first stage in root canal treatment and a necessary emergency procedure to render the patient pain-free.

Root canal treatment

Root canal treatment is needed for teeth with irreversible pulpitis or apical periodontitis. Treatment may be completed in a single visit if the tooth is not infected, the patient prefers and there is sufficient time available for this approach. Otherwise, the pulp may first have to be extirpated and another appointment scheduled for completion of the root canal treatment. If the tooth is infected or there is concern about being able to achieve predictable disinfection of the root canal system, then more than one visit may be necessary. A successful

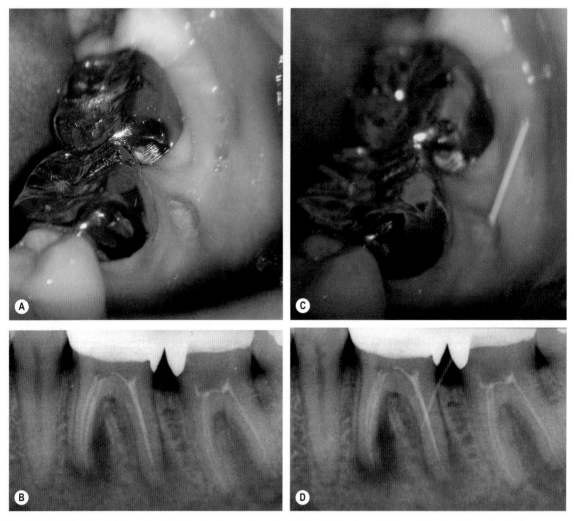

Figure 3.21 (A) A buccal sinus tract situated between two mandibular left molars. (B) A periapical radiograph showing both teeth with suboptimal root fillings. (C) A gutta-percha point is inserted into the sinus tract to trace the source and (D) a second radiograph taken confirmed the culprit is the mandibular left first molar. From Chong 2004,[71] with permission of Quintessence Publishing Co. Ltd.

treatment outcome should never be sacrificed for the sake of procedural expediency. The issue as to whether root canal treatment should be completed in one or more visits is discussed in Chapter 7.

Root canal retreatment

Although a tooth has already been root treated, if there are signs and symptoms indicative of treatment failure and the tooth is to be retained, then root canal retreatment is required[72] (Fig. 3.18). Retreatment may be via a non-surgical or a surgical approach. There is coverage on non-

surgical and surgical retreatment in Chapters 14 and 10 respectively.

LEARNING OUTCOMES

Following completion of this chapter, the reader should be able to understand and discuss the:

- systematic approach needed to achieving a diagnosis
- importance of deferring irreversible, invasive treatment until there is a clear diagnosis

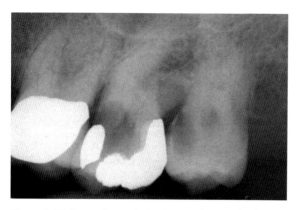

- special tests or additional investigations required to help confirm the provisional diagnosis
- conditions associated with pulpal or periapical diseases and their differential diagnosis
- general and specific endodontic treatment options
- process of formulating a treatment plan based on the diagnosis
- appropriate referral to a specialist if a diagnosis cannot be established or complex endodontic treatment is required.

Figure 3.22 A complex endodontic case that may be best referred to a specialist for management. Apart from extensive caries, especially in the second molar, both teeth have complicated root morphology and significant canal sclerosis; also, access to these teeth will not be easy.

REFERENCES

1. Roy R, Chandler NP. Tooth discolouration following dental trauma. ENDO (London England) 2007;1:181–187.
2. Petersson K, Söderström C, Kiani-Anaraki M, Lévy G. Evaluation of the ability of thermal and electrical tests to register pulp vitality. Endodontics and Dental Traumatology 1999;15:127–131.
3. Pitt Ford TR, Patel S. Technical equipment for assessment of dental pulp status. Endodontic Topics 2004;7:2–13.
4. Brännström M. A Hydrodynamic Mechanism in the Transmission of Pain-producing Stimuli in Dentine. In: Anderson DJ, editor. Sensory Mechanisms in Dentine. Oxford, UK: Pergamon Press; 1963. p. 73–79.
5. Brännström M. Hydrodynamic theory of dental pain: sensation in preparations, caries and dentinal crack syndromes. Journal of Endodontics 1986;12:453–457.
6. Trowbridge HO, Franks M, Korostoff E, Emling R. Sensory response to thermal stimulation in human teeth. Journal of Endodontics 1980;6:405–412.
7. Augsburger RA, Peters DD. In vitro effects of ice, skin refrigerant, and CO_2 snow on intrapulpal temperature. Journal of Endodontics 1981;7:110–116.
8. Ingram TA, Peters DD. Evaluation of the effects of carbon dioxide used as a pulpal test. Part 2. In vivo effect on canine enamel and pulpal tissue. Journal of Endodontics 1983;9:296–303.
9. Ehrmann EH. Pulp testers and pulp testing with particular reference to the use of dry ice. Australian Dental Journal 1977;22:272–279.
10. Seltzer S, Bender IB, Ziontz M. The dynamics of pulpal inflammation: Correlation between diagnostic data and actual histological findings in the pulp. Oral Surgery, Oral Medicine, Oral Pathology 1963;16:973–977.
11. Rickoff B, Trowbridge H, Baker J, et al. Effects of thermal vitality tests on human dental pulp. Journal of Endodontics 1988;14:482–485.
12. Närhi MVO. The characteristics of intradental sensory units and their responses to stimulation. Journal of Dental Research 1985;64:564–571.
13. Dummer PMH, Tanner M, McCarthy JP. A laboratory study of four electric pulp testers. International Endodontic Journal 1986;19:161–171.
14. Byers MR, Dong WK. Autoradiographic location of sensory nerve endings in dentin of monkey teeth, Anatomical Records 1983;205:441–454.
15. Byers MR. Dental sensory receptors. International Review of Neurobiology 1984;25:39–94.
16. Lilja J. Innervation of different parts of the predentine and dentine in young human premolars. Acta Odontologica Scandinavica 1979;37:339–346.
17. Bender IB, Landau MA, Fonsecca S, Trowbridge HO. The optimum placement-site of the electrode in electric pulp testing of the 12 anterior teeth. Journal of the American Dental Association 1989;118:305–310.
18. Rubach WC, Mitchell DF. Periodontal disease, age, and pulp status. Oral Surgery, Oral Medicine, Oral Pathology 1965;19: 482–493.
19. Pantera EA, Anderson RW, Pantera CT. Reliability of electric pulp testing after pulpal testing with dichlorodifluoromethane. Journal of Endodontics 1993;19:312–314.
20. Lin J, Chandler NP. Electric pulp testing: a review. International Endodontic Journal 2008;41: 365–374.

21. Manogue M, Patel S, Walker R. Diagnosis and treatment planning. Principles of Endodontics. Oxford UK: Oxford University Press; 2005. p. 31–45.

22. Eli I. Dental anxiety: A cause for possible misdiagnosis of tooth vitality. International Endodontic Journal 1993;26:251–253.

23. Klepac RK, Dowling J, Hauge G, McDonald M. Reports of pain after dental treatment, electrical tooth stimulation and cutaneous shock. Journal of the American Dental Association 1980;100:692–695.

24. Baume LJ. Diagnosis of diseases of the pulp. Oral Surgery, Oral Medicine, Oral Pathology 1970;29:102–116.

25. Dummer PMH, Hicks R, Huws D. Clinical signs and symptoms in pulp disease. International Endodontic Journal 1980;13: 27–35.

26. Garfunkel A, Sela J, Almansky M. Dental pulp pathosis: Clinicopathological correlation based on 109 cases. Oral Surgery, Oral Medicine, Oral Pathology 1973;35:110–117.

27. Hyman JJ, Cohen ME. The predictive value of endodontic diagnostic tests. Oral Surgery, Oral Medicine, Oral Pathology 1984;58:343–346.

28. Chambers IG. The role and methods of pulp testing in oral diagnosis: a review. International Endodontic Journal 1982;15:1–5.

29. Cameron CE. The cracked-tooth syndrome: additional findings. Journal of the American Dental Association 1976;93:971–975.

30. Calil E, Caldeira CL, Gavini G, Lemos EM. Determination of pulp vitality in vivo with pulse oximetry. International Endodontic Journal 2008;41:741–746.

31. Jafarzadeh H, Rosenberg P. Pulse oximetry: Review of a potential aid in endodontic diagnosis. Journal of Endodontics 2009;35: 329–333.

32. Jafarzadeh H, Udoye CI, Kinoshita J. The application of tooth temperature measurement in endodontic diagnosis: a review. Journal of Endodontics 2008;34: 1435–1440.

33. Gazelius B, Olgart L, Edwall B, Edwall L. Non-invasive recording of blood flow in human dental pulp. Endodontics and Dental Traumatology 1986;2:219–221.

34. Odor TM, Watson TF, Pitt-Ford TR, McDonald F. Pattern of transmission of laser light in teeth. International Endodontic Journal 1996;29:228–234.

35. Odor TM, Chandler NP, Watson TF, et al. Laser light transmission in teeth: a study of the patterns in different species. International Endodontic Journal 1999;32: 296–302.

36. Olgart L, Gazelius B, Lindh-Strömberg U. Laser Doppler Flowmetry in assessing vitality in luxated permanent teeth. International Endodontic Journal 1988;21:300–306.

37. Roy E, Alliot-Licht B, Dajean-Trutaud S, et al. Evaluation of the ability of Laser Doppler Flowmetry for the assessment of pulp vitality in general dental practice. Oral Surgery, Oral Medicine, Oral Pathology, Oral Radiology and Endodontology 2008;106: 615–620.

38. Emshoff R, Moschen I, Strobl H. Use of laser doppler flowmetry to predict vitality of luxated or avulsed permanent teeth. Oral Surgery, Oral Medicine, Oral Pathology, Oral Radiology and Endodontics 2004;98:750–755.

39. Emshoff R, Emshoff I, Moschen I, Strobl H. Laser doppler flow measurements of pulpal blood flow and severity of dental injury. International Endodontic Journal 2004b;37:463–467.

40. Patel S, Dawood A, Whaites E, Pitt Ford T. New dimensions in endodontic imaging: Part 1. Conventional and alternative radiographic systems. International Endodontic Journal 2009;42: 447–462.

41. Whaites E. Periapical radiography. Essentials of Dental Radiology and Radiography. 4th ed. Oxford, UK: Churchill Livingstone/Elsevier; 2007. p. 97–124.

42. Forsberg J, Halse A. Radiographic simulation of a periapical lesion comparing the paralleling and the bisecting-angle techniques. International Endodontic Journal 1994;27:133–138.

43. Forsberg J. Radiographic reproduction of endodontic 'working length' comparing the paralleling and the bisecting-angle techniques. Oral Surgery, Oral Medicine, Oral Pathology, Oral Radiology and Endodontics 1987;64:353–360.

44. Forsberg J. A comparison of the paralleling and bisecting-angle radiographic techniques in endodontics. International Endodontic Journal 1987;20: 177–182.

45. Arai Y, Tammisalo E, Iwai K, et al. Development of a compact computed tomographic apparatus for dental use. Dentomaxillofacial Radiology 1999;28:245–248.

46. Mozzo P, Procacci C, Tacconi A, et al. A new volumetric CT machine for dental imaging based on the cone-beam technique: preliminary results. European Radiology 1999;8:1558–1564.

47. Cotton TP, Geisler TM, Holden DT, et al. Endodontic applications of Cone-Beam Volumetric Tomography. Journal of Endodontics 2007;9:1121–1132.

48. Lofthag-Hansen S, Huumonen S, Gröndahl K, Gröndahl H-G. Limited cone-beam CT and intraoral radiography for the diagnosis of periapical pathology. Oral Surgery, Oral Medicine, Oral Pathology, Oral Radiology and Endodontology 2007;103: 114–119.

49. Scarfe WC, Farman AG, Sukovic P. Clinical applications of cone-beam computed tomography in dental practice. Journal of the Canadian Dental Association 2006;72:75–80.

50. Ludlow JB, Davies-Ludlow LE, Brooks SL, Howerton WB. Dosimetry of 3 CBCT devices for oral and maxillofacial radiology: CB Mercuray, NewTom 3G and i-CAT. Dentomaxillofacial Radiology 2006;35:219–226.

51. Mah J, Danforth RA, Bumann A, Hatcher D. Radiation absorbed in maxillofacial imaging with a new dental computed tomography device. Oral Surgery, Oral Medicine, Oral Pathology, Oral

Radiology and Endodontology 2003;96:508–513.

52. Ngan DCS, Kharbanda OP, Geenty JP, Darendeliler MA. Comparison of radiation levels from computed tomography and conventional dental radiographs. Australian Dental Journal 2003;19:67–75.

53. Nair MK, Nair UP. Digital and advanced imaging in endodontics: A Review. Journal of Endodontics 2007;33:1–6.

54. Patel S, Dawood A, Whaites E, Pitt Ford T. The potential applications of cone beam computed tomography in the management of endodontic problems. International Endodontic Journal 2007;40: 818–830.

55. Patel S. New dimensions in endodontic imaging: Part 2. Cone Beam Computed Tomography. International Endodontic Journal 2009;42:463–475.

56. White TC, Pharoah MJ. The evolution and application of dental maxillofacial imaging modalities. Dental Clinics of North America 2008;52:689–705.

57. Estrela C, Bueno MR, Leles CR, et al. Accuracy of Cone Beam Computed Tomography and panoramic radiography for the detection of apical periodontitis. Journal of Endodontics 2008;34: 273–279.

58. Low MTL, Dula KD, Bürgin W, von Arx T. Comparison of periapical radiography and limited Cone-Beam Tomography in posterior maxillary teeth referred for apical surgery. Journal of

Endodontics 2008;34: 557–562.

59. Patel S, Dawood A, Mannocci F, et al. The detection and management of root resorption lesions using intraoral radiography and cone beam computed tomography – an in vivo investigation. International Endodontic Journal 2009;42: 831–838.

60. Stavropoulos A, Wenzel A. Accuracy of cone beam dental CT, intraoral digital and conventional film radiography for the detection of periapical lesions: an ex vivo study in pig jaws. Clinical Oral Investigations 2007;11:101–106.

61. Tyndall DA, Rathore S. Cone-beam CT diagnostic applications: caries, periodontal bone assessment and endodontic applications. Dental Clinics of North America 2008;52: 825–841.

62. Thomas SL. Applications of cone-beam CT in the office setting. Dental Clinics of North America 2008;52:753–759.

63. Lundy T, Stanley HR. Correlation of pulpal histopathology and clinical symptoms in human teeth subjected to experimental irritation. Oral Surgery, Oral Medicine, Oral Pathology 1969;27: 187–201.

64. Michaelson PL, Holland GR. Is pulpitis painful? International Endodontic Journal 2002;35: 829–832.

65. Jyvasjarvi E, Kniffki DK. Cold stimulation of teeth: a comparison between the responses of cat intradental A- and C-fibers and

human sensations. Journal of Physiology 1987;391:193–207.

66. Mengel MK, Stiefenhofer AE, Jyvasjarvi E, Kniffki KD. Pain sensation during cold stimulation of the teeth: differential reflection of A delta and C fibre activity? Pain 1993;55:159–169.

67. Abbott PV. Assessing restored teeth with pulp and periapical diseases for the presence of cracks, caries and marginal breakdown. Australian Dental Journal 2004;49: 33–39.

68. McDonald A, Setchell D. Developing a tooth restorability index. Dental Update 2005;32: 343–348.

69. American Association of Endodontists. Endodontic Case Difficulty Assessment and Referral. Online. Available: <http://www. aae.org/NR/rdonlyres/CD6A4FE5-EEAC-47AE-8B53-6DF01D324E31/0/ casedifficultarticle.pdf>; 2005.

70. Canadian Academy of Endodontics. Case classification according to degrees of difficulty and risk. In: Standards of Practice. Online. Available: <http://www. caendo.ca/about_cae/standards/ standards_english.pdf>; 2006.

71. Ree MH, Timmerman MF, Wesselink PR. An evaluation of the usefulness of two endodontic case assessment forms by general dentists. International Endodontic Journal 2003;36:545–555.

72. Chong BS. Managing Endodontic Failure in Practice. London, UK: Quintessence Publishing Co. Ltd; 2004.

Chapter | 4 |

Pulp space anatomy and access cavities

A.D.M. Watson

CHAPTER CONTENTS

SUMMARY

Knowledge of pulp space anatomy is essential to achieving the objectives of endodontic treatment. The advent of newer imaging techniques including three-dimensional tomography has revealed and confirmed the complex and divergent anatomy of the pulp space. Classical, pre-conceptualized access cavity designs are informative in the understanding of pulp space anatomy. However, they have been replaced by emergent and customized access cavity designs, prepared according to treatment requirements. Unnecessary and excessive destruction of tooth tissue during access cavity preparation remains unwarranted. The wider adoption of magnification and enhanced illumination, especially the clinical use of an operating microscope, is invaluable, greatly aiding access cavity preparation and allowing the detailed examination of the pulp space.

INTRODUCTION

The major factors involved in the development of apical periodontitis are loss of integrity of coronal tooth substance and the entry of microorganisms into the dentine and pulp space. The primary aim of root canal treatment is the removal and exclusion of these microorganisms, their substrates and products from the pulp space and surrounding dentine. Current practice involves the chemomechanical cleaning, followed by the complete sealing of the pulp space. In addition, the need for a good coronal restoration is integral to reducing the risk of pulp space recontamination.

A clear understanding of the anatomy of human teeth is an essential prerequisite to achieving the objectives of adequate access, thorough cleaning, effective disinfection, and complete obturation of the pulp space. Many of the problems encountered during endodontic treatment occur because of the pulp response to irritation and an inadequate understanding of the pulp space anatomy. Both students and clinicians need to familiarize themselves with the intricacies, complexities and aberrations that are likely to occur within the pulp space. The importance of developing a visual picture of the expected locations and numbers of canals in a particular tooth cannot be overemphasized.

The internal anatomy of human teeth has been studied by many investigators, who have provided a valuable insight into the size, shape and form of the pulp space. Methods of study have included replication techniques,[1,2] ground sections,[3] clearing techniques[4,5,6] and radiography.[7–12] Clinical radiographs show the forms of roots and pulp canals in two planes only. A third plane exists in a buccolingual direction. The pulp space volume is invariably much greater than the clinical radiograph would suggest. Micro-computed tomography has allowed the appreciation of pulp space anatomy in three-dimensions (Fig. 4.1). More recently, Cone Beam Computed Tomography (CBCT) has increased our knowledge of the pulp space[13,14] and allowed the identification of missed anatomy.

NOMENCLATURE

Anatomically, the dental pulp space is surrounded by dentine to form the pulp-dentine complex. Dentine forms the bulk of the mineralized tissue of the tooth. The dentinal tubules, which are interconnected, make up 20–30% of the total volume of dentine.[15] The number of tubules per square millimetre more than doubles and the area occupied by tubules increases three-fold from the dentine near the amelodentinal junction, to that near the pulp.[16] These differences have a significant clinical effect on the permeability of dentine. It is now realized that the dentinal tubules are an important reservoir of microorganisms when pulpal necrosis occurs.[17] A direct route of contamination from unclean root canals into the periapical tissues may be created by the exposure of infected tubules following root-end resection during apical surgery.[18,19]

The pulp space is divided into two parts: the pulp chamber, which is usually described as that portion within the crown; and the pulp canal or root canal, which lies within the confines of the root. The pulp chamber is a single cavity, the dimensions of which vary according to the outline of the crown and the structure of the roots. Thus if the crown has well-developed cusps the pulp chamber projects into well-developed pulp horns. In multirooted teeth the depth of the pulp chamber depends upon the position of the root furcation and may extend beyond the anatomical crown. In young teeth, the outline of the pulp chamber resembles the shape of the exterior of the dentine. With age, the dentinal tubules and the pulp chamber become reduced in size by the laying down of intratubular dentine, secondary dentine and tertiary dentine, particularly in areas where there has been caries, tooth wear and exposure to operative treatment (Fig. 4.2). The pulp chamber may then become irregular in outline. With age, there is also a gradual decrease in pulp space volume, the number of nerves, blood vessels and cells within, but an increase in the fibrous and mineral components. The rate at which the pulps age varies from one tooth to another, and from one patient to another. Calcific changes can lead to the pulp space appearing entirely obliterated radiologically. A residual canal, although radiologically unidentifiable, almost certainly remains within the root as a pathway for microbes to reach the apex and cause periapical changes.

The pulp of root canals is continuous with the pulp chamber and normally the greatest diameter is at the pulp chamber level. Because roots tend to taper towards their apex, the canals also have a tapering form which is constricted at the end, the apical constriction, before emerging at the apical foramina, near the root end; rarely do the foramina open at the exact anatomical apex of the tooth. During root development, the pulp and periodontal tissues become separated, maintaining neural and vascular connections through the apical foramina.

The pulp space is complex and root canals may divide and rejoin, and possess forms that are considerably more involved than many textbooks of anatomy have implied. Many roots have additional canals and a variety of canal configurations. Eight separate pulp space configurations have been identified[6] (Fig. 4.3). In the simplest form, each root has a single canal and a single apical foramen (Type I). Commonly, however, other canal complexities are present and exit the root as one, two or more apical canals (Types II–VIII).

Since roots tend to be broader buccolingually than they are mesiodistally, the pulp space is similarly oval in cross-section. The diameter of the root canal decreases towards the apical foramen and reaches its narrowest point 1.0–1.5 mm from the foramen. This point, the apical constriction lies within dentine just prior to the first layers of cementum and is the narrowest point to which the canal tapers. During root development the apical part of the pulp is described as being 'open'. As the tooth matures, the funnel-shaped foramen closes and constricts to a normal root shape with a small apical foramen. The position of the apical foramen may also be altered, relative to the root apex with the deposition of secondary cementum.

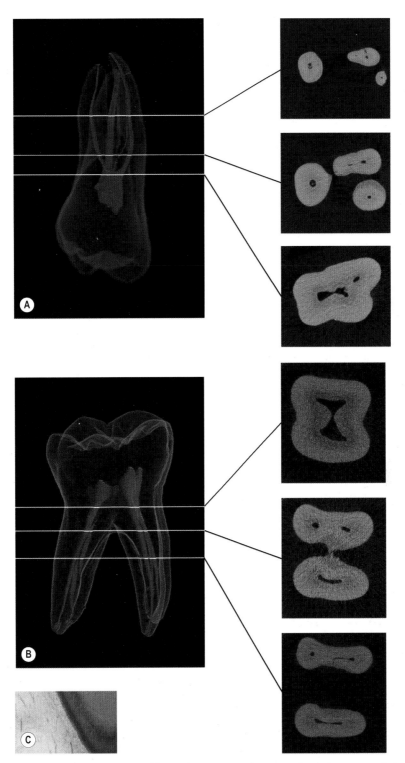

Figure 4.1 Three-dimensional images reconstructed from micro-computed tomography data; cross sections at various levels indicated by corresponding lines. (A) Maxillary molar. (B) Mandibular molar. (C) Cellular arrangement of odontoblast layer. From Peters 2008,[38] with permission of Quintessence Publishing Co. Ltd.

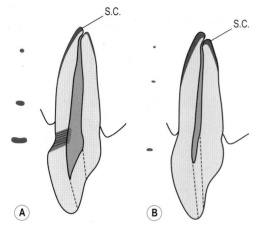

Figure 4.2 Alteration of pulp size with age. (A) Tooth of young adult; large pulp chamber with tertiary dentine under tubules affected by cervical abrasion; small amount of secondary cementum (SC) at apex. (B) Tooth of older patient showing smaller pulp space and greater amounts of secondary cementum that have altered the relationship of the apical constriction to the foramen. Access cavities are indicated by dotted lines. To the left: cross-sections of the root canals are shown at selected levels.

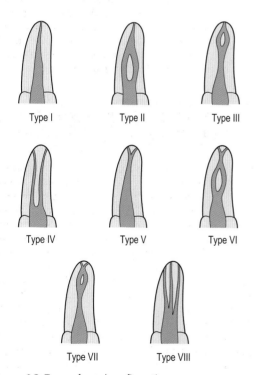

Figure 4.3 Types of canal configuration.

ACCESSORY AND LATERAL CANALS

The pulpal and periodontal tissues not only maintain connection through the apical foramina but also through accessory and lateral canals. A lateral canal can be found anywhere along the length of a root and tends to be at right angles to the main root canal. Accessory canals usually branch off the main root canal somewhere in the apical region. The presence of lateral canals in the furcation areas of molar teeth is well documented and their incidence is relatively high. Patent lateral canals are present in the coronal or middle third of 59% of molars;[20] 76% of molars are reported to have openings in the furcation.[21] It has been shown, using a vascular injection technique that these accessory canals often had a greater diameter than the apical foramina, and the blood vessels passing through them often had a greater diameter than those in the apical foramina.[22] The accessory and lateral canals may be demonstrated histologically, by clearing techniques, or clinically on radiographs (Fig. 4.4). The presence of these canals in teeth with necrotic pulps allows microbial toxins to stimulate inflammatory responses in the periapical tissues.

LOCATION OF APICAL FORAMINA

The majority of endodontists consider that the apical extent of canal preparation should be determined by the position of the apical constriction in the region of the dentine-cementum junction (Fig. 4.5). Provided that this constriction is not destroyed, the periapical tissues are not damaged during root canal preparation and obturation.

Studies indicate that the apical foramen rarely coincides in position with the anatomical apex. According to various radiological and morphological studies of different teeth,[23–28] the mean distance between the apical foramen and the most apical end of the root is between 0.2 and 2.0 mm. Furthermore, the apical constriction tends to occur about 0.5–1 mm from the apical foramen.[24] Ideally, the apical constriction should be used as a natural 'stop' or 'end point' in root canal treatment, and the integrity of the constriction should be maintained during treatment if complications are to be avoided. This position can usually be located accurately with an apex locator.[29,30,31]

VARIATIONS IN PULP SPACE ANATOMY

Variations in tooth form have interested scientists and anthropologists as well as dentists. These studies of

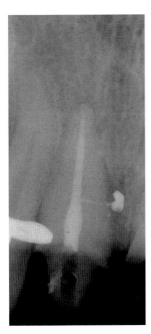

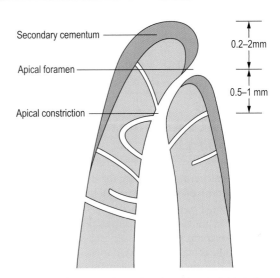

Figure 4.5 Diagrammatic section through apical third of root. The position of the apical foramen varies with age and may be 0.2–2.0 mm from the anatomical apex. The apical constriction may be 0.5–1.0 mm from the foramen.

Figure 4.4 Radiograph of a maxillary central incisor, a lateral canal is revealed after placement of the root filling.

variations have primarily been concentrated on the systematic description of dental crown morphology rather than root form. Variations in root form and number are likely to have a direct influence upon the configuration of the root canals in affected teeth. One variation, which has received some attention, is the three-rooted mandibular first molar; surveys of Mongoloid populations indicate a high prevalence.[32,33,34] The prevalence of other Mongoloid root traits has been less well studied. In clinical practice it is not always possible to observe these variations from radiographs.

In the condition *dens invaginatus*, the surface of the tooth formed with a deep pit into the pulp space during tooth development, which subsequently becomes a route for infection into the pulp. Depending on the severity of the condition, endodontic treatment will be difficult or very challenging. The most commonly affected tooth is the maxillary lateral incisor.[35,36] In the opposite condition *dens evaginatus*, the surface of the tooth formed into a very protuberant cusp during tooth development. There is a high risk of this cusp fracturing during function creating a route for infection of the pulp space. The mandibular premolar is most frequently affected and is more often found in Mongoloid people.[37] It is best managed by prophylactic treatment.[38]

The descriptions of the frequently occurring root and canal forms of permanent teeth are based largely on studies conducted in Europe and North America, and relate to teeth of predominantly Caucasoid origin. The descriptions may not be wholly applicable to teeth of non-Caucasoid origin. For example, the average lengths of teeth, around which there is wide variation, apply to Caucasoid populations. Practitioners who regularly treat Mongoloid populations are aware that roots are usually shorter. Racial differences and its influence on pulp space anatomy should always be kept in mind.

EFFECTS OF TERTIARY DENTINE ON PULP SPACE

Tertiary dentine is formed by odontoblasts in response to irritation from caries, restorative dentistry or tooth wear. The amount formed is dependent on the degree and duration of irritation. The function of this dentine is to wall off the pulp from the irritants; it is generally of great benefit to operative dentists. However, when root canal treatment becomes indicated, the coronal pulp is then exceedingly small and, therefore, difficult to locate. In addition, canal orifices become narrowed by deposition of tertiary dentine making their identification difficult.

There is no substitute for a good knowledge of pulpal anatomy; however, the clinician should be aided by a good quality preoperative radiograph from which the depth and direction of the root canals can be gauged. When inside the centre of the tooth and attempting to locate the pulp space, illumination and magnification are major assets. Whilst this can be provided by a headlamp and loupes, it is best achieved using an operating microscope. The increased illumination reveals the different colours of circumpulpal and tertiary dentine, so that the access to the root canals can be correctly orientated.

PULP SPACE ANATOMY AND ACCESS CAVITIES

Each line drawing accompanying the description of pulp space anatomy represents, from left to right:

- longitudinal mesiodistal section, viewed from the lingual in anterior teeth and from the buccal in posterior teeth;
- longitudinal buccolingual section viewed from the mesial, and also the axial angulation of the tooth relative to the horizontal occlusal plane;
- horizontal sections through the root(s): (above) 3 mm from apex; (below) at the cervical level;
- incisal or occlusal view.

The classical outline of the access cavity is shown as a dotted line. The size of the pulp cavity shortly after completion of root formation is as shown in pink, and in old age in brown. Line drawings are accompanied, where appropriate, by photographs of cleared specimens to give an insight into the variations of canal form that exist in the adult dentition.

Access cavity design should not be thought of as a one size fits all. Rather they should be developed to suit the specific pulpal anatomy of individual teeth.[39] The classical outline of access cavities is helpful in the appreciation of pulp space anatomy. However, it must be emphasized that rather than pre-conceptualized designs, access cavities should be prepared according to access requirements. Whilst unnecessary and excessive destruction of tooth tissue must be avoided it is important to remember that all caries and the roof of the pulp chamber must be completely removed. If and where necessary, following caries removal, a good temporary restoration should be placed to prevent coronal leakage.

Recently, several authors[40,41] have recognized the importance of the systematic development of the pulp space during tooth formation to the understanding of access cavity preparation. This recognition has led to a number of 'laws' being postulated, to serve as a guide to clinicians in developing the access cavity and locating accurately root canal orifices (Table 4.1).

Maxillary central and lateral incisors

The outlines and pulp cavities of these teeth are similar (Figs 4.6 & 4.7). Central incisors are larger with a mean length of 23 mm. Lateral incisors are smaller with a mean length of 21–22 mm. The canal form is usually Type I, and it is extremely rare for these teeth to have more than one

Table 4.1 Laws relating to pulp chamber anatomy (Adapted from Krasner & Rankow[37] and Peters[38])	
Law of centrality	The floor of the pulp chamber is always located in the centre of the tooth at the level of the cemento-enamel junction (CEJ).
Law of concentricity	At the level of the CEJ the shape of the pulp chamber mimics the external anatomy of the tooth.
Law of the CEJ	The distance from the external surface of the tooth to the wall of the pulp chamber is the same throughout the circumference of the tooth at the level of the CEJ. The CEJ is the most reliable and consistent feature for ascertaining the position of the pulp chamber.
First law of symmetry	With the exception of the maxillary molars, the orifices of the canals are equidistant either side of a line drawn mesial to distal through the floor of the pulp chamber.
Second law of symmetry	With the exception of the maxillary molars, the orifices of the canals lie on a line perpendicular to the line drawn mesial to distal through the floor of the pulp chamber.
The law of colour change	The dentine of the floor of the pulp chamber is, invariably a darker colour than the roof and walls. With good magnification and illumination this allows the clinician to differentiate and selectively remove tissue.
First law of orifice location	The orifices of the root canals are located where the walls and the floor meet.
Second law of orifice location	The orifices of the root canals are located at the angles in the floor/wall junctions.
Third law of orifice location	The orifices of the root canals are located at the ends of the root developmental fusion lines.

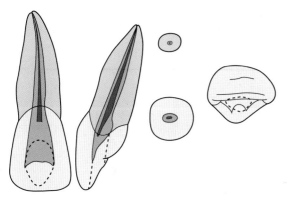

Figure 4.6 Maxillary central incisor with a Type I configuration.

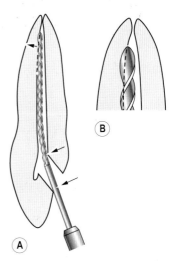

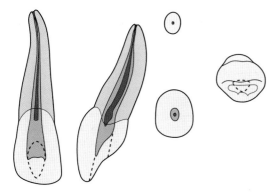

Figure 4.7 Maxillary lateral incisor with a Type I configuration.

Figure 4.8 (A) The access cavity is too small and close to the cingulum, therefore instruments do not lie passively in the canal and may create a ledge apically. The incorrect access also hinders cleaning of the pulp chamber and near the apex. (B) Enlargement of the apex showing labial ledge and uninstrumented palatal side.

root or more than one root canal. Where abnormalities do occur they seem to affect the maxillary lateral incisor, which may present with an extra root, second root canal, dens invaginatus, gemination or fusion.[42,43] The pulp chamber, when viewed labiopalatally, is seen to be pointed towards the incisal and widest at the cervical level. Mesiodistally both pulp chambers follow the general outline of their crowns and are thus widest at their incisal levels. The central incisors of young patients normally have three pulp horns. Lateral incisors usually have two pulp horns, and the incisal outline of the pulp chamber tends to be more rounded than that of central incisors.

The root canal differs greatly in outline when viewed mesiodistally and labiopalatally. The former view generally shows a fine straight canal that is seen on a radiograph. Labiopalatally the canal is very much wider and often shows a constriction just apical to the cervix; this view is rarely seen on radiographs and it is important to remember, during treatment, that all canals have this third dimension. The canal is tapered with an oval or irregular cross-section cervically that becomes round only very near

the apex. There is generally very little apical curvature in central incisors. The apex of lateral incisors is often curved in a distal/palatal direction. Sometimes the plane in which it lies means the apex is not easily discernible during radiographic canal length determination.

As the teeth age, the anatomy of the pulp space alters with the deposition of secondary dentine. The roof of the pulp chamber recedes, in some cases to the cervical level, and the canal appears very narrow mesiodistally on a radiograph. It is often possible to negotiate a canal that appears very fine or non-existent on a preoperative radiograph. When some incisors are traumatized, their pulps may mineralize, that is, the pulp canal becomes obliterated; subsequent root canal treatment is extremely difficult as mineralization frequently occurs throughout the length of the pulp space.

Access cavities to maxillary incisors

Access cavities in anterior teeth will vary in size and shape according to the dimension of the pulp. They should be designed so that a straight line approach is possible to the apical third of the root without the instruments bending, or binding against the walls of the access cavity or root canal. An access cavity that is too small and close to the cingulum leads to severe stresses in the instrument with binding against the access cavity walls and risks ledge formation apically (Fig. 4.8). The access cavity should extend far enough incisally to allow the instrument to reach the apical part of the canal. Sometimes the incisal edge must be involved if access is to be adequate.

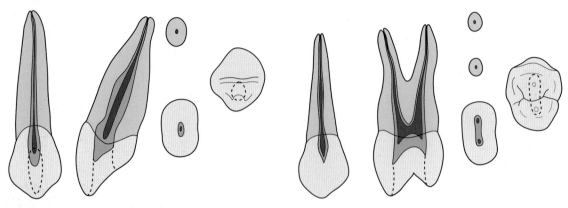

Figure 4.9 Maxillary canine with a Type I configuration.

Figure 4.10 Maxillary first premolar with two roots.

As the pulp is broader incisally than it is cervically, the outline should be triangular and must extend far enough mesially and distally to include the pulp horns. Once adequate access has been made into the pulp chamber, the cervical constriction should be removed to facilitate instrumentation of the apical part. The accuracy of initial access is particularly important in the older patient because the pulp space is more difficult to find. It is wise to begin the access cavity close to the incisal edge so that the pulp space can be approached in a straight line.

Maxillary canine

This is the longest tooth, mean length 26.5 mm, and therefore, longer root canal files are often required. It seldom has more than one root canal; the pulp chamber is quite narrow, and as there is only one pulp horn; the pulp is pointed incisally. The general shape of the pulp space is similar to the incisors (Fig. 4.9). The Type I root canal is oval and does not begin to become circular in cross-section until the apical third. The canal is usually straight but may show a distal apical curvature; the curvature depends on the movement of the tooth during eruption.

Maxillary first premolar

This tooth generally has two roots with two canals. The frequency of single-rooted maxillary first premolars ranges from 31–39% in Caucasians.[1,44] In people of Mongoloid origin, the frequency of maxillary first premolars with one root is in excess of 60%.[45,46,47] Three roots have been reported in 6% of cases.[1] A typical Caucasoid specimen has two well-developed fully formed roots that normally begin in the middle third of the roots (Fig. 4.10). The single-rooted condition prevalent in Mongoloid people represents a fusion of two separate roots.

Irrespective of origin, this tooth normally has two canals, and in the case of single-rooted specimens these canals may open through a common apical foramen. Many types of canal configuration are to be found in this tooth (Fig. 4.11) and the presence of lateral canals, particularly in the apical region can be as high as 49%.[44] The three-rooted form tends to have three canals, two located buccally and one palatally. Careful study of a preoperative radiograph should help reveal the root canal morphology. However, this morphology may be difficult to visualize radiologically, particularly when the apex is very fine.

The mean length of first premolars is 21 mm. The pulp chamber is wide buccopalatally with two distinct pulp horns, but is narrow mesiodistally. The floor is rounded with the highest point in the centre and generally just apical to the level of the cervix. The orifices into the root canals are funnel-shaped and lie buccally and palatally under the cusp tips. As the tooth ages, secondary dentine is deposited on the roof of the pulp chamber and this has the effect of bringing the roof very much closer to the floor. The floor level remains apical to the cervix and the thickened roof may reach apical to the cervix. The root canals are normally separate, and very rarely blend into the ribbon-like type of canal frequently seen in the second premolar. They are usually straight with a round cross-section.

Maxillary second premolar

The maxillary second premolar tends to be single-rooted. The Type I canal form is prevalent; however, over 25% of these teeth may present as Types II and III, and a further 25% may have Types IV-VII forms with two canals at the apex.[46,48] Thus, the typical maxillary second premolar may be envisaged as having one root with a single canal (Fig. 4.12). Less frequently two roots may be present, and while the outward appearance may be similar to the first premolar, the floor of the pulp chamber is well apical to the cervix. The mean length of the second premolar is slightly longer than the first premolar at 21.5 mm.

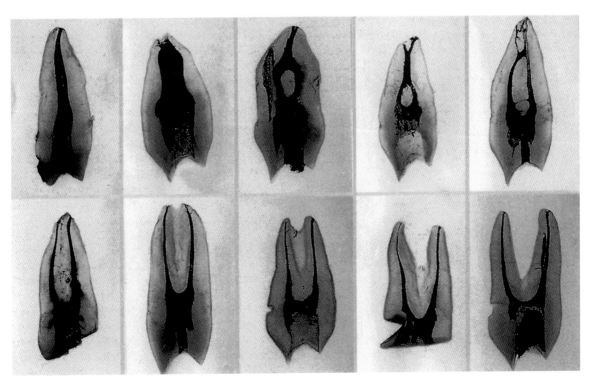

Figure 4.11 Cleared teeth showing various canal configurations in maxillary first premolars.

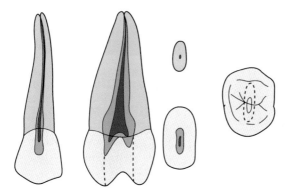

Figure 4.12 Maxillary second premolar with a Type I canal configuration.

The pulp chamber is wide buccopalatally and has two well-defined pulp horns. The root canal is also wide buccopalatally but narrow mesiodistally. It tapers apically but rarely develops a circular cross-section except in the apical 2–3 mm. Often, the root of this single-rooted tooth branches into two sections in the middle third of the root. These branches almost invariably join to form a common canal, which has a relatively large foramen. The canal is usually straight but the apex may curve to the distal. As the tooth matures, the roof of the pulp chamber recedes away from the crown.

Access cavities to maxillary premolars

Access should be through the occlusal surface, to allow files to negotiate the canals. The access cavity is a narrow slot in a buccolingual direction. In the case of the first premolar, the orifices of the root canal are readily visible as they lie just apical to the cervix. The second premolar root canal is ribbon-shaped and, because it lies well apical to the cervix, may not be readily visible. In preparing an access cavity, an inexperienced operator without magnification may easily mistake the pulp horns for the canal orifices.

Maxillary first molar

Maxillary first molars are generally three-rooted with four root canals (Fig. 4.13). The additional canal is located in the mesiobuccal root. The canal form of the mesiobuccal root has been extensively investigated. Studies in vitro indicate that a second canal is present in up to 90% of teeth.[3,11,49,50,51] Canal configuration is usually Type II (Fig. 4.14); however, the presence of a Type IV form with two separate apical foramina has been reported to be as

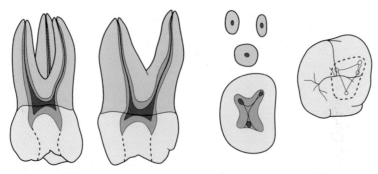

Figure 4.13 Maxillary first molar.

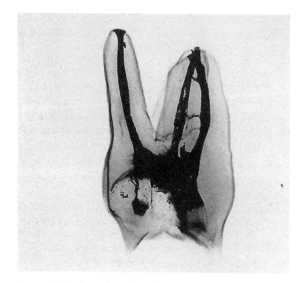

Figure 4.14 Cleared maxillary first molar with a Type II canal configuration in the mesiobuccal root.

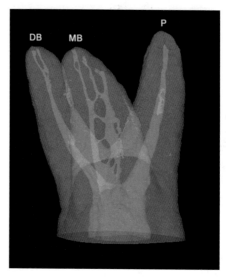

Figure 4.15 Micro-computed tomography of a maxillary first molar with three roots: mesiobuccal (MB), distobuccal (DB) and palatal (P); demonstrating the multiple and complicated intercanal connections between the first and second MB root canals; the MB and DB roots are further complicated by accessory canals in the apical third. From Somma et al 2009 with permission from Wiley-Blackwell.

high as 48%.[11] Studies in vivo[3,52,53,54] have, historically, reported a lower prevalence of the second mesiobuccal canal; however, as an operating microscope is used more routinely nowadays, unless otherwise proven, a second canal is assumed to be present. Three-dimensional tomographic radiography continues to reveal the complexity of root canal systems within the mesiobuccal root (Fig. 4.15). The palatal and distobuccal roots usually present a Type I configuration.

In Caucasians, the mean length of this tooth is 22 mm, the palatal root being slightly longer than the buccal roots. In Mongoloid teeth there is a tendency for the roots to be closer together and the average length slightly shorter. The pulp chamber is quadrilateral in shape and wider buccopalatally than mesiodistally. It has four pulp horns, of which the mesiobuccal is the longest and sharpest in outline. The distobuccal pulp horn is smaller than the mesiobuccal but larger than the two palatal pulp horns.

The floor of the pulp chamber is normally just apical to the cervix, and is rounded and dome-shaped. The orifices of the main pulp canals are funnel-shaped and lie, symmetrically in the middle of the appropriate root. The second mesiobuccal canal, if present, lies mesial to a line joining the main mesiobuccal and palatal canal orifices. It can be located anywhere between the two canals but is most frequently found adjacent to the main mesiobuccal canal under a lip of dentine. Further, the transverse cross-sectional shape of the pulp chamber 1 mm above the pulpal floor is trapezoidal in most teeth.[50] For this reason, the mesiobuccal canal opening is closer to the buccal wall than is the distobuccal orifice. The distobuccal root, and hence the opening into the root canal is closer to the middle of the tooth than to the distal wall. The palatal root canal orifice lies in the middle of the palatal root and is normally easy to identify.

The cross-section of the root canals varies considerably. The mesiobuccal canals are usually the most challenging to instrument as they leave the pulp chamber in a mesial direction before curving distopalatally. The second mesiobuccal canal is, generally, very fine and may join the main canal. The orifice of this canal may be concealed by a dentine lip, which needs to be removed to detect the orifice.[55] As both mesiobuccal canals lie in a buccopalatal plane they are often superimposed on radiographs. The distobuccal canal leaves the pulp chamber in a distal direction. It is ovoid in shape and again narrower mesiodistally. It tapers towards the apex and becomes circular in cross-section. The canal normally curves mesially in the apical half of the root. The palatal canal is the largest and longest of the three canals and leaves the pulp chamber as a round canal, which gradually tapers apically. In 50% of roots it is not straight but curves buccally in the apical 3–4 mm. This curvature may not be apparent on a clinical radiograph and unless appreciated, it may lead to incorrect length measurement and canal transportation following instrumentation.

As the tooth ages, secondary dentine is deposited chiefly on the roof of the pulp chamber; thus reducing the depth of the pulp chamber. The presence of tertiary dentine further complicates canal location. As the pulp chamber becomes progressively obliterated, access preparation becomes more challenging. It is relatively easy for the inexperienced operator, and particularly with high-speed handpieces, to perforate the floor of the pulp chamber. Access should be achieved patiently and with precision. The distance from cusp tips to roof of the pulp chamber should be measured on a preoperative radiograph, taken using the paralleling technique. This distance may then be marked on the bur to serve as a depth gauge. It is prudent to restrict the use of high-speed handpieces to removal of superficial tooth substance or restorative materials, and to complete the access cavity with round burs with low-speed handpieces or with ultrasound and special endodontic tips. The use of magnification and illumination, usually an operating microscope, allows better visualization of the pulp chamber. The variable nature of the pulp space anatomy of the maxillary first molar has received emphasis in recent clinical case reports. The occurrence of teeth with two palatal roots and multiple palatal canals has been reported.[56,57,58,59]

Maxillary second molar

The maxillary second molar is usually a smaller replica of the first molar (Fig. 4.16). The roots are less divergent, and fusion between two roots is much more frequent than in the maxillary first molar. Teeth with three canals and three apical foramina are prevalent, but a recent study has shown a high incidence of second mesiobuccal canals;[60] the mean length is 21 mm. Root fusion has been demonstrated in up to 55% of Caucasoid maxillary second molars, while in Mongoloid groups this figure may be up to 85%.[33,46] Where root fusion does occur, the canals and their orifices are much closer together (Fig. 4.17).

Maxillary third molar

The maxillary third molar displays a great deal of variability in terms of morphology. It may possess three separate roots, but more often partial or complete fusion occurs.[60] The pulp space anatomy is less predictable and these teeth may have a reduced number of canals.

Access cavities to maxillary molars

The traditional access cavity outline for maxillary teeth is normally in the mesial two-thirds of the occlusal surface leaving the oblique ridge intact, and is triangular with the base of the triangle towards the buccal, and the apex

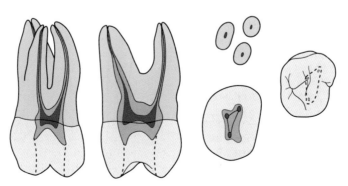

Figure 4.16 Maxillary second molar.

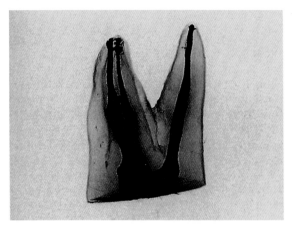

Figure 4.17 Cleared maxillary second molar with fused buccal roots.

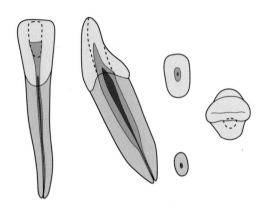

Figure 4.18 Mandibular central incisor with a Type I canal configuration.

palatally. It has been suggested that this traditional shape should be modified in the case of the first molar to a trapezoid shape.[54] Because the distobuccal canal is not as close to the buccal surface as the mesiobuccal canal, less tooth tissue removal is needed from this area.

Mandibular central and lateral incisors

Both types of teeth have a mean length of 21 mm, although the central incisor may be a little shorter than the lateral incisor. The root canal morphology may be placed into one of three configurations:[7]

- Type I – a single main canal extending from the pulp chamber to the apical foramen (Fig. 4.18).
- Type II/III – two main root canals that merge in the middle or apical third of the root into a single canal with one apical foramen (Fig. 4.19).
- Type IV – two main canals that remain distinct throughout the length of the tooth and exit through two major apical foramina (Fig. 4.20).

Studies indicate that the Type I canal form is most prevalent, Types II and III less prevalent, and Type IV least prevalent. The presence of two canals has been recorded to be as high as 41%;[7] however, the highest recorded figure for two separate apical foramina (Type IV) is 5%.[12] There is some evidence to suggest that there is a lower frequency of two canals in mandibular central and lateral incisors in Mongoloid people.[61]

The pulp chamber is a smaller replica of that in the maxillary incisors. It is pointed incisally with three pulp horns that are not well developed, is oval in cross-section, and wider labiolingually than it is mesiodistally. When the tooth has a single root canal it is normally straight but may curve to the distal and less often to the labial. The

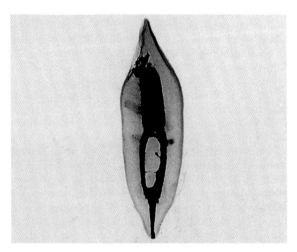

Figure 4.19 Cleared mandibular central incisor with a Type II canal configuration.

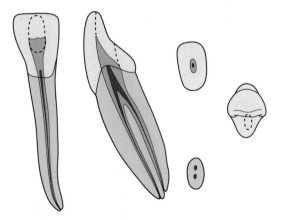

Figure 4.20 Mandibular lateral incisor with a Type IV canal configuration.

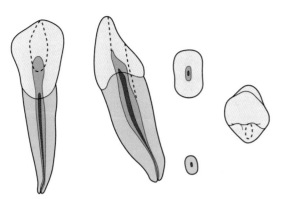

Figure 4.21 Mandibular canine with a Type I canal configuration.

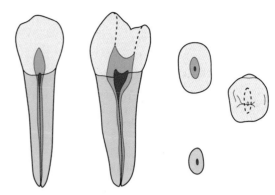

Figure 4.22 Mandibular second premolar with a Type I canal configuration.

tooth ages in a similar way to the maxillary incisors, and the incisal part of the pulp chamber may recede to a level apical to the cervix. The pulps of these teeth may mineralize in response to traumatic injury.

Mandibular canine

This tooth resembles the maxillary canine, although its dimensions are smaller. It rarely has two roots and the mean length is 22.5 mm. The Type I canal form is most prevalent (Fig. 4.21); the frequency of two canals is 14%.[8] However, less than 6% of mandibular canines display the Type IV canal form with two separate apical foramina.[5,11]

Access cavities to mandibular incisors and canines

Essentially, these cavities are similar to those in maxillary incisors. However, because of the more pronounced labial curvature of the crown and because the canals, particularly in older patients are so fine, it is sometimes necessary to involve the incisal edge of the tooth. However, it is important to be as conservative as possible and not remove more tooth tissue than necessary and the bulk of the cingulum should be retained.

Mandibular premolars

These teeth are usually single-rooted; however, the mandibular first premolar may present with a division of roots in the apical half. The Type I canal configuration is the most prevalent (Fig. 4.22). Where two canals are present, they are more likely in the first premolar and may involve up to one-third of teeth.[11,46,62,63,64] Additional canals may be suspected if a root canal that is visible radiologically in the coronal part of the root appears to stop abruptly as it is traced apically. Where division of canals occurs, the

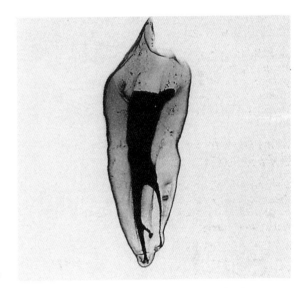

Figure 4.23 Cleared mandibular first premolar with a Type IV canal configuration and a lateral canal.

tendency is for them to remain separate, to produce a Type IV/V form (Fig. 4.23). The Type II/III forms are seen in less than 5% of these teeth (Fig. 4.24). The highest reported frequency of a second canal in second premolars is 11%. Less than 2% of first premolars have three canals.[11,46,64] The presence of multiple canals has been reported.[65,66,67,68] African Americans and the southern Chinese population of Hong Kong have a high prevalence of teeth with more than one canal.[46,63]

The pulp chamber is wide buccolingually, and while there are two pulp horns, only the buccal is well developed. The lingual pulp horn is very slight in the first premolar but better developed in the second premolar. The canals of these two teeth are similar, although smaller than the canines, and are thus wide buccolingually until they reach the middle third of the root, where they constrict.

Access cavities to mandibular premolars

These should be through the occlusal surface and wide buccolingually. In the first premolar with two canals it may be necessary to extend the cavity onto the buccal surface.

Mandibular first molar

The mandibular first molar usually has two roots, a mesial and a distal. The distal is smaller and usually rounder than the mesial. There is a variation with a supernumerary distolingual root; the reported frequency ranges from 6 to 44%.[69,70] The two-rooted molar usually has a canal configuration of three canals (Fig. 4.25), and the mean length is 21 mm. Two canals are usually located in the mesial root with one in the distal. The mesial root in 40–45% of cases has only one apical foramen.[2,11] These

canals may have a latticework arrangement of connections along their length[71,72,73,74] (Fig. 4.26). Specimens with three canals in the mesial root[75] and a total of five canals have also been observed (Fig. 4.27).

The single distal canal is larger, centrally placed buccolingually and more oval in cross-section than the mesial canals, and in 60% of cases, emerges on the distal side of the root surface short of the anatomical apex.[76] The incidence of two distal canals in mandibular first molars has been reported as 38%.[2] The orifices are sited buccal and lingual, and are small. The tendency for the mandibular first molar to have three roots appears to be associated with the frequency of the second distal canal, which approaches half of these teeth.[70]

The pulp chamber is wider mesially than it is distally and may have five pulp horns, the lingual pulp horns being longer and more pointed. The floor is rounded and convex toward the occlusal and lies just apical to the cervix. The root canals leave the pulp chamber through funnel-shaped openings of which the mesial tend to be much finer than the distal. Of the two mesial canals, the mesiobuccal is the more difficult canal to negotiate because of its tortuous path. It leaves the pulp chamber in a mesial direction, which alters to a distal direction in the middle third of the root. The mesiolingual canal is slightly larger in cross-section and generally follows a much straighter course, although it may curve mesially towards the apical part. When a second distal canal is present on the distolingual aspect it tends to curve towards the buccal. With age, the pulp chamber recedes from the occlusal surface and the canals become constricted.

Mandibular second molar

In Caucasoid populations the mandibular second molar presents as a smaller version of the mandibular first molar with a mean length of 20 mm. The mesial root has two canals and, unlike the first molar, there is usually only one distal canal. The mesial canals tend to fuse in the apical third to give rise to one main apical foramen (Fig. 4.28).

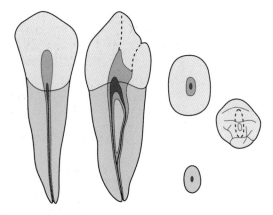

Figure 4.24 Mandibular first premolar with a Type II canal configuration.

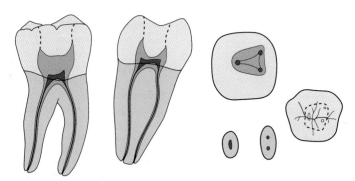

Figure 4.25 Mandibular first molar, with a Type IV canal configuration in the mesial root (second from left).

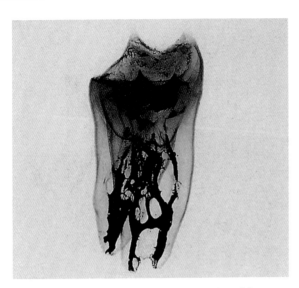

Figure 4.26 Cleared mandibular first molar viewed from the mesiobuccal showing connections between the mesial canals.

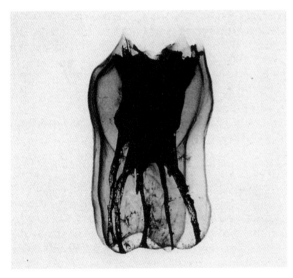

Figure 4.27 Cleared mandibular first molar viewed from the mesial showing five canals.

Studies[77-81] have highlighted the tendency for mandibular second molars to have fused roots in up to 52% of the Chinese population. The fusion gives rise to a horseshoe shape when the roots are viewed in cross-section. Where there is incomplete separation of roots there may also be incomplete division of canals giving rise to the C-shaped canal,[82,83,84] which increases the likelihood of canal interconnections and unpredictably placed canal orifices. One such orifice has now been termed the median buccal

canal orifice,[80] which leads to the median buccal canal (Fig. 4.29).

Mandibular third molar

The form of this tooth is often very varied. It generally has as many root canals as there are cusps. The roots are normally shorter than other molars. Root canal treatment on mandibular third molars may be relatively straight forward because access is facilitated by the mesial inclination of many of these teeth; however, aberrant forms of the pulp space do exist. Careful preoperative assessment is essential.

Access cavities to mandibular molars

The prevalence of the second distal canal in mandibular first molars may necessitate a rectangular outline. The access cavity should be placed in the mesial three-quarters of the occlusal surface. Care should always be taken to remove the roof of the pulp chamber completely without causing damage to the floor of the pulp chamber.

PULP SPACE ANATOMY OF PRIMARY TEETH

The object of endodontic treatment in primary teeth is to preserve the tooth in form and function (see Chapter 11); the endodontic techniques are modified from those for management of permanent teeth.

The pulp cavities in primary teeth have certain common characteristics:

- Proportionally, they are much larger than in permanent teeth.
- The enamel and dentine surrounding the pulp cavities are much thinner than in permanent teeth.
- There is no clear demarcation between the pulp chamber and the root canals.
- The pulp canals are more slender and tapering, and are longer in proportion to the crown than the corresponding permanent teeth.
- Multirooted primary teeth show a greater degree of interconnecting branches between pulp canals.
- The pulp horns of primary molars are more pointed than suggested by cusp anatomy.

Primary incisors and canines

The pulp chambers of both maxillary and mandibular incisors and canines follow closely their crown outlines. However, the pulp tissue is much closer to the surface of the tooth, and the pulp horns are not as sharp and pronounced as in permanent teeth (Fig. 4.30). The pulp

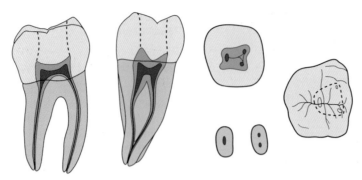

Figure 4.28 Mandibular second molar, with a Type II canal configuration in the mesial root (second from left).

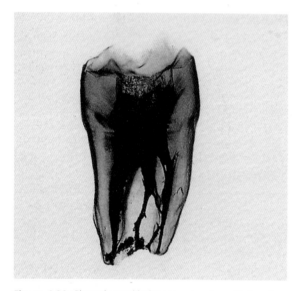

Figure 4.29 Cleared mandibular second molar with fused roots viewed from the buccal showing the median buccal canal.

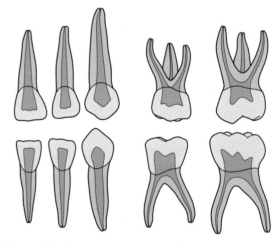

Figure 4.30 Pulpal space anatomy of the primary teeth.

canals are wide coronally and taper apically, and there is no clear demarcation between pulp chamber and root canal. Occasionally, the canals of mandibular incisors may be divided into two branches by a mesiodistal wall of dentine. Maxillary primary incisors have a mean length of 16 mm, while the laterals are slightly shorter. Mandibular central incisors are 14 mm, and mandibular lateral incisors are 15 mm. The canines are the longest primary teeth, the maxillary canines being 19 mm and the mandibular 17 mm.

Primary molars

As in the permanent dentition the maxillary molars are three-rooted (two buccal and one palatal) whilst the mandibular molars only have two roots (mesial and distal) (Fig. 4.30). The pulp chambers are large in relation to tooth size, and the pulp horns are well developed, particularly in the second molars. From a restorative point of view it is important to remember that the tip of the pulp horns may be as close as 2 mm from the enamel surface, and thus great care must be taken in preparing cavities in these teeth if pulpal exposure is to be avoided. Because of the relatively large size of the pulp chamber, there is relatively less hard tissue protecting the pulp.

The furcation of the roots is also very much closer to the cervical area of the crown and thus damage to the floor of the pulp chamber may lead to perforation. Mandibular molars normally have two root canals in each root, and the mesiobuccal root canal of the maxillary molars may divide into two. Thus both maxillary and mandibular primary molars frequently have four canals.

APICAL CLOSURE

While calcification and cementum deposition at the apex continue throughout life, apices can be considered as fully

Table 4.2 Ages when root apices are considered fully formed

TOOTH TYPE	AGE (YEARS)
Primary incisor	2
Primary canine and molar	3
Permanent first molar	9
Permanent central incisor	10
Permanent lateral incisor	11
Permanent premolar	15
Permanent second molar	17
Permanent third molar	21

formed several years after eruption, and approximate ages are shown in Table 4.2.

LEARNING OUTCOMES

After reading this chapter, the reader should be able to understand and discuss the:

- complex and divergent anatomy of the pulp space
- relationship between tooth development and pulp space anatomy
- design of access cavities for individual teeth and according to treatment requirements
- advantages of magnification and illumination in access cavity preparation and pulp space examination.

REFERENCES

1. Carns EJ, Skidmore AE. Configurations and deviations of root canals of maxillary first premolars. Oral Surgery, Oral Medicine, Oral Pathology 1973;36:880–886.
2. Skidmore AE, Bjorndal AM. Root canal morphology of the human mandibular first molar. Oral Surgery, Oral Medicine, Oral Pathology 1971;32:778–784.
3. Seidberg BH, Altman M, Guttuso J, Suson M. Frequency of two mesiobuccal root canals in maxillary permanent first molars. Journal of the American Dental Association 1973;87:852–856.
4. Madeira MC, Hetem S. Incidence of bifurcations in mandibular incisors. Oral Surgery, Oral Medicine, Oral Pathology 1973;36:589–591.
5. Vertucci FJ. Root canal anatomy of the mandibular anterior teeth. Journal of the American Dental Association 1974;89:369–371.
6. Vertucci FJ. Root canal anatomy of the human permanent teeth. Oral Surgery, Oral Medicine, Oral Pathology 1984;58:589–599.
7. Benjamin KA, Dowson J. Incidence of two root canals in human mandibular incisor teeth. Oral Surgery, Oral Medicine, Oral Pathology 1974;38:122–126.
8. Kaffe I, Kaufman A, Littner M, Lazarson A. Radiographic study of the root canal system of mandibular anterior teeth. International Endodontic Journal 1985;18:253–259.
9. Laws AJ. Prevalence of canal irregularities in mandibular incisors: a radiographic study. New Zealand Dental Journal 1971;67:181–186.
10. Miyoshi S, Fujiwara J, Tsuji Y, et al. Bifurcated root canals and crown diameter. Journal of Dental Research 1977;56:1425.
11. Pineda F, Kuttler Y. Mesiodistal and buccolingual roentgenographic investigation of 7,275 root canals. Oral Surgery, Oral Medicine, Oral Pathology 1972;33:101–110.
12. Rankine-Wilson RW, Henry P. The bifurcated root canal in lower anterior teeth. Journal of the American Dental Association 1965;70:1162–1165.
13. Somma F, Leoni D, Plotino G, et al. Root canal morphology of the mesiobuccal root of the maxillary first molar: a micro-computed tomographic analysis. International Endodontic Journal 2009;42:165–174.
14. Patel S, Dawood A, Pitt Ford T, Whaites E. The potential application of cone beam computed tomography in the management of endodontic problems. International Endodontic Journal 2007;40:818–830.
15. Garberoglio R, Brännström M. Scanning electron microscopic investigation of human dentinal tubules. Archives of Oral Biology 1976;21:355–362.
16. Dourda AO, Moule AJ, Young WG. A morphometric analysis of the cross-sectional area of dentine occupied by dentinal tubules in human third molar teeth. International Endodontic Journal 1994;27:184–189.
17. Oguntebi BR. Dentine tubule infection and endodontic therapy implications. International Endodontic Journal 1994;27:218–222.
18. Gutmann JL, Pitt Ford TR. Management of the resected root end: a clinical review. International Endodontic Journal 1993;26:273–283.
19. Tidmarsh BG, Arrowsmith MG. Dentinal tubules at the root ends of apicected teeth: a scanning electron microscopic study. International Endodontic Journal 1989;22:184–189.
20. Lowman JV, Burke RS, Pelleu GB. Patent accessory canals: incidence in molar furcation region. Oral Surgery, Oral Medicine, Oral Pathology 1973;36:580–584.
21. Burch JG, Hulen S. A study of the presence of accessory foramina and topography of molar furcations. Oral Surgery, Oral Medicine, Oral Pathology 1974;38:451–455.

22. Kramer IRH. The vascular architecture of the human dental pulp. Archives of Oral Biology 1960;2:177–189.

23. Burch JG, Hulen S. The relationship of the apical foramen to the anatomic apex of the tooth root. Oral Surgery, Oral Medicine, Oral Pathology 1972;34:262–268.

24. Chapman CE. A microscopic study of the apical region of human anterior teeth. Journal of the British Endodontic Society 1969;3:52–58.

25. Dummer PMH, McGinn JH, Rees DG. The position and topography of the apical canal constriction and apical foramen. International Endodontic Journal 1984;17: 192–198.

26. Kerekes K, Tronstad L. Morphometric observations on root canals of human anterior teeth. Journal of Endodontics 1977;3:24–29.

27. Levy AB, Glatt L. Deviation of the apical foramen from the radiographic apex. Journal of the New Jersey State Dental Society 1970;41:12–13.

28. Martos J, Ferrer-Luque CM, Gonzalez-Rodriguez MP, Castro LAS. Topographical evaluation of the major apical foramen in permanent human teeth. International Endodontic Journal 2009;42:329–334.

29. Jenkins JA, Walker WA, Schindler WG, Flores CM. An in vitro evaluation of the accuracy of the Root ZX in the presence of various irrigants. Journal of Endodontics 2001;27:209–211.

30. Shabahang S, Goon WW, Gluskin AH. An in vivo evaluation of Root ZX electronic apex locator. Journal of Endodontics 1996;22:616–618.

31. Wrbas KT, Ziegler AA, Altenburger MJ, Schirrmeister JF. In vivo comparison of working length determination with two electronic apex locators. International Endodontic Journal 2007;40: 133–138.

32. Tratman EK. Three rooted lower molars in man and their racial distribution. British Dental Journal 1938;64:264–274.

33. Turner CG. The dentition of the Arctic peoples. PhD thesis.

Madison, WI, USA: University of Wisconsin; 1967.

34. Turner CG. Three rooted mandibular first permanent molars and the question of American Indian origins. American Journal of Physical Anthropology 1971;34: 229–241.

35. De Sousa SM, Bramante CM. Dens invaginatus: treatment choices. Endodontics and Dental Traumatology 1998;14:152–158.

36. Hülsmann M. Dens invaginatus: aetiology, classification, prevalence, diagnosis, and treatment considerations. International Endodontic Journal 1997;30: 79–90.

37. Uyeno DS, Lugo A. Dens evaginatus: a review. ASDC Journal of Dentistry for Children 1996;63: 328–332.

38. Koh ET, Pitt Ford TR, Kariyawasam SP, et al. Prophylactic treatment of dens evaginatus using mineral trioxide aggregate. Journal of Endodontics 2001;27:540–542.

39. Patel S, Rhodes J. A practical guide to endodontic access cavity preparation in molar teeth. British Dental Journal 2007;203:133–140.

40. Krasner P, Rankow HJ. Anatomy of the pulp chamber floor. Journal of Endodontics 2004;30:5–16.

41. Peters OA. Accessing root canal systems: knowledge base and clinical techniques. ENDO (London, England) 2008;2:87–104.

42. Reid JS, Saunders WP, MacDonald DG. Maxillary permanent incisors with two root canals: a report of two cases. International Endodontic Journal 1993;26: 246–250.

43. Thompson BH, Portell FR, Hartwell GR. Two root canals in a maxillary lateral incisor. Journal of Endodontics 1985;11:353–355.

44. Vertucci FJ, Gegauff A. Root canal morphology of the maxillary first premolar. Journal of the American Dental Association 1979;99: 194–198.

45. Nelson CT. The teeth of the Indians of Pecos Pueblo. American Journal of Physical Anthropology 1938;23:261–293.

46. Walker RT. A comparative investigation of the root number and canal anatomy of permanent

teeth in a southern Chinese population. PhD thesis. Hong Kong: University of Hong Kong; 1987.

47. Walker RT. Root form and canal anatomy of maxillary first premolars in a southern Chinese population. Endodontics and Dental Traumatology 1987;3:130–134.

48. Vertucci F, Seelig A, Gillis R. Root canal morphology of the human maxillary second premolar. Oral Surgery, Oral Medicine, Oral Pathology 1974;38:456–464.

49. Imura N, Hata GI, Toda T, et al. Two canals in mesiobuccal roots of maxillary molars. International Endodontic Journal 1998;31: 410–414.

50. Thomas RP, Moule AJ, Bryant R. Root canal morphology of maxillary permanent first molar teeth at various ages. International Endodontic Journal 1993;26: 257–267.

51. Stropko J. Canal morphology of maxillary molars: clinical observations on canal configurations. Journal of Endodontics 1999;25:446–450.

52. Altman M, Guttuso J, Seidberg BH, Langeland K. Apical root canal anatomy of human maxillary central incisors. Oral Surgery, Oral Medicine, Oral Pathology 1970; 30:694–699.

53. Slowey RR. Radiographic aids in the detection of extra root canals. Oral Surgery, Oral Medicine, Oral Pathology 1974;37:762–772.

54. Weller RN, Hartwell GR. The impact of improved access and searching techniques on detection of the mesio-lingual canal in maxillary molars. Journal of Endodontics 1989;15:82–83.

55. Ting PCS, Nga L. Clinical detection of minor mesiobuccal canal of maxillary first molars. International Endodontic Journal 1992;25: 304–306.

56. Beatty RG. A five-canal maxillary first molar. Journal of Endodontics 1984;10:156–157.

57. Harris WE. Unusual root canal anatomy in a maxillary molar. Journal of Endodontics 1980;6: 573–575.

58. Stone LH, Stroner WF. Maxillary molars demonstrating more than one palatal root canal. Oral Surgery, Oral Medicine, Oral Pathology 1981;51:649–652.

59. Wong M. Maxillary first molar with three palatal canals. Journal of Endodontics 1991;17:298–299.

60. Ng YL, Aung TH, Alavi A, Gulabivala K. Root and canal morphology of Burmese maxillary molars. International Endodontic Journal 2001;34:620–630.

61. Walker RT. The root canal anatomy of mandibular incisors in a southern Chinese population. International Endodontic Journal 1988;21:218–223.

62. Cleghorn BM, Christie WH, Dong CCS. The root and root canal morphology of the human mandibular second premolar: A literature review. Journal of Endodontics 2007;33:1031–1037.

63. Trope M, Elfenbein L, Tronstad L. Mandibular premolars with more than one root canal in different race groups. Journal of Endodontics 1986;12:343–345.

64. Vertucci FJ. Root canal morphology of mandibular premolars. Journal of the American Dental Association 1978;97:47–50.

65. Chan K, Yew SC, Chao SY. Mandibular premolar with three root canals – two case reports. International Endodontic Journal 1992;25:261–264.

66. Rhodes JS. A case of unusual anatomy: a mandibular second premolar with four canals. International Endodontic Journal 2001;34:645–648.

67. Serman NJ, Hasselgren G. The radiographic incidence of multiple roots and canals in human mandibular premolars. International Endodontic Journal 1992;25:234–237.

68. Wong M. Four root canals in a mandibular second premolar. Journal of Endodontics 1991;17:125–126.

69. Gulabivala K, Aung TH, Alavi A, Ng YL. Root and canal morphology of Burmese mandibular molars. International Endodontic Journal 2001;34:359–370.

70. Walker RT. The root form and canal anatomy of mandibular first molars in a southern Chinese population. Endodontics and Dental Traumatology 1988;4:19–22.

71. Jafarzadeh H, Wu Y-N. The C-shaped root canal configuration: A review. Journal of Endodontics 2007;33:517–523.

72. Mannocci F, Peru M, Sherriff M, et al. The isthmuses of the mesial root of mandibular molars: a micro-computed tomographic study. International Endodontic Journal 2005;38:558–563.

73. Teixeira FB, Sano CL, Gomes BP, et al. A preliminary in vitro study of the incidence and position of the root canal isthmus in maxillary and mandibular first molars. International Endodontic Journal 2003;36:276–280.

74. von Arx T. Frequency and type of canal isthmuses in first molars detected by endoscopic inspection during periradicular surgery. International Endodontic Journal 2005;38:160–168.

75. Fabra-Campos H. Three canals in the mesial root of mandibular first permanent molars: a clinical study. International Endodontic Journal 1989;22:39–43.

76. Tamse A, Littner MM, Kaffe I, et al. Morphological and radiographic study of the apical foramen in distal roots of mandibular molars. Part 1. The location of the apical foramen on various root aspects. International Endodontic Journal 1988;21:205–210.

77. Cooke HG, Cox FL. C-shaped canal configurations in mandibular molars. Journal of the American Dental Association 1979;99:836–839.

78. Manning SA. Root canal anatomy of mandibular second molars. Part I. International Endodontic Journal 1990;23:34–39.

79. Manning SA. Root canal anatomy of mandibular second molars. Part II C-shaped canals. International Endodontic Journal 1990;23:40–45.

80. Walker RT. Root form and canal anatomy of mandibular second molars in a southern Chinese population. Journal of Endodontics 1988;14:325–329.

81. Yang ZP, Yang SF, Lin YC, et al. C-shaped root canals in mandibular second molars in a Chinese population. Endodontics and Dental Traumatology 1988;4:160–163.

82. Fan W, Fan B, Gutmann JL, Cheung GSP. Identification of C-shaped canal systems in mandibular second molars. Part I: Radiographic and anatomic features revealed by intraradicular contrast medium. Journal of Endodontics 2007;33:806–810.

83. Fan B, Gao Y, Fan W, Gutmann JL. Identification of a C-shaped canal system in mandibular second molars. Part II: The effect of bone image superimposition and intraradicular contrast medium on radiograph interpretation. Journal of Endodontics 2008;34:160–165.

84. Fan W, Fan B, Gutmann JL, Fan M. Identification of a C-shaped canal system in mandibular second molars. Part III: Anatomic features revealed by digital subtraction radiography. Journal of Endodontics 2008;34:1187–1190.

Chapter | 5 |

Maintaining dental pulp vitality

H.F. Duncan

SUMMARY

Maintaining pulp vitality and preventing apical periodontitis is a founding principle of operative dentistry and endodontics. The vital pulp as part of the pulp-dentine complex has an array of defensive attributes which aim to protect itself against irritation. Knowledge of these irritants and the pulpal response is essential to prevent damage and to harness the natural defences. Recent developments in material science and molecular biology have led to a better understanding of tertiary dentinogenesis and greater predictability in treating deep caries and pulpal exposures.

INTRODUCTION

Clinicians should be aware that the best root canal filling is healthy pulp tissue. It should not be assumed that every damaged pulp must be extirpated and that pulp conservation is an unsatisfactory procedure. Therefore, preserving the pulp should be encouraged within the discipline of modern endodontics; it is more conservative, more biologically acceptable and less technically demanding than pulpectomy.

PULP-DENTINE COMPLEX

The dental pulp is in the centre of the tooth and is the tissue from which the dentine was formed during tooth development. It remains throughout life and provides nourishment for the odontoblasts that line its surface. These odontoblasts have long processes that may extend partly[1] or completely to the amelodentinal junction.[2] The tubules around and beyond the odontoblast processes are normally patent and filled with tissue fluid. When irritants are applied to the distal ends of the dentinal tubules, the odontoblasts will form more dentine, within tubules as intratubular dentine, leading to tubular sclerosis, or within the pulp as tertiary dentine. Sclerosis is a mechanism designed to protect the pulp and results in a more highly mineralized dentine at the distal extremities of the odontoblast processes. Two types of tertiary dentine are recognized, reactionary dentine formed by existing odontoblasts in response to mild irritation, or reparative dentine formed by newly recruited odontoblasts in response to severe irritation and odontoblast death.[3,4] Reparative dentine formation also occurs after pulp exposure when a dentine bridge is formed. If tertiary dentine is formed quickly, in response to more severe stimuli, the tubular pattern is less regular than if it is formed slowly, in response to mild stimuli. The tertiary dentine formed is, generally, confined to the tubules affected by the carious lesion. In addition to hard tissue deposition, another defensive feature in response to irritation is outward movement of fluid through the tubules during pulpal inflammation; this will reduce the inward movement of toxins.

The pulp and dentine can thus be regarded as one interconnected tissue, the pulp-dentine complex. This is normally protected from irritation by an intact layer of enamel. When enamel is breached by caries, erosion or operative procedures, the pulp is at risk. In a young patient, the tubules are wider and the pulp closer to the surface, so a similarly sized breach of enamel will have a greater effect on the pulp than that in an older patient. The greater the area of exposed dentine, the greater is the effect on the pulp. Therefore, the potential damage of crown preparations, extensive tooth wear and large cavities is greater.

PULP RESPONSE TO IRRITANTS

The pulp response to irritation is inflammation and formation of tertiary dentine and tubular sclerosis; these hard tissues attempt to wall off the irritants from the pulp, which will then become less inflamed. It has been shown that if buccal cavities are prepared in otherwise sound teeth and are left open to salivary microbial contamination, the pulp underneath the exposed tubules becomes inflamed.[5] If the irritant is removed and a restoration which prevents microleakage is placed, the pulpal inflammation subsides and tertiary dentine is formed; therefore, damaged pulps have the capacity to recover.[6]

PULP IRRITANTS

The dental pulp may be affected by a variety of stimuli, which can be broadly classified as being either microbial,

chemical or mechanical in origin. These irritants, for example mechanical and microbial, may act in combination to provoke pulpal inflammation.

Microbial

Dental caries

This has been regarded as the main cause of pulpal injury as it has been classically demonstrated that in the absence of bacteria, pulpal inflammation does not occur.[7] In the early carious lesion the odontoblasts respond by hard tissue deposition.[8,9]

As the carious lesion progresses, the enamel surface breaks down and bacteria enter the dentine. The rate of decay usually then accelerates. The lesion may be divided into zones: an outer zone of destruction, a middle zone of bacterial penetration and an inner zone of demineralization. The zone of destruction contains dentine partially destroyed by proteolytic enzymes from the mixed microbiota. The dentinal tubules and shrinkage clefts are filled with microorganisms. This carious dentine can be readily removed with hand excavators in active lesions and often has a light colour. In slowly progressing or arrested lesions, this dentine is darker and has a harder consistency.

The next zone, the zone of bacterial penetration, contains microorganisms within the dentinal tubules. The structure of the dentine, when examined in a demineralized histological section, is otherwise normal. Some tubules are deeply infected while others contain no microorganisms. A variety of microorganisms from this zone have been identified by culturing techniques – *Lactobacilli*, *Streptococci* and *Actinomyces* species.[10,11] More recently, molecular techniques have suggested that the microbiota is more complex than previously thought with many uncultivable species.[12] Deep carious dentine has been shown to contain predominantly anaerobic bacteria including *Propionibacteria*, *Prevotella*, *Eubacteria*, *Arachnia* and *Lactobacilli*.[13,14,15] Ahead of the zone of microorganism penetration is a zone of demineralization, frequently considered to be devoid of bacteria because the conditions for bacterial survival are too unfavourable; however, small numbers of anaerobic bacteria have been demonstrated in this zone.[16]

When dental caries affects the superficial dentine, initially localized inflammation is evident in the pulp. The dentine-pulp complex responds by intratubular dentine deposition leading to tubular sclerosis and by tertiary dentine deposition. Therefore, after a short interval the pulp is likely to recover and be of normal histological appearance.[17] No foci of inflammatory cells can be observed in the pulp until caries has penetrated to within 0.5 mm.[18] As the early dentine carious lesion progresses, the sclerotic zone of dentine becomes demineralized and the lesion subsequently advances into the tertiary dentine. When bacteria invade this dentine, severe pulp changes such as abscess formation often occur. Therefore, until the caries is very deep, the pulp is likely to be no more than reversibly damaged. Treatment should normally consist of removal of carious dentine and insertion of an effective restoration. This has been shown to result in recovery of the pulp.[6] Since it is difficult to assess accurately the histological state of the pulp from signs and symptoms, it is important to monitor teeth with deep caries.

The pulp is not infected until late in the carious process, typically when the tertiary dentine is invaded. Infection of the inflamed pulp is localized to necrotic tissue in a pulp abscess.[19] Wider infection of the pulp only occurs after necrosis.

Bacterial microleakage

Bacterial microleakage occurs around all restorations to a greater or lesser degree.[20] The bacteria from the oral cavity colonize the space around the restoration after its placement, rather than surviving from the time it was placed. The lack of importance of bacterial contamination at the time of cavity preparation has been shown in studies of pulpal exposures.[21,22] There is a good correlation between bacterial leakage around restorations and pulpal inflammation.[23,24]

The pulpal responses to irritation from bacterial microleakage are inflammation, tubular sclerosis and formation of tertiary dentine, so that after some months the bacteria ceases to irritate.[25] Nevertheless, measures should be taken to prevent pulp damage during this initial period. These consist of placing a cavity lining or base, the application of cavity varnish if appropriate, the use of a dentine-bonding agent and etching of enamel, or the use of an adhesive cement. In operative dentistry, the main reason for placing a cavity lining is to prevent damage to the pulp from bacterial leakage around restorations. Former reasons such as material irritancy or thermal protection have been severely criticized.[26,27]

In many instances, the choice of lining material in deep cavities without pulpal exposures would appear to be a matter of operator preference. Cements based on calcium hydroxide, glass ionomer, zinc phosphate or zinc oxide-eugenol would all appear to be satisfactory under amalgam, and have been widely used. Zinc oxide-eugenol cement has the benefit of prolonged antibacterial activity. Under resin-based restorative materials, linings are rarely placed as dentine-bonding agents are often adequate; zinc oxide–eugenol cement is inappropriate, unless separated by a covering layer of alternative cement (e.g. glass ionomer), as otherwise the eugenol may plasticize the resin. The durability of some calcium hydroxide cements has been questioned, particularly if the overlying restoration has an imperfect seal.[28,29]

Chemical

Dental materials

Historically, dental materials have been considered to exert an irritant effect on the pulp.[30,31,32] However, during the last 25 years, much of the earlier work on the irritancy of various materials has been brought into question.[20,24,33,34,35,36] For example, composite resin has been regarded as irritant to the pulp, but the blandness of this material has now been demonstrated together with the important contribution of bacterial leakage to pulp reaction.[36,37] Composite resin contracts when polymerized causing a gap to occur between the resin and the tooth, into which bacteria penetrates; inflamed pulps have been found in teeth with bacteria in the gap.[20,38] From a clinical standpoint, both etching enamel margins and dentine bonding are considered necessary to prevent a pulpal inflammatory reaction. Composite resins are continually evolving and appear to prevent leakage if carefully placed, demonstrating good clinical success.[39,40,41] However, some concern remains regarding their long-term bond to tooth substance.[42] Generally, it is accepted that most restorations 'leak' to varying degrees so prevention of microleakage is more important than the chemical irritancy of the material itself. Clinically, a restoration should be placed which either bonds to tooth tissue or if not, a lining should be placed under the restoration which prevents leakage.

Pulp damage may occur in relation to temporary crown materials, again not because of their inherent toxicity but more as a result of marginal leakage and bacterial invasion of dentinal tubules. Temporary crowns should not be used for long periods and they must always be adequately cemented.[26,43] Another way to reduce pulp damage during temporary crown placement is to 'block' the dentinal tubules and prevent bacterial ingress, by placing bonding agent prior to cementation of the temporary crown.

Although there is now considerable evidence to show the blandness of restorative materials, many, particularly when freshly mixed, have been shown to be toxic to cell cultures[44] but, dentine has a moderating effect.[45]

Bleaching

Vital bleaching procedures are an increasingly prominent aspect of modern dentistry and tooth sensitivity is a common side-effect of such procedures. Sensitivity was experienced in 15–65% of patients undergoing bleaching[46,47] but only a small number of patients experienced severe symptoms.[48] Chairside bleaching procedures, which are often associated with a rise in pulpal temperature, are associated with a higher incidence of sensitivity than home bleaching.[49] The symptoms are usually reversible and generally resolve 1–2 weeks after the end of the procedure[46,48,50] but it may be more severe if the patient has a previous history of sensitivity.[46,48] The mechanism appears to be that the peroxide diffuses through the enamel and down the dentinal tubules into the pulp resulting in inflammation. However, irreversible pulp damage has not been observed[51] even when heat-generating bleaching techniques were employed.[52]

Mechanical

Operative dentistry

The preparation of dentine with rotary instruments can have a damaging effect on the pulp unless measures are taken to minimize injury. Cavity preparation without water-spray causes significantly more pulp damage than when water-spray is used.[53,54] The operator must verify that the water-spray is continuously directed at the revolving bur. If the spray is obstructed by tooth structure or excess pressure is applied to the bur during use, pulp damage may occur.[55] High speed instrumentation is acceptable provided adequate water coolant is used; the use of air coolant alone is considered unsatisfactory.

The area of dentine prepared can have a profound effect on the pulp response. The more tubules exposed, the more routes there are for irritants to reach the pulp. Therefore, pulpal damage results not because of the operative procedure per se, but because the preparation exposes avenues for microbial penetration. Dentinal fluid outflow counteracts this by acting as a flushing mechanism to prevent the inward movement of irritants. Small cavities are likely to be less damaging to the pulp than large ones. In addition, in a small cavity prepared to treat a carious lesion, most of the exposed dentinal tubules would have been blocked by tubular sclerosis as a result of the caries. The deeper the cavity, the greater is the potential for damage: the pulp is closer, odontoblast processes may have been cut, more tubules will have been exposed, and the deeper dentinal tubules have a larger diameter. However, no correlation between thickness of remaining dentine and pulp damage has been shown.[53,56] Only when cavities are very deep, with the remaining dentine less than 0.3mm thick, does some pulp damage occur.[54] Prolonged drying of cavities causes odontoblast aspiration, i.e. their cell bodies move into the dentinal tubules, but there is no permanent damage to the pulp.[57]

Crown preparations, due to the number of tubules exposed, are potentially the most damaging to the pulp, with irreversible damage the occasional result;[33] 10 and 15% of crowned teeth have been shown to lose vitality over a 10 year period.[58,59] When local anaesthetics containing adrenaline are used for crown preparation, the pulp is at particular risk of damage because of vasoconstriction and reduced blood flow.[60,61] The reduction in blood flow means that the pulp is unable to regulate its temperature control and other physiological defences.

The pulp response to the use of lasers for cavity preparation has been reported to have no long-term adverse effects.[62,63,64,65] Many of the beneficial properties of a laser are due to its thermal properties, so unless rigorous safety parameters are established for every type of laser equipment, there is a substantial risk of pulpal damage when they are used to treat the exposed pulp. Damage has been reported when lasers were used directly on the pulp.[66] Whilst other studies have suggested that lasers have no detrimental effects.[67,68,69]

Trauma

The extent of the damage may range from infraction of enamel through lost cusps to a split tooth that cannot be restored. Direct trauma to the anterior teeth often results in fractures that are horizontal or oblique;[70] while with indirect trauma, fractures are, generally, longitudinal. Trauma to anterior teeth most commonly affects children. These teeth frequently have large pulps and wide dentinal tubules so any injury which exposes dentine can potentially damage the pulp and early treatment is important. Traumatic injuries may also damage the blood supply to the pulp, which as a result may calcify or die.

Exposure of dentine

This may occur due to fracture of part of the tooth, by a defective restoration which fails to cover the entire area of the prepared cavity, or by attrition, abrasion or erosion of the overlying cementum or enamel. In the early period after exposure of dentine by trauma, parafunction or cavity preparation, the pulp is sensitive to stimuli and may become inflamed, particularly if bacteria colonize the exposed dentine and enter the tubules. The pulp responds to the low-grade irritation, as previously described, by hard tissue formation, thereby protecting itself over time and making it less sensitive to stimuli.[71]

Cervical sensitivity can occur in undamaged or non-restored teeth, where the gingival tissues have receded and the root dentine is exposed; this is often as a result of vigorous tooth brushing. Without protection the exposed tubules are open and communicate with the pulp. Sensitivity may be reduced by application of potassium oxalate or bonding resins, which not only occludes the tubules but also reduces nerve activity.[71,72] The repair process can be undermined by further assault either by parafunction, further abrasion or erosion. This is particularly problematic in patients who continue to erode their teeth either with acid from drinks and foods, or from regurgitation.[26,73]

Function/parafunction

The effects of occlusion on the pulp are negligible as long as a protective covering of enamel remains intact. When enamel is breached, the dentine is exposed and irritants have a direct pathway to the pulp via the dentinal tubules.

The pulp will protect itself from damage by tubular sclerosis and tertiary dentine deposition. Loss of enamel and exposure of dentine is unlikely during normal function but can occur by attrition after extended periods of parafunction. If the parafunction is particularly severe, continued sensitivity can result due to continual wear of the dentine, rather than due to any direct irritation by occlusal forces. Parafunction can also result in cuspal flexure which stimulates the pulp by outward movement of dentinal fluid; this is exaggerated considerably if a 'crack' in the tooth develops.[74]

MANAGEMENT OF DEEP CARIES

With the treatment of any carious cavity in dentine, it is accepted that the margins and the amelodentinal junction in particular, must be caries-free. However, there has been less agreement over whether all carious dentine overlying the pulp should be removed.[75,76,77] In a tooth with a deep carious lesion, which is considered to have a healthy pulp, partial caries removal appears to be preferable to complete caries removal and the risk of pulp exposure.[78]

A traditional view prevails that if any carious dentine remains, the carious process will continue. An opposite view, supported by clinical evidence, is that if a small amount of caries is left on the pulpal aspect of the cavity and the margins are clear, the lesion can arrest. It appears that the change in environmental conditions and a reduction in bacterial load render the remaining carious lesion inactive. Visually, the yellow carious dentine will darken and dry over time.[79,80] However, the latter technique is subjective and lacks precision as the definition of a small amount of caries will vary from one operator to another, and when does a little become an unacceptably large amount?

There are two recognized approaches to partial caries removal, indirect pulp therapy and stepwise excavation. The former is a one-stage procedure in which most, but not all of the caries is removed prior to placement of a permanent restoration. This technique is gaining momentum as the treatment of choice for advanced caries in deciduous teeth.[81–83] In comparison, stepwise excavation is a two-step approach in which a small amount of carious dentine is left at the first visit and the tooth dressed, prior to the tooth being re-entered after a period of several months. This technique has also been shown to be successful in reducing the frequency of pulpal exposure.[76,84] The principal of a two-stage approach is that the reaction to the treatment can be visually assessed and the remaining decay removed without an increased risk of pulp exposure. This is dependent on tertiary dentine deposition over the intervening period but this may be difficult to assess, as the volume of tertiary dentine deposited will vary from patient to patient. These differing approaches raise the question as to whether a second intervention is really necessary. At present, this is yet to be fully clarified, as indirect pulp therapy is principally carried out in the United States and stepwise excavation mainly in Scandinavia. In addition, although indirect pulp therapy can be carried out on permanent teeth, most of the research to date has been on deciduous teeth. Therefore, data comparing the two techniques are not available.

Clinical opinion is in conflict with scientific evidence when deciding if a cavity is caries-free. In one study, only 64% of clinically hard dentine was bacteria-free;[85] therefore, in a third of teeth where the clinician thought there was a clean cavity floor, the diagnosis was wrong. Dyes which stain the superficial infected dentine but not the deeper demineralized non-infected dentine have been advocated to address this problem.[86] However, the use of dye may lead to excessive removal of carious dentine, as all the remineralizable dentine may not be conserved.[87]

Light coloured dentine is usually indicative of more active caries but a deep lesion may extend into dentine modified by tubular sclerosis, dead tracts or into tertiary dentine. These are darker than normal dentine, but must not be regarded as carious simply because of their colour. If carious dentine is left in a cavity, the clinician may be unaware as to whether it has invaded the pulp. If the pulp is already inflamed, placing a permanent coronal restoration such as a crown will be an expensive mistake as the crown may need to be modified or destroyed when root canal treatment is needed later. If removal of all the cariously infected dentine leads to the pulp, then root canal treatment is appropriate and should not be deferred, except in certain situations where pulpotomy may be indicated (see later).

Following removal of the carious dentine, a protective lining may be placed in a very deep cavity; hard-setting calcium hydroxide materials, which stimulate pulp repair, have traditionally been used. The use of a liner is dependent on the proposed restorative material and the thickness of dentine remaining over the pulp. The previously held view that liners/bases prevented thermal and chemical damage to the pulp have been discredited with the main reason for failure and sensitivity attributed to microleakage around the restoration.[20] Linings are rarely placed under resin restorations as the entire cavity can be etched and a dentine bonding agent placed to seal the cavity.[38] However, doubts remain regarding the long-term efficacy of resins in preventing microleakage[41] and, therefore, whether they provide an adequate seal in deep cavities. Due to their biological properties as pulp capping agents, calcium hydroxide cements are still the material of choice if the thickness of dentine remaining over the pulp is judged to be less than 0.5 mm. However, substantial washout of calcium hydroxide linings/bases under amalgam restorations occurs;[28,29] this may be due to the surface seal not offering long-term protection against bacterial microleakage. For this reason, an antibacterial liner/base should be placed over the calcium hydroxide; zinc oxide–eugenol or glass ionomer cements are both effective for this purpose.

MANAGEMENT OF PULP EXPOSURE

Exposure of the dental pulp can occur as a result of caries, trauma or accidently during cavity preparation. In traumatic and accidental exposures, the pulp can be regarded as being normal prior to the injury. Treatment is usually by pulp capping or partial pulpotomy and provided that treatment is not unnecessarily delayed, a good outcome can be achieved.[88] With a carious exposure, there will be varying degrees of inflammation present in the pulp. This is due to the sustained bacterial onslaught. Inflammation of the pulp has a marked effect on the outcome of vital pulp therapy.[89,90]

Pulp capping

Direct pulp capping is as a procedure in which the pulp is covered with a protective material directly over the site of the exposure. The pulp wound should be cleansed of debris and the haemorrhage arrested by applying pressure using sterile paper points or cotton wool; saline and sodium hypochlorite solution can also be useful. When the wound is dry, the pulp capping agent should be placed over the exposure, followed by a zinc oxide–eugenol or glass ionomer as a base and then a permanent restoration. Delay in placing the permanent restoration reduces the prognosis of the procedure[91] due to the likelihood of microleakage.[20]

Partial pulpotomy

The traditional method involves removing the coronal pulp and placing the pulp dressing on the radicular pulp. A variation of pulpotomy was developed for treatment of traumatized anterior teeth[22] which is more conservative and involves removal of the superficial layer of damaged and/or inflamed pulp tissue prior to application of the base/liner. This is advantageous as the superficial damaged tissue is removed, which should encourage healing, and also space is created which allows the pulp dressing to be retained within the dentine. The procedure is similar to pulp capping. It involves cutting a small 2 mm deep cavity into the pulp with an air turbine under water-spray, placing the pulp dressing and covering it with a base and then a coronal restoration (Fig. 5.1).

In recent years, partial pulpotomy has been practised in carious as well as traumatic exposures with favourable outcomes, indicating that rather than pulp capping, it may be used in traumatic and carious pulpal exposures.[22,92,93]

Choice of material

Calcium hydroxide has been established as the gold standard pulp capping/ partial pulpotomy material over the last 50 years.[94–99] Resins have been investigated as alternatives but they have, generally, been dismissed as not matching the performance of calcium hydroxide.[100,101] Over the last 10 years, Mineral Trioxide Aggregate (MTA) has emerged as the material of choice for vital pulp therapy.[102,103]

The mechanism of both calcium hydroxide and MTA appears to be the dampening of pulpal inflammation, providing an environment conducive to repair. Thereafter, bioactive molecules are liberated in the dentine which stimulate differentiation of pulpal stem cells and also further control the inflammatory response; this allows the pulp to repair.[97,104] Pulpal stem cells have the ability to develop into odontoblast-like cells which allows the pulp to regenerate and form dentine bridges across the deficit. The dentine bridge is not formed by calcium from the material, but instead from the underlying tissues.[105,106] With resin-based composite, MTA and hard-setting calcium hydroxide, the bridge forms close to the material; however, with calcium hydroxide powder and water mixes the barrier is formed with an intervening zone of necrosis.[99] The dentine bridges formed under calcium hydroxide are often imperfect with numerous tunnel defects;[107,108] this is in contrast to MTA where tunnel defects are not seen[102] (Figs 5.2 & 5.3).

Although the material choice may favour the outcome of treatment, healing of pulpal exposures is critically dependent on the capacity of the material or surface restoration to prevent microleakage.[25,35] Therefore, regardless of the capping agent used, prevention of microleakage is critical.

REGENERATIVE DEVELOPMENTS

The aim of a regenerative approach is to reconstitute a normal tissue at the pulp-dentine border, capable of regulating tertiary dentinogenesis.[109] If the pulpal injury is not too severe, the dental pulp stem cells have the ability to develop into odontoblast-like cells, this gives pulp tissue considerable scope to regenerate and form dentine bridges at the site of exposure. The exact mechanism of differentiation of new odontoblasts has not been fully elucidated, but bioactive molecules released from the dentine matrix when the pulp/dentine complex is damaged have a key role. Cytokines such as the TGF-β family[110,111,112] and bone morphogenic proteins,[113,114] which are incorporated into the dentine matrix during formation, are released and diffuse into the pulp; this stimulates odontoblast differentiation and tertiary dentinogenesis. The interaction of bioactive molecules is complex and the exact mechanisms involved are unclear.[115] Recent developments have not

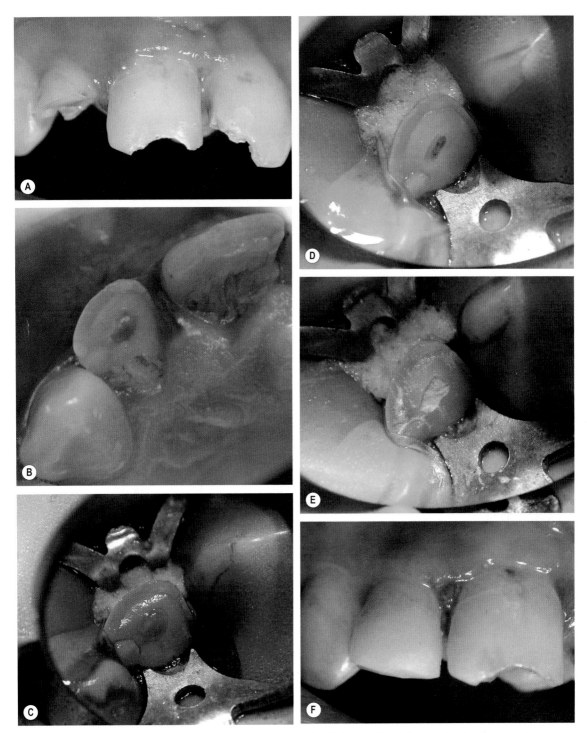

Figure 5.1 (A) Traumatized, fractured maxillary incisors. (B) The pulp of the maxillary right lateral incisor is exposed. (C) Rubber dam placed to isolate the maxillary right lateral incisor. (D) Partial pulpotomy, 2 mm of pulp tissue was removed with a diamond bur in a high-speed handpiece. (E) MTA placed into the partial pulpotomy 'cavity'. (F) Immediately after placement of a permanent restoration. From Duncan et al 2008[88] with permission of Quintessence Publishing Co Ltd.

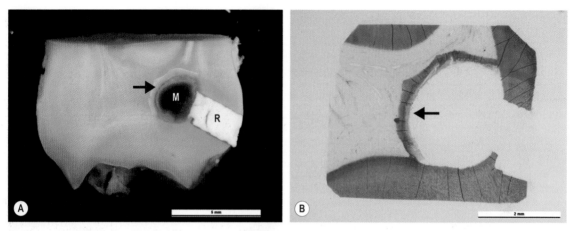

Figure 5.2 MTA pulp cap 3 months after placement (A) Macrophotograph showing remnants of the restorative material (R) and MTA capping material (M). A distinct hard tissue bridge (arrowed) can be seen (original magnifications ×6). (B) Microphotograph of part of the same histological section. Note again the thick mineralized barrier (arrowed) stretched across the entire length of the exposed pulp (original magnification ×8). From Nair et al 2008,[102] with permission of Wiley-Blackwell.

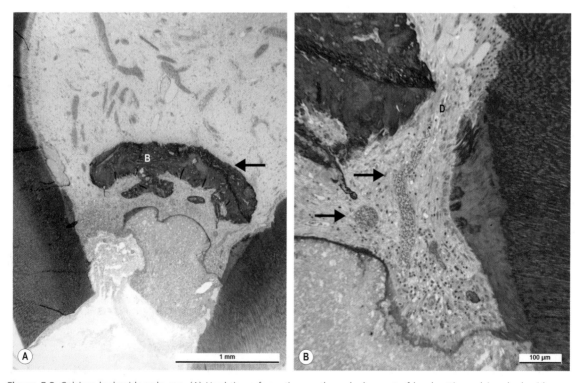

Figure 5.3 Calcium hydroxide pulp cap. (A) Hard tissue formation on the pulpal aspect of hard-setting calcium hydroxide capping material (arrowed) and a thick, calcified hard tissue barrier (B) at a distance from the capping material with gaps at the periphery (original magnification ×25). (b) Higher magnification. A 'tunnel' defect (D) is evident peripherally, associated with engorged blood vessels (arrowed) and surrounded by acute and chronic inflammatory cells (original magnification ×100). From Nair et al 2008,[102] with permission of Wiley-Blackwell.

only aided future treatment techniques, but also revealed possible mechanisms for defensive dentinogenesis during pulpal irritation.

Regenerative therapies have introduced growth factors, within a suitable carrier, placed directly on the pulpal interface.[112,114] A possible benefit of bioactive pulp capping agents is that they may be an improvement over conventional materials such as calcium hydroxide or composite resin that only produces a small amount of reparative dentine at the exposure site.[113] It has been postulated that a greater quantity of dentine would offer better pulp protection;[114] however, overproduction of dentine could lead to future problems during endodontic treatment.[116] These techniques although promising, are expensive, require a suitable carrier and may have damaging side-effects.[109] Other critical questions such as dose-response effects and the short biological half-life of the growth factors clinically remain unanswered.[44] Another approach has been to investigate the release of dormant bioactive molecules already present within the dentine and develop ways of liberating them in a controlled manner. The use of etchants[110] or dental materials such as MTA appear to be effective in harnessing these cytokines. More traditional materials such as calcium hydroxide may not be as effective in this role, or in providing the necessary environment for repair to occur.

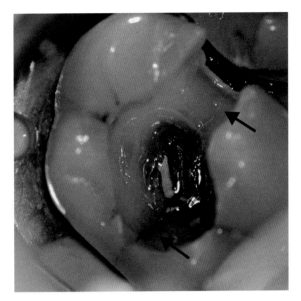

Figure 5.4 A maxillary molar tooth after removal of an amalgam restoration. A crack (arrowed) is sited centrally, the distal extension is stained.

PULP RESPONSE AND MAINTAINING PULP VITALITY

Cracked teeth

A patient may complain of poorly localized pain from an unidentified posterior tooth on biting or from hot or cold drinks. Clinically and radiologically, there is often no evidence of caries, and the offending tooth although it is restored, the restoration may not be deep. Mandibular molars are the most frequently affected.[117] The patient's pain is due to the crack exposing multiple dentinal tubules, bacteria and their byproducts pass down the exposed tubules to elicit pulpal inflammation.[26,118] Biting on the cracked tooth creates a wedging effect stimulating fluid movement in the crack and communicating tubules; this provokes a painful response in an already inflamed tooth.

Treatment of cracked teeth can be unpredictable due to the difficulty in accurately assessing the true extent of the crack. Generally, cracks which are centrally placed in the axial plane are more difficult to treat than those eccentrically placed as the latter tend to exit the tooth laterally. Centrally-placed cracks lead into the pulp and with time can split the tooth (Fig 5.4). Treatment will depend on whether there have been symptoms of reversible or irreversible pulpitis. In the case of reversible pulpitis and if there is a loose cusp, any restoration should be removed together with the loose cusp and a new restoration placed as appropriate. If no loose cusp is detected, the tooth may be crowned, initially with a temporary crown. Following placement of the temporary crown, relief from pain is normally achieved. Where there have been symptoms of irreversible pulpitis, pulpal extirpation and root canal filling will be required. During root canal treatment, it is advisable to place a band (e.g. stainless steel orthodontic band) to splint the tooth together, preventing further crack propagation and to reduce the tooth out of occlusion other than in the intercuspal position.

Orthodontics

Application of orthodontic forces will provoke a haemodynamic response in the pulp which varies in intensity depending on several factors. Orthodontic movements such as tipping lead to an initial decrease in blood supply,[119] before a reactive hyperaemia increases the pulp perfusion.[120,121] However, intrusive movements can lead to a sustained reduction in blood flow,[122,123] which is generally reversible, but may jeopardize vitality if the tooth has been previously compromised. Pulp necrosis is considered a rare event. However, teeth with closed apices and pulps which have been compromised particularly by previous trauma, but also by caries, restorations, or periodontal disease are more susceptible to irreversible damage and necrosis.[124,125,126]

Orthodontic forces have other pulpal effects including a reduction in respiration, altered metabolism and localized cell death; these changes are probably as a result of the haemodynamic alterations described and are, similarly, likely to be reversible.[127,128,129] In a small number of cases orthodontic movement can stimulate an increase in calcification within the root canal which can, in extreme cases, obstruct the entire root canal.[130] This can lead to problems if the tooth requires root canal treatment at a later date.

Periodontal disease and treatment

Periodontal disease does not cause pathological change in the pulp unless the disease extends all the away to the tooth apex;[131,132,133] therefore, pulp necrosis is rare. The normality of the pulp is maintained during periodontal disease because of the intact layer of cementum on the root surface. If this layer is destroyed during treatment or disease then pulpal inflammation under the affected tubules occurs.[134] The pulp responds to the stimuli by formation of tubular sclerosis and tertiary dentine.[135] Therefore, even extensive periodontal disease causes little or no inflammatory changes in the pulp.[136]

It has been shown that scaling or root planing procedures, which remove cementum, may cause pulpal inflammation, and frequently the formation of tertiary dentine.[134,135] However, the response to scaling is not severe and does not adversely affect pulp vitality. Following scaling, dentinal tubules become opened and the teeth are hypersensitive; after several weeks the sensitivity decreases, presumably as the tubules become blocked by mineral deposits.[26]

Intra-alveolar surgery and implants

Implants have become a popular replacement for missing teeth. Loss of vitality can occur during implant placement due to the root being damaged directly or indirectly if the neurovascular bundle apically is severed.[137] If the quantity of bone is unacceptable for a satisfactory result, bone will have to be augmented by grafts, often from the mandible or iliac crest. A common site for mandibular bone harvesting is the chin region which due to the proximity of the incisor apices can lead to a reduction of blood supply, reduction of pulpal sensitivity or pulpal necrosis.[137] The loss of pulpal sensitivity varies depending on the level of the osteotomy.[138,139] It has usually been considered that pulp necrosis and abscess formation will follow surgical cutting or severance of a root near its apex. A distance of 3–10 millimetres between the root apex and the osteotomy has been recommended to avoid pulpal degeneration or necrosis.[138,140] However, this has been disputed in an experimental study which demonstrated that no undesirable pulp sequelae occurred even when the roots were surgically cut.[141]

LEARNING OUTCOMES

At the end of this chapter the reader should have knowledge of the:

- response of the pulp-dentine complex to irritation;
- different types of pulpal irritant and their relative importance;
- ways to harness the pulp-dentine complex when treating deep caries lesions and pulpal exposures;
- impact of new regenerative research and how it has altered our understanding of tertiary dentinogenesis and the treatment of pulpal exposures;
- precautions necessary in order to maintain vitality during various dental procedures.

REFERENCES

1. Brännström M, Garberoglio R. The dentinal tubules and the odontoblast processes. A scanning electron microscopic study. Acta Odontologica Scandinavica 1972;30:291–311.

2. Holland GR. The odontoblast process: form and function. Journal of Dental Research 1985;64(special issue):499–514.

3. Smith AJ, Cassidy N, Perry H, Bègue-Kirn C, Ruch JV, Lesot H. Reactionary dentinogenesis. International Journal of Developmental Biology 1995;39: 273–280.

4. Smith AJ, Lumley PJ, Tomson PL, Cooper PR. Dental regeneration and materials: a partnership. Clinical Oral Investigations 2008; 12:103–108.

5. Mjör IA, Tronstad L. Experimentally induced pulpitis. Oral Surgery, Oral Medicine, Oral Pathology 1972;34:102–108.

6. Mjör IA, Tronstad L. The healing of experimentally induced pulpitis. Oral Surgery, Oral Medicine, Oral Pathology 1974; 38:115–121.

7. Kakehashi S, Stanley HR, Fitzgerald RJ. The effects of surgical exposures of dental pulps in germ-free and conventional laboratory rats. Oral Surgery, Oral Medicine, Oral Pathology 1965; 20:340–349.

8. Smith AJ, Murray PE, Lumley PJ. Preserving the vital pulp in operative dentistry: 1. A biological approach. Dental Update 2002;29:64–69.

9. Trowbridge HO. Pathogenesis of pulpitis resulting from dental caries. Journal of Endodontics 1981;7:52–60.

10. Bowden GHW. The microbial ecology of dental caries. Microbial Ecology in Health and Disease 2000;12:138–148.

11. Edwardsson S. Bacteriological studies on deep areas of carious dentine. Odontologisk Revy 1974;25(supplement 32):1–143.

12. Munson MA, Banerjee A, Watson TF, Wade WG. Molecular analysis of the microflora associated with dental caries. Journal of Clinical Microbiology 2004;42: 3023–3029.

13. Chhour KL, Nadkarni MA, Byun R, et al. Molecular analysis of microbial diversity in advanced caries. Journal of Clinical Microbiology 2005;43:843–849.

14. Hoshino E. Predominant obligate anaerobes in human carious dentin. Journal of Dental Research 1985;64:1195–1198.

15. Nadkarni MA, Caldon CE, Chhour KL, et al. Carious dentine provides a habitat for a complex array of novel Prevotella-like bacteria. Journal of Clinical Microbiology 2004;42: 5238–5244.

16. Hoshino E, Ando N, Sato M, Kota K. Bacterial invasion of non-exposed dental pulp. International Endodontic Journal 1992;25:2–5.

17. Warfvinge J, Bergenholtz G. Healing capacity of human and monkey dental pulps following experimental-induced pulpitis. Endodontics and Dental Traumatology 1986;2, 256–262.

18. Reeves R, Stanley HR. The relationship of bacterial penetration and pulpal pathosis in carious teeth. Oral Surgery, Oral Medicine, Oral Pathology 1966;22:59–65.

19. Massler M, Pawlak J. The affected and infected pulp. Oral Surgery, Oral Medicine, Oral Pathology 1977;43:929–947.

20. Bergenholtz G, Cox CF, Loesche WJ, Syed SA. Bacterial leakage around dental restorations: its effect on the dental pulp. Journal of Oral Pathology 1982;11: 439–450.

21. Cox CF, Bergenholtz G, Fitzgerald M, et al. Capping of the dental pulp mechanically exposed to the oral microflora – a 5-week observation of wound healing in the monkey. Journal of Oral Pathology 1982;11:327–339.

22. Cvek M. A clinical report on partial pulpotomy and capping with calcium hydroxide in permanent incisors with complicated crown fracture. Journal of Endodontics 1978;4: 232–237.

23. Browne RM, Tobias RS. Microbial microleakage and pulpal inflammation: a review. Endodontics and Dental Traumatology 1986;2:177–183.

24. Browne RM, Tobias RS, Crombie IK, Plant CG. Bacterial microleakage and pulpal inflammation in experimental cavities. International Endodontic Journal 1983;16:147–155.

25. Tobias RS, Plant CG, Browne RM. Reduction in pulpal inflammation beneath surface-sealed silicates. International Endodontic Journal 1982;15: 173–180.

26. Brännström M. The cause of postrestorative sensitivity and its prevention. Journal of Endodontics 1986;12:475–481.

27. Brännström M, Vojinovic O, Nordenvall KJ. Bacteria and pulpal reactions under silicate cement restorations. Journal of Prosthetic Dentistry 1979;41: 290–295.

28. Novickas D, Fiocca VL, Grajower R. Linings and caries in retrieved permanent teeth with amalgam restorations. Operative Dentistry 1989;14:33–39.

29. Pereira JC, Manfio AP, Franco EB, Lopes ES. Clinical evaluation of Dycal under amalgam restorations. American Journal of Dentistry 1990;3:67–70.

30. Frank RM. Reactions of dentin and pulp to drugs and restorative materials. Journal of Dental Research 1975;54:B176–B187.

31. Plant CG, Jones DW. The damaging effects of restorative materials. Part 1 – Physical and chemical properties. British Dental Journal 1976;140: 373–377.

32. Plant CG, Jones DW. The damaging effects of restorative materials. Part 2 – Pulpal effects related to physical and chemical properties. British Dental Journal 1976;140:406–412.

33. Bergenholtz G. Iatrogenic injury to the pulp in dental procedures: aspects of pathogenesis, management and preventive measures. International Dental Journal 1991;41:99–110.

34. Brännström M. Communication between the oral cavity and the dental pulp associated with restorative treatment. Operative Dentistry 1984;9:57–68.

35. Cox CF, Keall CL, Keall HJ, et al. Biocompatibility of surface-sealed dental materials against exposed pulps. Journal of Prosthetic Dentistry 1987;57:1–8.

36. Brännström M, Nordenvall KJ. Bacterial penetration, pulpal reaction and the inner surface of Concise enamel bond. Composite fillings in etched and unetched cavities. Journal of Dental Research 1978;57:3–10.

37. Cox CF, Hafez AA, Akimoto N, et al. Biocompatibility of primer, adhesive and resin composite systems on non-exposed and exposed pulps of non-human primate teeth. American Journal of Dentistry 1998;11: S55–S63.

38. Brännström M, Nyborg H. The presence of bacteria in cavities filled with silicate cement and composite resin materials. Swedish Dental Journal 1971;64: 149–155.

39. Baratieri LN, Ritter AV. Four-year clinical evaluation of posterior resin-based composite restorations placed using the total etch technique. Journal of Esthetic and Restorative Dentistry 2001;13:50–57.

40. Felton D, Bergenholtz G, Cox CF. Inhibition of bacterial growth under composite restorations following GLUMA pretreatment. Journal of Dental Research 1989;68:491–495.

41. Sturdevant JR, Lundeen TF, Sluder TB, et al. Five-year study of two light-cured posterior composite resins. Dental Materials 1988;4: 105–110.

42. Kato G, Nakabayashi N. The durability of adhesion to phosphoric acid etched, wet dentin substrates. Dental Materials 1998;14:347–352.

43. Brännström M. Reducing the risk of sensitivity and pulpal complications after the placement of crowns and fixed partial dentures. Quintessence International 1996;27:673–678.

44. Browne RM. The in vitro assessment of the cytotoxicity of dental materials – does it have a role? International Endodontic Journal 1988;21:50–58.

45. Meryon SD. The model cavity method incorporating dentine. International Endodontic Journal 1988;21:79–84.

46. Haywood VB, Leonard RH, Nelson CF, Brunson WD. Effectiveness, side effects and long-term status of nightguard vital bleaching. Journal of the American Dental Association 1994;125:1219–1226.

47. Schulte JR, Morrissette DB, Gasior EJ, Czajewski MV. The effects of bleaching application time on the dental pulp. Journal of the American Dental Association 1994;125:1330–1335.

48. Jorgensen MG, Carroll WB. Incidence of tooth sensitivity after home whitening treatment. Journal of the American Dental Association 2002;133:1076–1082.

49. Nathanson D, Parra C. Bleaching vital teeth: a review and clinical study. Compendium of Continuing Education in Dentistry 1987;8:490–497.

50. Leonard Jr RH, Smith LR, Garland GE, et al. Evaluation of side effects and patients' perceptions during tooth bleaching. Journal of Esthetic and Restorative Dentistry 2007;19:355–364.

51. Baumgartner JC, Reid DE, Pickett AB. Human pulpal reaction to the modified McInnes bleaching technique. Journal of Endodontics 1983;9:527–529.

52. Robertson WD, Melfi RC. Pulpal response to vital bleaching procedures. Journal of Endodontics 1980;6:645–649.

53. Morrant GA. Dental instrumentation and pulpal injury. Part II clinical considerations. Journal of the British Endodontic Society 1977;10:55–63.

54. Swerdlow H, Stanley Jr HR. Reaction of the human dental pulp to cavity preparation. Part II at 150,000 rpm with an air-water spray. Journal of Prosthetic Dentistry 1959;9:121–131.

55. Langeland K. Prevention of pulpal damage. Dental Clinics of North America 1972;16:709–732.

56. Plant CG, Anderson RJ. The effect of cavity depth on the pulpal response to restorative materials. British Dental Journal 1978;144:10–13.

57. Brännström M. The effect of dentin desiccation and aspirated odontoblasts on the pulp. Journal of Prosthetic Dentistry 1968;20:165–171.

58. Cheung GS, Lai SC, Ng RP. Fate of vital pulps beneath a metal-ceramic crown or a bridge retainer. International Endodontic Journal 2005;38:521–530.

59. Valderhaug J, Jokstad A, Ambjørnsen E, Norheim PW. Assessment of the periapical and clinical status of crowned teeth over 25 years. Journal of Dentistry 1997;25:97–105.

60. Kim S. Ligamental injection: a physiological explanation of its efficacy. Journal of Endodontics 1986;12:486–491.

61. Pitt Ford TR, Seare MA, McDonald F. Action of adrenaline on the effect of dental local anaesthetic solutions. Endodontics and Dental Traumatology 1993;9:31–35.

62. Miserendino LJ, Levy GC, Abt E, Rizoiu IM. Histologic effects of a thermally cooled Nd : YAG laser on the dental pulp and supporting structures of rabbit teeth. Oral Surgery, Oral Medicine, Oral Pathology 1994;78:93–100.

63. Takamori K. A histopathological and immunohistochemical study of dental pulp and pulpal nerve fibers in rats after the cavity preparation using Er : YAG laser. Journal of Endodontics 2000;26:95–99.

64. Tanabe K, Yoshiba K, Yoshiba N, et al. Immunohistochemical study on pulpal response in rat molars after cavity preparation by Er : YAG laser. European Journal of Oral Sciences 2002;110:237–245.

65. White JM, Goodis HE, Setcos JC, et al. Effects of pulsed Nd : YAG laser energy on human teeth: a three-year follow-up study. Journal of the American Dental Association 1993;124:45–51.

66. Jukić S, Anić I, Koba K, et al. The effect of pulpotomy using CO2 and Nd : YAG lasers on dental pulp tissue. International Endodontic Journal 1997;30:175–180.

67. Moritz A, Schoop U, Goharkhay K, Sperr W. The CO_2 laser as an aid in direct pulp capping. Journal of Endodontics 1998;24:248–251.

68. Olivi G, Genovese MD, Maturo P, Docimo R. Pulp capping: advantages of using laser technology. European Journal of Paediatric Dentistry 2007;8:89–95.

69. Shoji S, Nakamura M, Horiuchi H. Histopathological changes in dental pulps irradiated by CO_2 laser: a preliminary report on laser pulpotomy. Journal of Endodontics 1985;11:379–384.

70. Andreasen JO, Andreasen FM, Tsukiboshi M. Crown-Root Fractures. In: Andreasen JO, Andreasen FM, Andersson L, editors. Textbook and Color Atlas of Traumatic Injuries to the Teeth, 4th edn. Munksgaard: Copenhagen, Denmark; 2007. p. 314–336.

71. Pashley DH. Dentin permeability, dentin sensitivity and treatment through tubule occlusion. Journal of Endodontics 1986;12:465–474.

72. Pollington S, van Noort R. A clinical evaluation of a resin composite and a compomer in non carious Class V lesions. A 3-year follow-up. American Journal of Dentistry 2008;21:49–52.

73. Barbour ME, Rees GD. The role of erosion, abrasion and attrition in tooth wear. Journal of Clinical Dentistry 2006;17:88–93.

74. Cameron CE. Cracked-tooth syndrome. Journal of the

American Dental Association 1964;68:405–411.

75. Bjørndal L. Indirect pulp therapy and stepwise excavation. Journal of Endodontics 2008; 34(supplement 7):S29–S33.

76. Bjørndal L, Thylstrup A. A practice-based study on stepwise excavation of deep carious lesions in permanent teeth: a 1-year follow-up study. Community Dentistry and Oral Epidemiology 1998;26:122–128.

77. Fisher FJ. The treatment of carious dentine. British Dental Journal 1981;150:159–162.

78. Ricketts DN, Kidd EA, Innes N, Clarkson J. Complete or ultraconservative removal of decayed tissue in unfilled teeth. Cochrane Database of Systematic Reviews 2006;3:CD003808.

79. Bjørndal L, Larsen T, Thylstrup A. A clinical and microbiological study of deep carious lesions during stepwise excavation using long treatment intervals. Caries Research 1997;31:411–417.

80. Fairbourn DR, Charbeneau GT, Loesche WJ. Effect of improved Dycal and IRM on bacteria in deep carious lesions. Journal of the American Dental Association 1980;100:547–552.

81. Al-Zayer MA, Straffon LH, Feigal RJ, Welch KB. Indirect pulp treatment of primary posterior teeth: a retrospective study. Pediatric Dentistry 2003;25:29–36.

82. Coll JA. Indirect pulp capping and primary teeth: is the primary tooth pulpotomy out of date? Journal of Endodontics 2008;34(supplement 7):S34–S39.

83. Marchi JJ, de Araujo FB, Fröner AM, et al. Indirect pulp capping in the primary dentition: a 4 year follow-up study. Journal of Clinical Pediatric Dentistry 2006;31:68–71.

84. Magnusson BO, Sundell SO. Stepwise excavation of deep carious lesions in primary molars. Journal of the International Association of Dentistry for Children 1977;8:36–40.

85. Shovelton DS. A study of deep carious dentine. International Dental Journal 1968;18:392–405.

86. Fusayama T. Two layers of carious dentin: diagnosis and treatment. Operative Dentistry 1979;4:63–70.

87. Kidd EA, Joyston-Bechal S, Beighton D. The use of a caries detector dye during cavity preparation: a microbiological assessment. British Dental Journal 1993;174:245–248.

88. Duncan HF, Nair PNR, Pitt Ford TR. Vital pulp treatment: clinical considerations. ENDO (London, England) 2009;3:7–17.

89. Matsuo T, Nakanishi T, Shimizu H, Ebisu S. A clinical study of direct pulp capping applied to carious-exposed pulps. Journal of Endodontics 1996;22:551–556.

90. Mejàre I, Cvek M. Partial pulpotomy in young permanent teeth with deep carious lesions. Endodontics and Dental Traumatology 1993;9:238–242.

91. Barthel CR, Rosenkranz B, Leuenberg A, Roulet RF. Pulp capping of carious exposures: treatment outcome after 5 and 10 years: a retrospective study. Journal of Endodontics 2000;26:525–528.

92. Barrieshi-Nusair KM, Qudeimat MA. A prospective clinical study of mineral trioxide aggregate for partial pulpotomy in cariously exposed permanent teeth. Journal of Endodontics 2006;32:731–735.

93. Mass E, Zilberman U. Clinical and radiographic evaluation of partial pulpotomy in carious exposure of permanent molars. Pediatric Dentistry 1993;15:257–259.

94. Glass RL, Zander HA. Pulp healing. Journal of Dental Research 1949;28:97–107.

95. Pitt Ford TR, Roberts GJ. Immediate and delayed direct pulp capping with the use of a new visible light-cured calcium hydroxide preparation. Oral Surgery, Oral Medicine, Oral Pathology 1991;71:338–342.

96. Schröder U. Evaluation of healing following experimental pulpotomy of intact human teeth and capping with calcium hydroxide. Odontologisk Revy 1972;23:329–340.

97. Schröder U. Effects of calcium hydroxide-containing pulp-capping agents on pulp cell migration, proliferation and differentiation. Journal of Dental Research 1985;64(special issue):541–548.

98. Stanley HR, Lundy T. Dycal therapy for pulp exposures. Oral Surgery, Oral Medicine, Oral Pathology 1972;34:818–827.

99. Tronstad L. Reaction of the exposed pulp to Dycal treatment. Oral Surgery, Oral Medicine, Oral Pathology 1974;38:945–953.

100. Bergenholtz G. Evidence for bacterial causation of adverse pulpal responses in resin-based dental restorations. Critical Reviews in Oral Biology and Medicine 2000;11:467–480.

101. Fernandes AM, Silva GAB, Lopes Jr N, et al. Direct capping of human pulps with a dentin bonding system and calcium hydroxide: an immunohistochemical analysis. Oral Surgery, Oral Medicine, Oral Pathology, Oral Radiology and Endodontics 2008;105:385–390.

102. Nair PNR, Duncan HF, Pitt Ford TR, Luder HU. Histological, ultrastructural and quantitative investigations on the response of healthy human pulps to experimental capping with mineral trioxide aggregate: a randomised controlled trial. International Endodontic Journal 2008;41:128–150.

103. Pitt Ford TR, Torabinejad M, Abedi HR, et al. Using mineral trioxide aggregate as a pulp-capping material. Journal of the American Dental Association 1996;127:1491–1494.

104. Mjör IA, Dahl E, Cox CF. Healing of pulp exposures: an ultrastructural study. Journal of Oral Pathology and Medicine 1991;20:496–501.

105. Pisanti S, Sciaky I. Origin of calcium in the repair wall after pulpal exposure in the dog. Journal of Dental Research 1964;43:641–644.

106. Sciaky I, Pisanti S. Localization of calcium placed over amputated pulps in dogs' teeth.

Journal of Dental Research 1960;39:1128–1132.

107. Cox CF, Sübay RK, Ostro E, et al. Tunnel defects in dentin bridges: their formation following direct pulp capping. Operative Dentistry 1996;21:4–11.

108. Langeland K, Dowden WE, Tronstad L, Langeland LK. Human pulp changes of iatrogenic origin. Oral Surgery, Oral Medicine, Oral Pathology 1971;32:943–980.

109. Tziafas D. The future role of a molecular approach to pulp-dentinal regeneration. Caries Research 2004;38:314–320.

110. Cassidy N, Fahey M, Prime SS, Smith AJ. Comparative analysis of transforming growth factor-β isoforms 1–3 in human and rabbit dentine matrices. Archives of Oral Biology 1997;42: 219–223.

111. Rutherford RB, Wahle J, Tucker M, et al. Induction of reparative dentine formation in monkeys by recombinant human osteogenic protein-1. Archives of Oral Biology 1993;38:571–576.

112. Tziafas D, Alvanou A, Papadimitriou S, et al. Effects of recombinant basic fibroblast growth factor, insulin-like growth factor-II and transforming growth factor-β1 on dog pulp cells in vivo. Archives of Oral Biology 1998;43:431–444.

113. Iohara K, Nakashima M, Ito M, et al. Dentin regeneration by dental pulp stem cell therapy with recombinant human bone morphogenetic protein 2. Journal of Dental Research 2004;83: 590–595.

114. Nakashima M. Induction of dentin formation on canine amputated pulp by recombinant human bone morphogenetic proteins (BMP) -2 and -4. Journal of Dental Research 1994;73:1515–1522.

115. Mitsiadis TA, Rahiotis C. Parallels between tooth development and repair: conserved molecular mechanisms following carious and dental injury. Journal of Dental Research 2004;83: 896–902.

116. Goldberg M, Smith AJ. Cells and extracellular matrices of dentin and pulp: a biological basis for repair and tissue engineering. Critical Reviews in Oral Biology and Medicine 2004;15:13–27.

117. Cameron CE. The cracked tooth syndrome: additional findings. Journal of the American Dental Association 1976;93:971–975.

118. Brännström M. The hydrodynamic theory of dentinal pain: sensation in preparations, caries and the dentinal crack syndrome. Journal of Endodontics 1986;12:453–457.

119. McDonald F, Pitt Ford TR. Blood flow changes in permanent maxillary canines during retraction. European Journal of Orthodontics 1994;16:1–9.

120. Kvinnsland S, Heyeraas K, Snorre Øfjord E. Effect of experimental tooth movement on periodontal and pulpal blood flow. European Journal of Orthodontics 1989; 11:200–205.

121. Nixon CE, Saviano JA, King GJ, Keeling SD. Histomorphometric study of dental pulp during orthodontic tooth movement. Journal of Endodontics 1993;19: 13–16.

122. Guevara MJ, McClugage Jr SG. Effects of intrusive forces upon the microvasculature of the dental pulp. Angle Orthodontist 1980;50:129–134.

123. Sano Y, Ikawa M, Sugawara J, Horiuchi H, Mitani H. The effect of continuous intrusive force on human pulpal blood flow. European Journal of Orthodontics 2002;24:159–166.

124. Årtun J, Urbye KS. The effect of orthodontic treatment on periodontal bone support in patients with advanced loss of marginal periodontium. American Journal of Orthodontics and Dentofacial Orthopedics 1988;93:43–148.

125. Bauss O, Röhling J, Rahman A, Kiliaridis S. The effect of pulpal obliteration on pulpal vitality of orthodontically intruded traumatized teeth. Journal of Endodontics 2008;34: 417–420.

126. Rotstein I, Engel G. Conservative management of a combined endodontic-orthodontic lesion. Endodontics and Dental Traumatology 1991;7:266–269.

127. Hamersky PA, Weimer AD, Taintor JF. The effect of orthodontic force application on the pulpal tissue respiration rate in the human premolar. American Journal of Orthodontics 1980;77: 368–378.

128. Hamilton RS, Gutmann JL. Endodontic-orthodontic relationships: a review of integrated treatment planning challenges. International Endodontic Journal 1999;32:343–360.

129. Perinetti G, Varvara G, Festa F, Esposito P. Aspartate aminotransferase activity in pulp of orthodontically treated teeth. American Journal of Orthodontics and Dentofacial Orthopedics 2004;125:88–92.

130. Delivanis HP, Sauer GJ. Incidence of canal calcification in the orthodontic patient. American Journal of Orthodontics 1982; 82:58–61.

131. Harrington GW, Steiner DR, Ammons WF. The periodontal-endodontic controversy. Periodontology 2000 2002;30: 123–130.

132. Langeland K, Rodrigues H, Dowden W. Periodontal disease, bacteria, and pulpal histopathology. Oral Surgery, Oral Medicine, Oral Pathology 1974;37:257–270.

133. Rotstein I, Simon JH. Diagnosis, prognosis and decision making in the treatment of combined periodontal-endodontic lesions. Periodontology 2000 2004;34: 165–203.

134. Bergenholtz G, Lindhe J. Effect of experimentally induced marginal periodontitis and periodontal scaling on the dental pulp. Journal of Clinical Periodontology 1978;5:59–73.

135. Hattler AB, Listgarten MA. Pulpal response to root planing in a rat model. Journal of Endodontics 1984;10:471–476.

136. Torabinejad M, Kiger RD. A histologic evaluation of dental pulp tissue of a patient with periodontal disease. Oral Surgery, Oral Medicine, Oral Pathology 1985;59:198–200.

137. Margelos JT, Verdelis KG. Irreversible pulpal damage of teeth adjacent to recently placed osseointegrated implants. Journal of Endodontics 1995;21: 479–482.

138. Nkenke E, Schultze-Mosgau S, Radespeil-Tröger M, et al. Morbidity of harvesting of chin grafts: a prospective study. Clinical Oral Implant Research 2001;12:495–502.

139. Raghoebar GM, Meijndert L, Kalk WW, Vissink A. Morbidity of mandibular bone harvesting: a comparative study. The International Journal of Oral and Maxillofacial Implants 2007;22:359–365.

140. Duran S, Güven O, Günhan Ö. Pulpal and apical changes secondary to segmental osteotomy in the mandible-an experimental study. Journal of Cranio-Maxillo-Facial Surgery 1995;23:256–260.

141. Hitchcock R, Ellis E, Cox CF. Intentional vital root transection: a 52-week histopathologic study in Macaca mulatta. Oral Surgery, Oral Medicine, Oral Pathology 1985;60:2–14.

Chapter | 6 |

Basic instrumentation in endodontics

B.S. Chong

SUMMARY

Clinicians have to remain up-to-date in the fast evolving world of everyday practice. Newer materials, innovative techniques and novel devices are continually being developed by manufacturers to facilitate the clinical practice of endodontics. Released onto the market, often promising simpler, quicker and better results, the hope is that it will allow the management of even the most challenging cases. In this chapter, the basic instruments and essential devices needed in clinical endodontic practice are identified and described. The equipment necessary for rubber dam application, instruments for access cavity and root canal preparation, devices to determine working length and deliver irrigants, instruments for retrieving broken instruments and posts, and for filling root canals are covered. Storage

© 2009 Elsevier Ltd, Inc, BV
DOI: 10.1016/B978-0-7020-3156-4.00009-7

and sterilization of endodontic instruments, and the advantages of enhanced illumination and magnification are also explained.

INTRODUCTION

The principles of root canal treatment consist of thorough cleaning, adequate shaping and complete filling of the root canal system. In order to accomplish these objectives, many different instruments are available. Some of the instruments are common to all branches of dentistry while others have been modified or are specifically designed for endodontics.

BASIC INSTRUMENT PACK

For convenience, a basic selection of instruments should be packaged or set-up in a tray, ready to use (Fig. 6.1). A front-surfaced mouth mirror produces an undistorted image for good visibility deep within the pulp chamber. The endodontic explorer is a double-ended, extra-long, sharp instrument designed to help in the location of canal entrances and for detecting fractures. A long spoon excavator is required to remove pulpal contents and soft caries where present. Locking tweezers are ideal for handling paper points, gutta-percha points, cotton wool pellets and root canal instruments. Both Briault and periodontal probes are necessary for the initial assessment of the tooth for caries and the localized periodontal condition. A flat plastic instrument and an amalgam plugger are needed for placement of an inter-appointment restoration. A millimetre ruler or other measuring device should be available for measuring purposes. A surgical haemostat may be

used to position X-ray films, for radiography during treatment.

RUBBER DAM

It is a prerequisite that the tooth being treated must be isolated; this is effectively and efficiently achieved by the use of rubber dam. There are many good reasons for using rubber dam:

- It protects the patient from inhalation or ingestion of instruments, medicaments and debris.
- It prevents infection by providing a clean, dry, aseptic working field, free from salivary contamination.
- It allows retraction of soft tissues and the tongue so as not to obstruct the operating field and also protect them from injury.
- It enhances access thereby improving the efficiency of treatment.
- It provides better patient comfort without the oral cavity being flooded with water and/or debris.

Rubber dam is available in pre-cut (commonly 150 mm) squares and also in a roll. The sheets come in different colours and thickness (thin, medium, heavy, extra heavy and special heavy); some are even scented. The thicker material has the advantage of a tighter fit around the neck of the tooth, thus providing a more hermetic seal, so floss ligatures may not be required[1] and offers better protection for the underlying soft tissues. If there is a small amount of seepage around the margins between the tooth and the rubber dam, temporary filling material (e.g. Cavit, 3M ESPE, Neuss, Germany) or a non-setting caulking agent (Oraseal, Ultradent, South Jordan, UT, USA) (Fig. 6.2) may be placed to seal off the leakage. For patients allergic to latex, non-latex rubber dam, made of silicone (e.g. Flexi Dam, Roeko, Coltène/Whaledent, Langenau, Germany) (Fig. 6.3) is also obtainable. The other items for the application of rubber dam include the following.

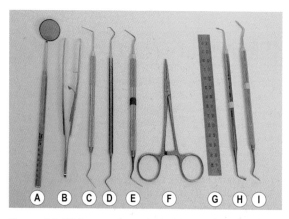

Figure 6.1 (A) Front surface mirror; (B) endodontic locking tweezers; (C) DG16 endodontic explorer; (D) Briault probe; (E) long-shank excavator; (F) surgical haemostat; (G) millimetre ruler; (H) amalgam plugger; (I) flat plastic.

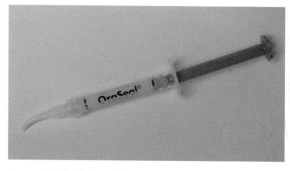

Figure 6.2 OraSeal caulking agent, a non-setting sealant.

Rubber dam punch

A punch is used to make the required numbers of holes depending on the teeth to be isolated. Usually single tooth isolation is all that is required for endodontic treatment. Single-hole punches (Dentsply Ash, Weybridge, Surrey, UK) are available which will cut a neat hole (1.63 or 1.93 mm), while those with a rotatable table (Ainsworth pattern) will cut different sized holes ranging in diameter from 0.5 to 2.5 mm (Fig. 6.4). Whichever is chosen, it is important to ensure that the punch is sharp, so as to produce a clean hole without any residual tags on the rubber dam. Otherwise, the rubber dam will tear when stretched and applied to the tooth. The size of hole that is punched is also important; the ease of application with

a larger hole must be balanced by the quality of the seal at the cervical margin.

Rubber dam clamp

There are many different designs of rubber dam clamp to cater for every possible situation. However, there are no standards governing the manufacture of rubber dam clamps.[2]

Clamps have two uses: first, they anchor the rubber dam to the tooth, and second, they retract the gingivae. In endodontics, anchorage is the main requirement. Most clamps are made from stainless steel; some are made from plated steel, which may be more susceptible to corrosion by sodium hypochlorite. There are also non-metallic clamps made of plastic (SoftClamp, KerrHawe, Bioggio, Switzerland) on the market. Clamps are winged or wingless, retentive or bland (Fig. 6.5). A winged clamp allows the attachment of the rubber dam to the clamp so that both clamp and rubber dam may be applied to the tooth together. Retentive clamps are designed to make a four-point contact with the tooth; they have narrow, curved and slightly inverted jaws, which may displace gingival tissue to grip the tooth below the level of greatest circumference; they are very useful on partly erupted teeth. Bland clamps are less likely to impinge on the gingivae as they have flat jaws, which grip the tooth around its entire circumference. However, they can only be used where a tooth is fully erupted and has a cervical constriction that prevents the clamp from slipping off.

A basic assortment of clamps may consist of the following (Fig. 6.6): Ivory pattern 00, 0, 1, 2A, 9, W8A, 14 and 14A. The wingless W8A, the winged 14 and 14A are for molars, the 2A and 1 for premolars, and the 9 for incisors. A range of lettered Ash clamps, which are generally smaller,

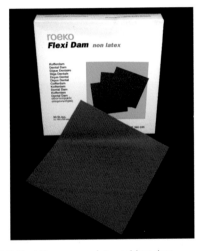

Figure 6.3 Flexi Dam, a non-latex rubber dam.

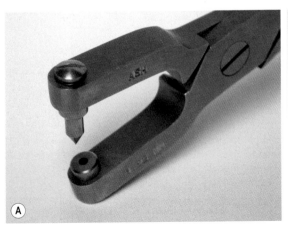 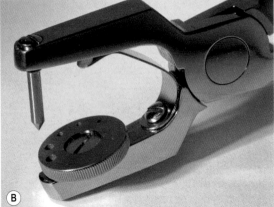

Figure 6.4 Rubber dam punch: (A) Ash single hole; (B) Ainsworth.

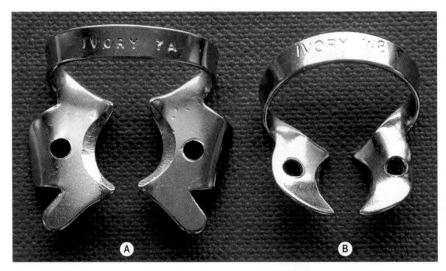

Figure 6.5 Rubber dam clamps: (A) winged clamp with bland jaws (7A); (B) wingless clamp with retentive jaws (W8).

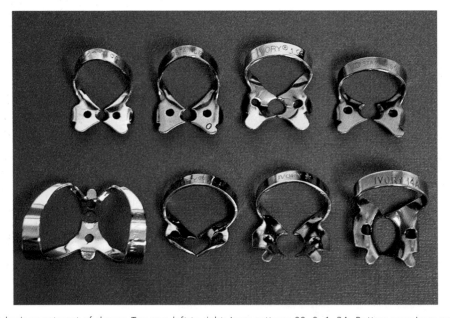

Figure 6.6 A basic assortment of clamps. Top row, left to right: Ivory patterns 00, 0, 1, 2A. Bottom row: Ivory patterns 9, W8A, 14, 14A.

may also be used; the winged K and E for molars and premolars respectively, and the wingless EW for incisors and broken down premolars. The EW clamp gives better access than the 9 clamp. The fracture or unexpected dislodgement of a rubber dam clamp is probably the only serious risk associated with rubber dam usage. The risk of inhaling or swallowing the fractured or dislodged clamp may be minimized if it can be retrieved. A length of floss

should be tied to one of the holes in the jaw of the clamp and then knotted, it is then wound around the bow of the clamp, threaded through the other hole in the opposite jaw and tied again (Fig. 6.7).

In anterior teeth, it is sometimes possible to secure the rubber dam without the use of clamps. The interproximal spaces may be wedged with wooden wedges, strips of rubber dam or short lengths of specially made latex or

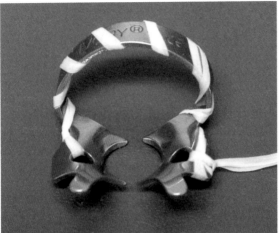

Figure 6.7 Dental floss tied onto the rubber dam clamp to aid retrieval in case of fracture or dislodgement.

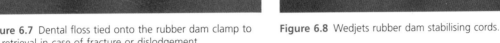

Figure 6.8 Wedjets rubber dam stabilising cords.

non-latex cords (Wedjets, Hygenic, Coltène/Whaledent, Cuyahoga Falls, OH, USA) (Fig. 6.8).

Clamp forceps

Several types are available including the University of Washington/Stoke, Ivory (Heraeus Kulzer, South Bend, IN, USA) (Fig. 6.9) and Brewer (Dentsply Ash) patterns; the choice is a matter of personal preference. The forceps are used to place, adjust and remove the rubber dam clamp. Some forceps may require adjustment to their working ends prior to first use. If the ends are too large, they need to be reshaped so that it is less difficult to disengage the clamp on the tooth.

Rubber dam frame

The corners of the rubber dam are held apart on a frame, stretched over the patient's mouth, so as not to obscure the operator's vision and not to be uncomfortable for the patient. Rubber dam frames come in various sizes and designs; they are shaped so that they do not impinge on the patient's face. Rubber dam frames are made from either metal or plastic; the latter is lighter, more comfortable and being radiolucent, removal is not always necessary when taking radiographs (Fig. 6.10). Plastic, foldable rubber dam frames (Dentsply Ash) with an articulated joint to facilitate radiography are also available.

Methods of application

Basically, there are three methods of application. In the first method, the rubber dam is attached to the clamp, with or without the frame beforehand, and the whole

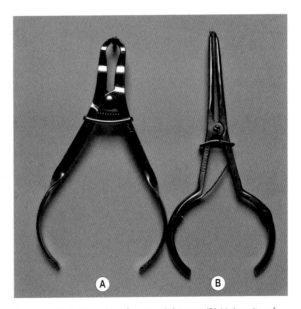

Figure 6.9 Rubber dam forceps: (A) Ivory; (B) University of Washington/Stokes.

assembly placed onto the tooth. In this method, only winged clamps can be used. Once the clamp is firmly seated, a plastic instrument is used to lift the rubber off the wings to fit against the side of the tooth (Fig. 6.11). In the second method, winged or wingless clamps may be used. The clamp is placed on the tooth and the dam is then stretched over the clamp. If this technique is used, as mentioned earlier, the clamp should be wrapped in dental floss as a precaution against clamp fracture or dislodgement. In the third method, the dam is stretched over the tooth and the clamp, winged or wingless, then placed on

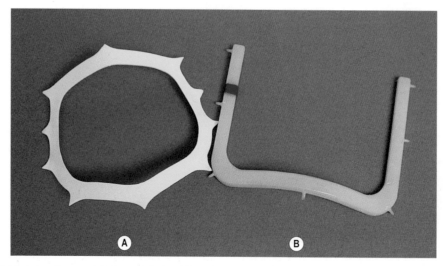

Figure 6.10 Rubber dam frames: (A) Nygaard-Ostby; (B) Starlite VisiFrame.

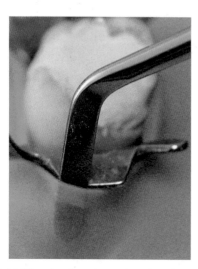

Figure 6.11 After the clamp is positioned on the tooth, the rubber is lifted off the wings with a flat plastic instrument.

the tooth. The assistance of a dental nurse is normally required for this method of application.

If more than one tooth is to be isolated, the rubber is knifed through each succeeding contact point. The rubber is stretched, positioned vertically above the contact point and gently forced through the point. It is important that the rubber remains as a single layer and does not fold over on contact with the teeth. Sometimes knifing is insufficient and the rubber must be forced through the contacts using dental floss. Techniques for placing rubber dam have been reviewed.[3,4,5] The use of a lubricant on the undersurface of the dam will aid placement; brushless shaving cream or water-soluble tasteless gels are suitable lubricants.

If a tooth is broken-down and there is insufficient tooth structure for clamp placement, there are several ways of managing the problem. It is normally possible to cement an orthodontic band onto the tooth; this transforms a tooth that is difficult to isolate into one that is straightforward. It may alternatively be possible to remove enough soft tissue surgically, or by electrosurgery, to allow a clamp to be placed. Another method is the 'split-dam' technique in which clamps are placed on the teeth mesial and distal to it. Three holes are punched in the rubber dam and these holes are joined by cutting through with a pair of scissors. The dam is then stretched over both the mesial and distal clamps, isolating the broken-down tooth. Protection against salivary contamination is aided by the use of a cotton-wool roll placed beneath the dam buccally and an aspirator lingually, plus a caulking agent to stop any seepage. This technique may also be used for cases where bridgework is present.

INSTRUMENTS FOR ACCESS CAVITY PREPARATION

The first stage of root canal treatment is to gain entry into the pulp chamber. Several types of bur will be required for access cavity preparation (Fig. 6.12).

Burs

Friction grip burs

Friction grip tapered or cylindrical fissure burs, ISO 010 or ISO 012, are used in the initial stages of access preparation to establish the correct outline form. For penetrating

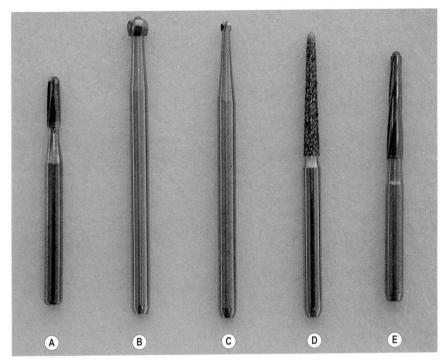

Figure 6.12 Access cavity burs (left to right): (A) FG 557 ISO 010 (TC); (B) FG ISO round 018 (long); (C) FG ISO round 010 (long); (D) FG safe-ended diamond 332 ISO 018; (E) FG safe-ended TC, Endo Z (Dentsply Maillefer).

ceramic or composite materials, diamond-coated burs are needed.

Round burs

Round burs, normal and extra-long, sizes ISO 010, 014 and 018, in a contra-angle handpiece are used to lift the roof off the pulp chamber and eliminate overhanging dentine. If a standard length bur is too short, burs with longer shanks, up to 28 mm, are available. So as not to obstruct vision when in use, some long neck burs have a slender shank (Hager & Meisinger, Neuss, Germany). The longer and smaller sizes of burs may be used to remove dentine when opening calcified canals.

Safe-ended burs

Following initial access to the pulp space, a safe-ended or non-cutting tip, tapered diamond or tungsten-carbide bur (e.g. Endo Z bur, Dentsply Maillefer, Ballaigues, Switzerland) (Fig. 6.12), can be used to remove the entire roof of the pulp chamber. The non-cutting tip prevents 'gouging' of the pulpal floor.

Gates-Glidden burs

The Gates-Glidden bur has a slender shank with a cutting bulb and a pilot-tip. It is designed so that if it fractures,

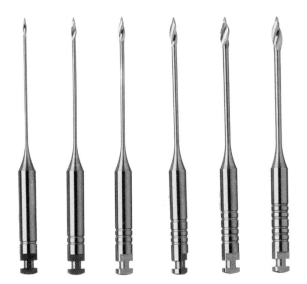

Figure 6.13 A set of Gates-Glidden drills, sizes 1–6.

this will occur near the hub rather than between the shank and the cutting bulb. Gates-Glidden burs are made of stainless steel and the set of six different sizes of burs have cutting bulbs with diameter ranging 0.5–1.5 mm (Fig. 6.13). They are also available in different lengths, a standard 32 mm, a shorter 24 mm and a longer 36 mm. The Gates-Glidden bur is operated at low-speed. It may be used for coronal root canal enlargement but there is a risk of furcal perforation in mandibular molars;[6] they have largely been superseded by rotary nickel-titanium instruments (see later) for this purpose. In retreatment cases, Gates-Glidden burs may also be used to remove gutta-percha in the coronal part of the root canal.

INSTRUMENTS FOR ROOT CANAL PREPARATION

Hand instruments

Hand instruments are grouped according to usage and to the classification established by the International Organization for Standardization (ISO). The terminology, dimensions, physical properties, measuring systems and quality control of endodontic instruments and materials are defined by these standards. As a result, endodontic hand instruments, i.e. files, reamers and barbed broaches, are standardized in relation to size, colour coding and physical properties.[7] The relevant information on sizing and colour coding for files and reamers are listed in Table 6.1; d_1 is an assessment of the diameter of the working part at the tip end, and is its nominal size; d_3 represents a point at 16 mm from d_1 where the cutting part of the instrument ends. The taper is a constant 0.02 mm per mm of cutting flute; hence also referred to as 0.02 taper. The shape of the tip is variable. The lengths of instruments available are normally 21, 25 and 31 mm. Endodontic hand instruments have been reviewed.[8]

Barbed broaches

Barbed broaches are used mainly for the removal of pulp tissue from wide root canals, and cotton wool dressings from the pulp chamber. Provided the instrument is loose within the canal and is used to engage soft tissue or dressings, the risk of fracture is minimal. Barbed broaches are made from soft steel wire (Fig. 6.14). The barbs are formed by cutting into the metal and distending the cut portion away from the shaft. The cuts are made eccentrically around the shaft so that it is not weakened excessively at any one point.

Reamers

Reamers (Fig. 6.14) are manufactured by twisting a tapered stainless steel blank to form an instrument with sharp cutting edges along the spiral. They are used with a half-turn twist and pull action, which shaves the canal wall, removing dentine chips from the root canal. Nominally they have a triangular cross-section, but the smaller sizes may be manufactured from a square blank.

Table 6.1 Nominal sizes, diameters, and colour coding of standardized root canal files and reamers

SIZE	d_1 (mm)	COLOUR	
006	0.06	Orange	●
008	0.08	Grey	○
010	0.10	Purple	●
015	0.15	White	○
020	0.20	Yellow	○
025	0.25	Red	●
030	0.30	Blue	○
035	0.35	Green	○
040	0.40	Black	●
045	0.45	White	○
050	0.50	Yellow	○
055	0.55	Red	●
060	0.60	Blue	○
070	0.70	Green	○
080	0.80	Black	●
090	0.90	White	○
100	1.00	Yellow	○
110	1.10	Red	●
120	1.20	Blue	○
130	1.30	Green	○
140	1.40	Black	●

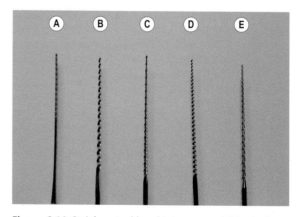

Figure 6.14 Stainless steel hand instruments: (A) barbed broach; (B) reamer; (C) K-flex file; (D) Flexofile; (E) Hedstrom file.

Files

There are various types of root canal file, and they are mostly made from stainless steel. Files are predominantly used with a filing or rasping action, in which there is little or no rotation of the instrument in the root canal. The properties of different files are related to their design features.[9,10,11] The common types of files on the market are:

- K-file
- K-flex file
- Flexofile
- Hedstrom file.

K-file

This file (Fig. 6.14) is so named as it was introduced by the Kerr Company. These files are made, like reamers, by twisting a triangular or square blank, but into a tighter series of spirals to produce from 0.9 to 1.9 cutting edges per millimetre length. They will work either in a reaming or a push-and-pull filing motion.

K-flex file

The K-flex file (Fig. 6.14) was developed in an effort to improve on the original K-file design. It has a rhomboid-shaped cross-section. As a result, when the blank is twisted to form the instrument, it has a series of cutting flutes with alternate sharp (<60°) cutting edges and obtuse non-cutting edges. The high and low flute configuration is designed to endow the instrument with greater flexibility, and provide a reservoir for the dentinal debris. A disadvantage of the K-Flex file is that it tends to lose its cutting efficiency quicker.

Flexofile

This file (Fig. 6.14) is manufactured by Dentsply Maillefer in the same way as the K-file but using a more flexible stainless steel alloy. The alloy used in file manufacture has a bearing on its cutting efficiency[12] and resistance to fracture.[13] The Flexofile has a non-cutting (Batt) tip and a triangular cross-section so the cutting flutes are sharper and there is more room for debris removal; it was reported to produce good instrumentation results.[14]

Hedstrom file

The Hedstrom file (Fig. 6.14) is made by a milling process from a steel blank of round cross-section to produce elevated cutting edges. The tapering effect appears to form a series of intersecting cones. Although the design leads to a sharp and flexible instrument, the file is inherently weaker due to the reduced shaft diameter and is therefore slightly more prone to breakage. It is most effective when used in a pull motion.[15] With sharp cutting flutes, it is also used to engage and remove retained instruments, gutta-percha and silver points.

Nickel-titanium instruments

There have been a number of newer developments in instrument design and technology. Instead of stainless steel, nickel-titanium (NiTi) alloys have been introduced in the manufacture of endodontic instruments.[16] The NiTi alloys have many interesting properties: a shape memory effect (ability to return perfectly to its original shape), superelasticity (low modulus of elasticity), good biocompatibility and high corrosion resistance. The concept of using NiTi for endodontic instruments came from orthodontics, where its properties have been utilized in the archwires of fixed appliances. The NiTi alloy used in root canal instruments is known generically as Nitinol (Ni for nickel, ti for titanium and nol for Naval Ordinance Laboratory). The manufacture of NiTi endodontic instruments is more complicated than that of stainless steel; the majority of the instruments are machined.[17]

Compared with stainless steel, NiTi instruments have greater flexibility in bending[18] and better resistance to torsional fracture[19] (see later). NiTi instruments have a non-cutting tip and they cannot be easily precurved. Their cutting efficiency is dependent on cross-sectional shape,[20] but is less aggressive compared with stainless steel instruments.[21,22] NiTi instruments tend to straighten curved root canals less than stainless steel instruments,[23] producing a more centered, tapered and acceptable preparation.[24,25] They also have different wear characteristics compared with stainless steel instruments.[26]

Power-assisted root canal instruments

Many different power-assisted root canal instruments have been developed over the years in the hope of making root canal preparation quicker and to reduce operator fatigue.

Reciprocating handpieces

These handpieces impart a mechanical action to the root canal instrument to cut dentine. An early example is the Giromatic, a mechanized handpiece in which the continuous rotation of the driveshaft is transformed into an alternating quarter-turn movement of the file. A later example is the M4 Safety handpiece (SybronEndo, Orange, CA, USA) (Fig. 6.15). This handpiece has a push button-type chuck mechanism to accommodate plastic handled root canal instruments. The handpiece imparts a watch-winding oscillatory movement to the attached root canal instrument.

Rotary NiTi instruments

With the advent of instruments made from NiTi, the endodontic market has become dominated by many new rotary

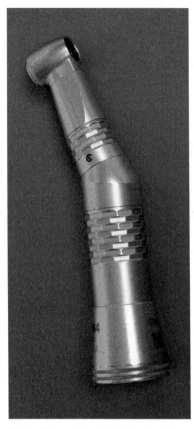

Figure 6.15 The SybronEndo M4 Safety handpiece.

Table 6.2 Rotary NiTi instrument systems
ProFile (Dentsply Maillefer, Ballaigues, Switzerland)
System GT (Dentsply Maillefer)
Quantec (SybronEndo, Orange, CA, USA)
Lightspeed LSX (Discus Dental, Culver City, CA, USA)
Hero 642 (Micro-Mega, Besançon, France)
K3 (SybronEndo)
RaCe and BioRaCe (FKG Dentaire, La Chaux-de-Fonds, Switzerland)
ProTaper Universal (Dentsply Maillefer)
Twisted Files (SybronEndo)

root canal instrument systems (Table 6.2); many consist of a combination of rotary and hand NiTi files. It is impossible to detail all the different rotary NiTi systems but many newer and unique design features have been incorporated by manufacturers.

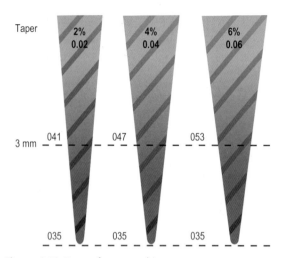

Figure 6.16 Taper of root canal instruments.

Variable taper

The concept of taper variation is to maximize the cutting efficiency by minimizing the contact area between the surface of the instrument and the canal wall. Instead of having to flare a canal using different sizes of standard 0.02 taper files to achieve the desired shape, the preparation is produced by using files of the desired taper straightaway. The larger the taper, the more conical the shape of the instrument (Fig. 6.16). For ease of use, many rotary instrument systems have matching variable taper hand files, paper points and gutta-percha points.

Flute design

The shape of the flutes in cross-section determines cutting efficiency and the ability to remove debris. A design incorporating a reservoir for the dentine debris will help effective evacuation as the debris is transported coronally.

Rake angle

The rake or cutting angle of most conventional instruments is negative so the cutting blade scrapes rather than cuts the dentine, and this is inefficient. A positive rake angle results in more effective cutting but if the rake angle is excessively positive, the cutting blade will dig into the dentine substrate. Therefore, the rake angle should be only slightly positive.

Helical flute angle

This is the angle at which the cutting flutes spiral around the shaft of the instrument. If there are too few spirals, the dentine debris will accumulate quickly before being removed, and the instrument will become clogged. On the other hand, if there are too many spirals, the dentine debris has too great a distance to travel before being evacuated and frictional resistance may trap and compress the debris. The ideal helical ⬛⬛⬛ allows efficient removal of dentinal debris witho⬛⬛⬛⬛ g the instrument. Also, increasing the helical fl⬛⬛⬛⬛ along the length of the file, from tip to handle, ⬛⬛⬛⬛ debris removal.

Core diameter/flute ⬛

The core strength and ⬛⬛⬛ of an instrument is dependent on its core c⬛⬛⬛⬛al diameter; the larger the core diameter, the more robust and rigid the instrument. The core diameter is inversely related to the flute depth. The proportion of the core diameter to the outside diameter should be greatest at the tip, where strength is most important. By uniformly decreasing this proportion as the fluting moves up the taper, resulting in greater flute depth, the flexibility increases while the strength of the instrument is maintained. An additional advantage is that dentine debris is also removed more efficiently.

Non-cutting tip

A non-cutting, safe-ended or Batt tip helps to pilot the instrument down the canal so that it follows the canal shape. Rather than gouging into the canal wall, the tip will help guide the instrument and this reduces the risk of apical transportation.

Surface treatment

The majority of rotary NiTi instruments are produced using a milling process. As a result, defects and adherent debris are present on the instrument's surface, which may act as stress concentration and crack initiation sites. Electropolishing reduces these defects and produces a surface free of contaminants, thereby increasing the instrument's fatigue resistance.[27,28] Milling grooves, cracks, pits and areas of metal rollover are less evident on electropolished instruments. A variety of other surface treatments have also been investigated to improve the hardness and wear resistance, hence the cutting efficiency of rotary NiTi instruments. They include ionic implantation of boron[29] and creation of a titanium nitride layer via thermal nitridation, ionic implantation,[30] physical and chemical vapour deposition.[31,32]

Rotary NiTi handpiece and motor

Rotary NiTi instruments are normally operated at low torque and low speed (150–350 rpm). Therefore, these instruments must be used with a speed-reducing handpiece, which is driven by either an air or electric motor (Fig. 6.17). Handpieces driven by electric motors have the advantage of being smoother, vibration-free and better at maintaining the selected speed. There are also cordless, motorized handpieces, which are powered by rechargeable batteries on the market (e.g. Endo-Mate TC, NSK, Tochigi, Japan and EndoTouch TC, SybronEndo) (Fig. 6.18). To improve access, some of these handpieces are available

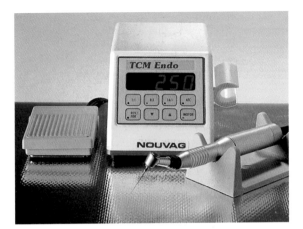

Figure 6.17 Electric motor and handpiece for rotary NiTi root canal instruments.

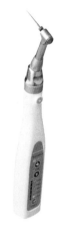

Figure 6.18 A cordless motorized handpiece for rotary NiTi root canal instruments.

with a reduced size head. Many rotary files are also made with shorter handles or lengths to facilitate access in posterior teeth.

Some rotary handpieces and motors, particularly electric motors, have control units, which allow for different speed and torque settings. The risk of instrument breakage can be reduced by selecting lower speeds[33] and setting the torque lower, to the limit of elasticity of each instrument.[34,35] The control units may also have a built-in auto-reverse feature so that the instrument will run in reverse when a pre-set torque is exceeded. Some sophisticated units have programmable memory, for storing different instrumentation protocols that will automatically alter the speed and torque settings depending on the type, size and brand of rotary NiTi file used.

The susceptibility of a rotary NiTi instrument to fracture is related to root curvature and becomes greater as the angle of curvature increases and the radius of curvature decreases;[36,37,38] severely curved canals with an angle of curvature greater than 30° are the most risky.[39,40] Used rotary NiTi instruments examined revealed signs of deterioration including surface cracks[41,42] and are significantly more susceptible to fracture than new ones.[35,43] Recently issued advice against reuse of endodontic instruments (see later) should help reduce the incidence of instrument fracture as they are discarded after one patient.

It was found that torsional failures caused by using too much apical force during instrumentation occur slightly more frequently than flexural failures due to cyclic fatigue, which may result from usage in curved canals.[44] The susceptibility of NiTi instruments to cyclic fatigue is dependent on its cross-sectional designs, diameters and tapers.[45] Recently, a series of papers on defects in NiTi instruments has been published; the type and location of defects and the factors involved;[46] the mode of failure of different brands of NiTi instruments,[47] including one that had been electropolished;[48] the incidence and mode of NiTi instrument separation after being used by undergraduate students.[49]

The incidence of fracture can be reduced if clinicians are more aware of this possibility and take avoidance measures.[50] The prevalence, causes and management of rotary NiTi instrument fracture, and its impact on prognosis have been reviewed.[51] Ways of preventing instrument fracture have been recommended.[52] In general, rotary NiTi instruments are safe, able to respect canal anatomy, effective in terms of shaping and cleaning, and preparation time is reduced compared with stainless steel hand instruments.[53,54,55,56]

Manufacturers are continuing in their quest to improve the fracture resistance of NiTi instruments; possible strategies include newer manufacturing processes or the use of alloys with better mechanical properties. M-Wire, a new NiTi alloy produced using a proprietary thermal process was developed, and is used for the manufacture of GT series X instruments (GTX) (Dentsply Tulsa Dental Specialties, Tulsa, OK, USA). The manufacturer claimed that instruments produced from M-Wire alloy have comparatively greater flexibility and increased resistance to cyclic fatigue.

The traditional production of NiTi instruments by grinding across the crystalline grain structure creates microfracture points along the length of the instruments. A completely different manufacturing process was developed to produce Twisted Files (TF) (SybronEndo) (Fig. 6.19). A NiTi blank in the austenitic phase is transformed into a different crystalline structure (R-phase) by a process of heating and cooling. In the R-phase, the NiTi blank is twisted and then heated and cooled again to maintain its new shape and converted back to the austenitic phase. The manufacturer claimed that as a result, TF have enhanced superelasticity and increased cyclic fatigue resistance. TF was found to be more flexible[57] and more

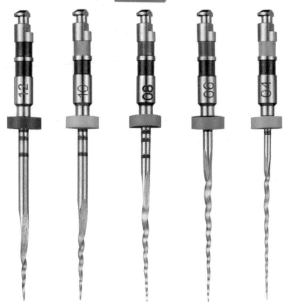

Figure 6.19 Twisted Files (TF).

resistant to cyclic fatigue compared with NiTi instruments produced by grinding.[58] However, studies comparing the resistance to cyclic fatigue of TF with GTX have reported conflicting results[58,59] so further investigations are needed.

DEVICES TO DETERMINE WORKING LENGTH

The objectives of endodontic treatment cannot be achieved without knowing the canal length; therefore, the accurate determination of root canal length is important to ensure success of root canal treatment. The two commonest ways of verifying canal length are by radiography and by the use of an electronic apex locator.

Radiographic method

In this method of verifying canal length, an instrument is placed into the root canal and then a conventional or digital radiograph taken. The length of the instrument, marked with a rubber/silicone stop, is recorded. Depending on whether the desired depth is reached, as shown radiographically, adjustments are made accordingly. When determining the working length using this method, the X-ray film or digital sensor must be positioned and kept in place. With an X-ray film, this is achieved with the aid of a surgical haemostat rather than the patient's finger. Alternatively, specially designed X-ray film (e.g. Endoray

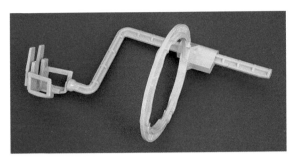

Figure 6.20 Endoray II beam-aiming device used for taking working length radiographs.

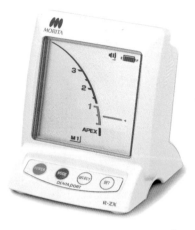

Figure 6.21 Root ZX apex locator with a digital visual display.

II, Dentsply Rinn, Elgin, IL, USA) (Fig. 6.20) and digital sensor holders are available (XCP-DS, Dentsply Rinn).

Electronic apex locators

A method of estimating root canal length based on the different electrical conductivity in a root canal and the oral mucosa was reported[60] and developed.[61] The operation of electronic apex locators (EALs) has evolved from measuring the electrical resistance with direct, alternating or high frequency currents to measuring the voltage gradients and calculating the ratio between impedances.[62] The fundamental operating principles of electronic root canal length measurement devices have been reviewed.[63]

A typical EAL has a meter or digital display and two electrodes. One electrode, the ground electrode, is fashioned into a hook and placed into the oral cavity. The other electrode, in the form of a spring-loaded clip or probe is attached to the endodontic instrument, which is inserted into the root canal. As the instrument is advanced apically, a visual display will show, and often an audio signal will also be emitted, to indicate when the apical foramen is reached. The depth is marked on the instrument and the length measured following its removal from the root canal.

Newer generations of EALs measure opposition to the flow of alternating current or impedance using multiple frequencies to determine the distance from the end of the canal[64,65] and the canal does not need to be dry. An example, the popular Root ZX (Morita, Suita City, Osaka, Japan) (Fig. 6.21) works on the feedback variation impedance of two frequencies (0.4 and 8 kHz) and has a powerful microprocessor to process the mathematical quotient and algorithm calculations required for greater accuracy. Another, the Elements Diagnostic Unit and Apex Locator (SybronEndo) uses a composite waveform of two signals (0.5 and 4 kHz); the impedance information is not processed as a mathematical algorithm, but instead the resistance and capacitance measurements are taken separately and compared with a database to determine the distance to the apex of the root canal.[64]

While these devices are useful in determining root canal length, they must be used carefully to avoid errors.[64,66] A major influencing factor is the size of the apical foramen; when this is large, the apex locator may give a reading short of the apex. However, when the apex is small, an accurate reading within 0.5 mm of the apical foramen is likely. Newer generations of EALs are less susceptible to inaccuracies caused by the presence of fluid (blood, exudate or sodium hypochlorite irrigant) in the root canal. The Root ZX has been exhaustively tested for accuracy in many clinical conditions and was reported to be reliable.[64,65,67,68] The use of an EAL is invaluable in assessing the root canal working length; combined with radiographic confirmation, this should reduce the number of X-ray exposures.[69]

A cordless, combined motorized handpiece and EAL (Tri Auto ZX, Morita)[70] that will measure root canal length and also drive rotary instruments for canal preparation is available (Fig. 6.22). Powered by a rechargeable battery, the motor is capable of a speed of up to 400 rpm without load and one of eight speed settings may be selected. Other features of this dual-function handpiece/EAL include auto-apical reverse when the instrument is inserted deeper than the set depth and auto-torque reverse when more than the set torque is applied. A more recent handpiece/EAL combination[71] consists of the addition of a motor and handpiece module to the Root ZX to form the Dentaport ZX system (Morita) (Fig. 6.23).

Measuring devises

Devices for measuring file lengths range from a simple metal ruler, obtainable from a hardware shop, to specially designed gauges and measuring blocks. Silicone stops, as markers, are usually already placed on hand instruments by most manufacturers. The ruler incorporated into

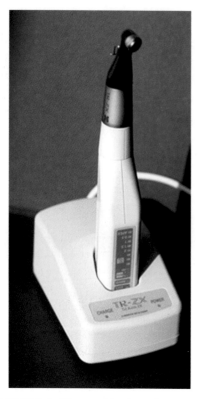

Figure 6.22 Tri Auto ZX, a combined, cordless, motorized handpiece and electronic apex locator.

combination devices like a silicone stop dispenser and a file-bending instrument may also be used for measuring.

IRRIGANT DELIVERY DEVICES

Irrigants are used to wash out canal debris, dissolve pulpal remnants and lubricate the canal, thus improving the efficiency of canal preparation. Irrigants may be delivered into the root canal using either a needle and syringe, or an ultrasonic device. Endodontic irrigation needles are blunt-ended with either a hole or the side cut out (Fig. 6.24). They come in different gauges[72] and are secured to the syringes using a Luer-lok twist mechanism so the needle will not be dislodged when the plunger of the syringe is depressed.

Ultrasonic devices to irrigate root canals can be very effective, as large volumes of irrigant can be dispensed with ease, to flush out the root canal system thoroughly; the irrigant cleans by acoustic microstreaming.[73,74] These units (e.g. Piezon-Master 400, EMS, Le Sentier, Switzerland) (Fig. 6.25) in which the ultrasound is generated by the piezo-electric effect are supplied with a multifunctional handpiece into which different tips may be fitted. A file-holding tip is used for ultrasonic irrigation. Other tips (Fig. 6.26) are also available for controlled removal of dentine during the location of calcified canals, to break up the cement lute when removing cemented posts, and for root-end cavity preparation during apical surgery. The use of ultrasound in endodontics has been reviewed.[75,76]

Hydrodynamic systems for irrigating root canals in the form of pressure alternation devices have come on the market; they include RinsEndo (Dürr Dental, Bietigheim-

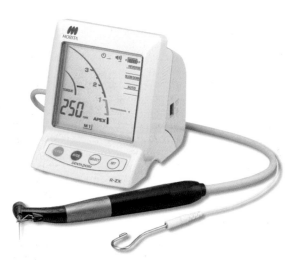

Figure 6.23 Dentaport ZX - the addition of a motor and handpiece module to the Root ZX.

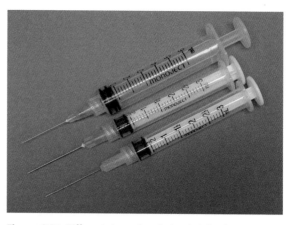

Figure 6.24 Different sizes of endodontic irrigating syringes and needles; the blunt-ended, notched needles are attached to the syringes using a Luer-lok mechanism.

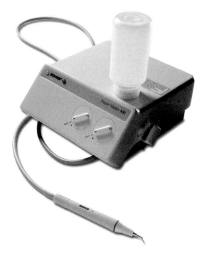

Figure 6.25 The Piezon-Master 400 unit; the ultrasonic vibration is generated by the piezo-electric effect.

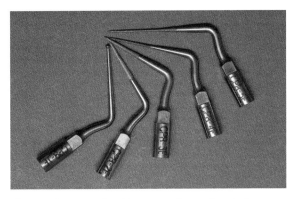

Figure 6.26 A set of multi-purpose diamond-coated ultrasonic micro-tips.

Bissingen, Germany)[77,78] and Endo-Vac (Discus Dental, Culver City, CA, USA).[79,80]

INSTRUMENTS FOR RETRIEVING BROKEN INSTRUMENTS AND POSTS

All root canal instruments should be used with care to prevent breakage. Prevention is better than cure. However, if breakage does occur it may be possible to remove the fragment with one of a number of different devices and techniques.[81]

Forceps

Fine-beaked haemostats or Steiglitz forceps (Hu-Friedy, Chicago, IL, USA) can be used to remove a broken instrument (Fig. 6.27). However, this is only possible if the end

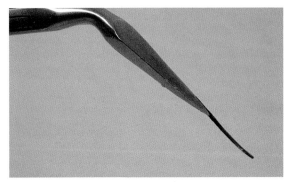

Figure 6.27 Steiglitz forceps, fine-beaked, for removal of retained instruments or metal filling points.

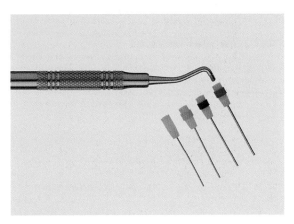

Figure 6.28 Cancellier kit consisting of a set of extractors and a handle.

of the fractured instrument is accessible and not jammed firmly within the canal.

Cancellier kit

If the fractured file is loose but not free, a Cancellier extractor (SybronEndo) (Fig. 6.28) may be used. The extractors are a set of hollow tubes, which fit into a handle; the assembly resembles a hollow plugger. The appropriately sized extractor is chosen to fit over the file. A drop of cyanoacrylate glue is placed into the hollow end of the extractor so that it adheres when fitted over the file. A drop of acrylic monomer liquid is then used to accelerate the setting of the cyanoacrylate glue so that the file is retrieved when the extractor is removed. The Cancellier extractors can be cleaned with a solvent, e.g. Xylol, and reused.

Masserann kit

The technique using the Masserann instrument (Micro-Mega, Besançon, France) (Fig. 6.29) to remove a broken metal post or retained instrument is well documented.[82,83] A hollow trepan bur is chosen whose internal diameter corresponds to the diameter of the obstruction. The principle of the technique is to create a trough around the top of the post or instrument to be removed using the trepans, which are rotated in an anticlockwise direction; this action frees the obstruction around its periphery enabling its removal.

Meitrac endo safety system

The Meitrac system (Hager & Meisinger, Neuss, Germany) (Fig. 6.30) is a similar but reduced version of the Masserann kit; consisting of trepans and extractors intended for removal of intraradicular objects of different diameters. In the system are: Meitrac I (0.15–0.5 mm diameter) for broken instruments, Meitrac II (0.5–0.9 diameter) for silver points and Meitrac III (0.9–1.5 mm diameter) for posts.

Post removal devices

Many techniques have been devised to remove cemented metal posts. These include the use of ultrasound to disrupt the cement lute and loosen the post or simple drilling with burs. There are also dedicated post removal devices; examples are the Post Puller,[84] the Eggler post remover[85] and the Gonon post removal system[86] (Fig. 6.31). The principle behind all these devices is the same and is akin to a corkscrew in which opposing forces are created to extract the post from the root canal. The Ruddle Post Removal System (SybronEndo) is meant to be an improved version of the Gonon system. Non-metal posts, e.g. fibre posts are not amenable to removal using these post removal devices (see Chapter 14).

INSTRUMENTS FOR FILLING ROOT CANALS

The instruments needed are dependent on the technique employed to fill the root canal. For more information on root canal filling, including materials other than gutta-percha, please refer to Chapter 9.

Lateral condensation

In this technique, a well-fitting master gutta-percha point is chosen and combined with sealer to fill the root canal. A hand or finger spreader (Fig. 6.32), designed with a pointed tip, is used to condense the gutta-percha, creating space for placement of accessory gutta-percha points. The gutta-percha is added sequentially until the canal is completely filled. Spreaders are available in a variety of different lengths and widths; they are usually made of stainless steel but there are also NiTi versions. The NiTi fingers spreaders are reported to penetrate to a significantly greater depth in curved canals[87,88] compared with stainless steel spreaders. Depending on the manufacturer, spreaders are available with matching sizes of non-standardized (Fig. 6.32), standardized and variable taper accessory gutta-percha points. However, there may be a degree of variation between sizes of finger spreaders and their corresponding accessory gutta-percha points.[89,90]

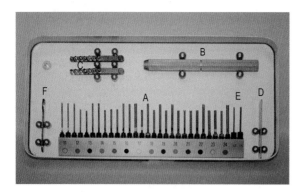

Figure 6.29 Masserann kit containing a range of trepans (A), handle (B), gauges (C,D), extractor (E) and spanner (F).

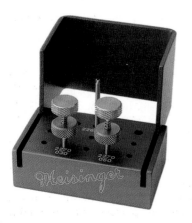
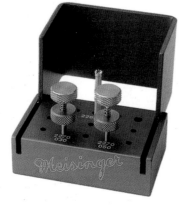
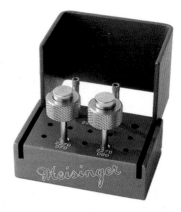

Figure 6.30 The Meitrac Endo safety system.

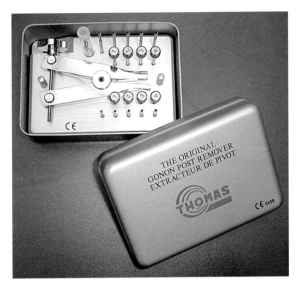

Figure 6.31 The Gonon post remover system.

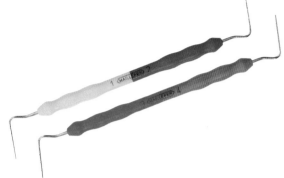

Figure 6.33 A set of double-ended hand pluggers.

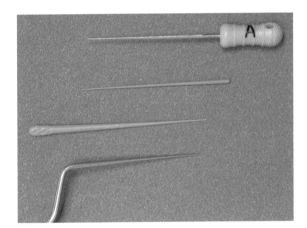

Figure 6.32 Hand and finger spreaders with matching accessory gutta-percha points.

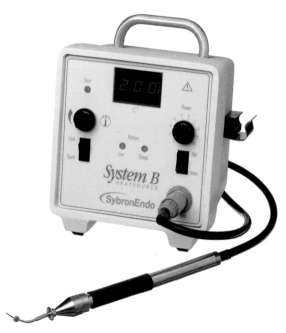

Figure 6.34 System B heat source for warm condensation of gutta-percha.

Vertical condensation

In this technique, hand or finger pluggers (Fig. 6.33), which have blunt, flat ends, are used to apply vertical pressure to condense the gutta-percha and sealer. Hand pluggers of different diameters are usually marked with reference lines to allow the assessment of plugger depth. In the classic Schilder technique, small segments of gutta-percha are added, heat is applied using heat carriers to soften the gutta-percha and then condensed with the aid of a series of different sized pluggers; the sequence is repeated until the canal is completely filled. Double-ended instruments, with one end a heat carrier and the other a plugger, are available. Electrically heated carriers fitted with spreaders or pluggers have been developed for warm gutta-percha

filling techniques (Touch 'n Heat and System B Heat Source, SybronEndo) (Fig. 6.34). The tips of these carriers are heated rapidly and internally so that the heat is concentrated at the tip. A contact spring on the front of the handle acts as a switch to activate the heater. Different temperatures may be chosen for different stages of the filling sequence; with the System B, the chosen temperature will be maintained throughout when activated. The System B is used for the Buchanan 'Continuous Wave' filling technique, which is a modification of the Schilder technique. The root surface temperature produced varies depending on the heat source and technique used.[91,92]

Thermomechanical compaction

In this technique, an engine-operated compactor e.g. Gutta-Condensor (Dentsply Maillefer) (Fig. 6.35), designed with reverse turning screw threads, is rotated in a forward direction alongside a fitted gutta-percha point or several points. The heat created by the friction plasticizes the gutta-percha and, at the same time, the centrifugal forces generated compacts the gutta-percha onto the canal walls. The higher the speed of rotation the greater the heat generated.[93] As the bulk of gutta-percha in the canal builds up, the compactor is forced out of the canal. The result can be a well-condensed root canal filling that is more homogeneous compared with lateral condensation.[94] If the compactor is used accidentally in reverse, it screws into the root canal and will break. Another disadvantage is that it is possible to extrude gutta-percha through the apex with this technique; to prevent this, the hybrid technique was developed, in which an apical gutta-percha plug is first created by lateral condensation prior to thermomechanical compaction.[95]

A modified technique of thermomechanical compaction involves coating the condenser with already plasticized gutta-percha of a different viscosity (e.g. Microseal, SybronEndo). The ultra-low fusing gutta-percha for this technique comes in cartridges, which are heated in an oven and delivered with a syringe. A master gutta-percha point is placed beforehand and as previously, when the coated condensor is operated in the canal, plasticized gutta-percha is compacted onto the canal walls. Without the reliance on friction to plasticize the gutta-percha, the condensor can be operated at a lower speed lessening the risk of instrument fracture and potential heat damage to the periodontium.

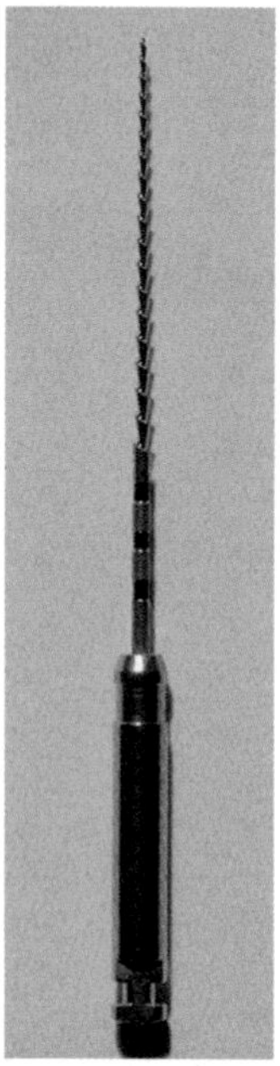

Thermoplasticized injectable gutta-percha

The concept of injecting softened gutta-percha into the root canal was introduced many years ago[96] as a development of vertical condensation. An example is the Obtura III Max (Obtura Spartan, Earth City, MO, USA) (Fig. 6.36), a high temperature system capable of taking the temperature of gutta-percha in the heating chamber to 200°C. It consists of a delivery unit with an electrical cord connected to a temperature control box with a digital display. The gutta-percha is loaded into the heating chamber. When the trigger of the delivery unit is squeezed, the softened gutta-percha is extruded through a 20, 23 or 25 gauge needle; the needles are reusable, bendable and sterilizable. Thermal protectors are used to insulate the heating unit and to prevent burning the patient's lip. This technique is useful when filling large and irregular canals. The root filling produced is well adapted to the prepared canal.[97] It is also used for back filling canals after an apical plug has been established.

Other manufacturers have brought out similar thermoplasticized injectable gutta-percha delivery devices including a cordless version (HotShot, Discus Dental) (Fig. 6.37) and a dual-function combination of a System B-type heated spreader with a motor-driven warm gutta-percha extruder (Elements Obturation Unit, SybronEndo) (Fig. 6.38).

Figure 6.35 Gutta-Condensor (Dentsply Maillefer) for thermomechanical compaction of gutta-percha.

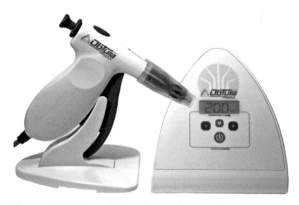

Figure 6.36 Obtura III Max thermoplasticized injectable gutta-percha system. The heated delivery gun extrudes gutta-percha through the fine needle; the temperature is controlled by the main unit.

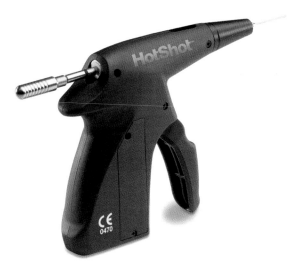

Figure 6.37 HotShot, a cordless thermoplasticized injectable gutta-percha delivery device.

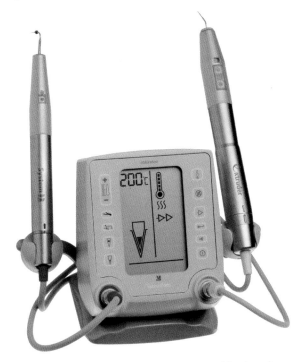

Figure 6.38 Elements Obturation Unit, a combination of a System B-type heated spreader with a motor-driven warm gutta-percha extruder.

Gutta-percha carrier devices

The Thermafil system (Dentsply Maillefer) is an example of a gutta-percha carrier device. This commercial product originated from a technique of moulding heated gutta-percha to a root canal file, which was then used to fill the

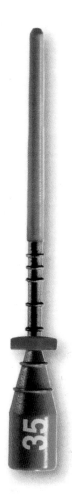

Figure 6.39 Thermafil obturator, a plastic carrier-based device coated with gutta-percha.

root canal.[98] The Thermafil obturators have a 0.04 taper, V-shaped cross-section plastic core, which is coated with alpha-phase gutta-percha that has excellent flow properties (Fig. 6.39). The obturators are colour-coded and come in ISO sizes 20–140. The size of the Thermafil obturator required is first determined with the aid of a set of Verifier files. The chosen obturator is warmed by placement in a special oven (ThermaPrep Plus oven). When warmed, the obturator is removed from the oven and inserted, with force, into the root canal. After cooling, the handle, if already pre-notched is twisted off; otherwise it is cut off with a bur. A Thermafil Post Space bur is available if post space preparation is required.

The Thermafil system is intended to make filling easier and faster.[99] However, a minor disadvantage of leaving a plastic core filling material in situ is the problem of removal, should retreatment be required. The retained obturator is not easy to remove.[100] Many rotary NiTi systems include similar carrier-based devices that correspond to the size of their instruments and are marketed as a comprehensive package (e.g. System GT obturators and ProTaper Universal obturators, Dentsply Maillefer).

STORAGE AND STERILIZATION OF ENDODONTIC INSTRUMENTS

Instrument stands and storage systems

Root canal instruments such as files, unless labelled sterile when supplied, should be cleaned and sterilized beforehand. They may be stored in small boxes with stands (e.g. Endo-Stand, Dentsply Maillefer), or in Pyrex glass test tubes with different coloured covers for instrument identification (Fig. 6.40). Complete sets of instruments can be pre-arranged, sterilized and kept, ready for use. Metal or plastic boxes with lids, in a variety of sizes are available. Some can house all the basic instruments required for endodontic treatment; there is also a file stand, a medicament dish and a cotton wool pellet container. Alternatively, instruments can be sterilized and stored in transparent autoclave bags and laid out on an open plastic tray, with a sponge for files.

Another instrument-holding device, the Endoring II system (Jordco, Beaverton, OR, USA) comprises a triangular disposable sponge for root canal instruments, which is inserted into an autoclavable thermoplastic resin sponge holder, with a snap-on finger ring handle (Fig. 6.41). Disposable wells (Gelwells) for medicaments and canal lubricants, may be attached to the sponge holder; there is also a ruler incorporated. The Endoring II system allows easy access to root canal instruments within the operating field, eliminating the time-consuming action of picking up instruments from the bracket table.

Sterilization of endodontic instruments

Infection control is of paramount importance and the responsibility of every member of the dental team. Recommended, universal methods of infection control must be employed to prevent the risk of transmission of infection within the dental surgery.[101] All instruments and equipment must be cleaned thoroughly and sterilized. However, concerns regarding the re-use of endodontic instruments and the possible transmission of variant Creutzfeldt-Jakob Disease (vCJD) led to current United Kingdom guidelines[102,103,104,105] advising dentists to ensure that endodontic files and reamers are treated as single use. Prions, the abnormal proteins associated with vCJD are more resistant than other types of infectious agent to conventional clean-

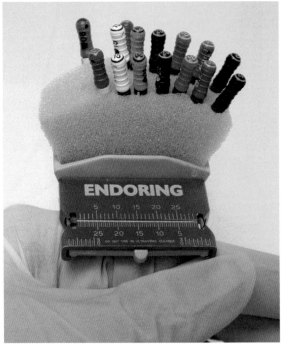

Figure 6.41 Endoring II, comprising a sponge for instruments in a plastic holder incorporating a ruler.

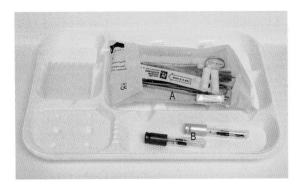

Figure 6.40 (A) Plastic tray containing instruments in a transparent sterile bag; (B) files can be stored and sterilized in Pyrex glass test tubes.

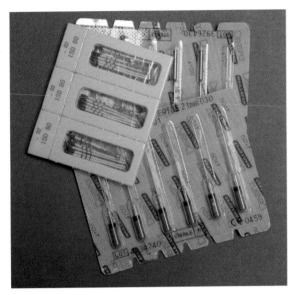

Figure 6.42 Sterilized paper points, files and burs in blister packs.

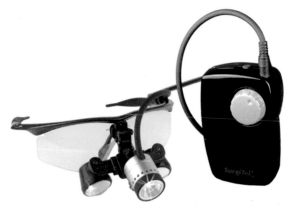

Figure 6.43 Telescopes and portable headlight attached to spectacle frame for enhanced vision and illumination.

ing and sterilization procedures normally used to decontaminate dental instruments.[106]

For convenience, and if available, single-use, disposable items are recommended. Sterile packs of files, burs and blister packs of paper points are produced by many manufacturers (Fig. 6.42) and are often available at no extra cost.

LOUPES, FIBRE-OPTIC LIGHTS AND OPERATING MICROSCOPES

Endodontic procedures are often performed in areas of limited access and reduced visibility. The use of magnification and better illumination can certainly be extremely helpful in these situations. Magnifying binocular loupes (e.g. SurgiTel, Ann Arbor, MI, USA) (Fig. 6.43) can help enhance vision while fibre-optic lighting provides better illumination. Dedicated dental operating microscopes (e.g. Global Microscope, Global Surgical Corp., St. Louis, MO, USA) (Fig. 6.44) provide the combined benefits of magnification and illumination.[107] They allow greater magnification and facilitate canal orifice location in difficult cases; they are widely used by specialist practitioners. A fibre-optic endoscope, to provide magnified intracanal visualization was also developed for use in endodontics.[108]

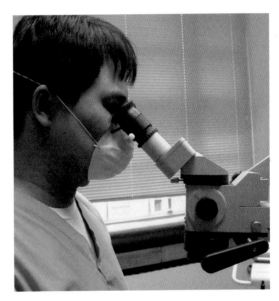

Figure 6.44 Dental operating microscope provides a range of magnifications and improved illumination.

- basic selection of instruments required for endodontic treatment
- reasons and equipment for rubber dam application
- instruments for root canal preparation
- devices for delivering root canal irrigants
- instruments for retrieving broken instruments and posts
- instruments for filling root canals
- storage, sterilization and guidelines on re-use of endodontic instruments
- uses and advantages of magnification and additional illumination.

LEARNING OUTCOMES

At the end of this chapter, the reader should be able to recognize and discuss the:

REFERENCES

1. Svec TA, Powers JM, Ladd GD, Meyer TN. Tensile and tear properties of dental dam. Journal of Endodontics 1996;22: 253–256.

2. Svec TA, Powers JM, Ladd GD. Hardness and stress corrosion of rubber dam clamps. Journal of Endodontics 1997;23:397–398.

3. Antrim DD. Endodontics and the rubber dam: a review of techniques. General Dentistry 1983;31:294–299.

4. Bhuva B, Chong BS, Patel S. Rubber Dam in Clinical Practice. ENDO (London, England) 2008;2:131–141.

5. Reuter JE. The isolation of teeth and the protection of the patient during endodontic treatment. International Endodontic Journal 1983;16:173–181.

6. Wu M-K, van der Sluis LWM, Wesselink PR. The risk of furcal perforation in mandibular molars using Gates-Glidden drills with anticurvature pressure. Oral Surgery, Oral Medicine, Oral Pathology, Oral Radiology, Endodontics 2005;99:378–382.

7. International Organization for Standardization (ISO). Dental Root Canal Instruments – Part 1: Specification for Files, Reamers, Barbed Broaches, Rasps, Paste Carriers, Explorers and Cotton Broaches. ISO 3630-1: 1992. London, UK: British Standards Institution; 1992.

8. Schäfer E. Root canal instruments for manual use: a review. Endodontics and Dental Traumatology 1997;13:51–64.

9. Schäfer E. Relationship between design features of endodontic instruments and their properties. Part 1. Cutting efficiency. Journal of Endodontics 1999;25:52–55.

10. Schäfer E. Relationship between design features of endodontic instruments and their properties. Part 2. Instrumentation of curved canals. Journal of Endodontics 1999;25:56–59.

11. Schäfer E, Tepel J. Relationship between design features of endodontic instruments and their properties. Part 3. Resistance to bending and fracture. Journal of Endodontics 2001;27:299–303.

12. Brau-Aguade E, Canalda-Sahli C, Berastegui-Jimeno E. Cutting efficiency of K-files manufactured with different metallic alloys. Endodontics and Dental Traumatology 1996;12:286–288.

13. Canalda-Sahli C, Brau-Aguade E, Berastegui-Jimeno E. A comparison of bending and torsional properties of K-files manufactured with different metallic alloys. International Endodontic Journal 1996;29: 185–189.

14. Schäfer E, Tepel J, Hoppe W. Properties of endodontic hand instruments used in rotary motion. Part 2. Instrumentation of curved canals. Journal of Endodontics 1995;21:493–497.

15. Tepel J, Schäfer E. Endodontic hand instruments: cutting efficiency, instrumentation of curved canals, bending and torsional properties. Endodontics and Dental Traumatology 1997;13:201–210.

16. Thompson SA. An overview of nickel-titanium alloys used in dentistry. International Endodontic Journal 2000;33: 297–310.

17. Serene TP, Adams JD, Saxena A. Nickel-Titanium Instruments: Applications in Endodontics. St. Louis MO, USA: Ishiyaku Euro America, Inc; 1995.

18. Kazemi RB, Stenman E, Spångberg LS. A comparison of stainless steel and nickel-titanium H-type instruments of identical design: torsional and bending tests. Oral Surgery, Oral Medicine, Oral Pathology, Oral Radiology, Endodontics 2000;90:500–506.

19. Tepel J, Schäfer E, Hoppe W. Properties of endodontic hand instruments used in rotary motion. Part 3. Resistance to bending and fracture. Journal of Endodontics 1997;23: 141–145.

20. Camps JJ, Pertot WJ. Machining efficiency of nickel-titanium K-type files in a linear motion. International Endodontic Journal 1995;28:279–284.

21. Schäfer E, Tepel J. Cutting efficiency of Hedstrom, S and U files made of various alloys in filing motion. International Endodontic Journal 1996;29: 302–308.

22. Tepel J, Schäfer E, Hoppe W. Properties of endodontic hand instruments used in rotary motion. Part 1. Cutting efficiency. Journal of Endodontics 1995;21: 418–421.

23. Glosson CR, Haller RH, Dove SB, Del Rio CE. A comparison of root canal preparations using Ni-Ti hand, Ni-Ti engine-driven, and K-Flex endodontic instruments. Journal of Endodontics 1995;21: 146–151.

24. Bishop K, Dummer PMH. A comparison of stainless steel Flexofiles and nickel-titanium NiTiFlex files during the shaping of simulated canals. International Endodontic Journal 1997;30: 25–34.

25. Zmener O, Balbachan L. Effectiveness of nickel-titanium files for preparing curved root canals. Endodontics and Dental Traumatology 1995;11:121–123.

26. Bonetti Filho I, Miranda Esberard R, De Toledo Leonardo R, Del Rio CE. Microscopic evaluation of three endodontic files pre- and postinstrumentation. Journal of Endodontics 1998;24:461–464.

27. Anderson ME, Price JW, Parashos P. Fracture resistance of electropolished rotary nickel-titanium endodontic instruments. Journal of Endodontics 2007;33: 1212–1216.

28. Tripi TR, Bonaccorso A, Condorelli GG. Cyclic fatigue of different nickel-titanium endodontic rotary instruments. Oral Surgery, Oral Medicine, Oral Pathology, Oral Radiology, Endodontics 2006;102: 106–114.

29. Lee DH, Park B, Saxena A, Serene TP. Enhanced surface hardness by boron implantation in Nitinol

alloy. Journal of Endodontics 1996;22:543–546.

30. Rapisarda E, Bonaccorso A, Tripi TR, et al. The effect of surface treatments of nickel-titanium files on wear and cutting efficiency. Oral Surgery, Oral Medicine, Oral Pathology, Oral Radiology, Endodontics 2000;89:363–368.

31. Schäfer E. Effect of physical vapor deposition on cutting efficiency of nickel-titanium files. Journal of Endodontics 2002;28:800–802.

32. Tripi TR, Bonaccorso A, Condorelli GG. Fabrication of hard coatings on NiTi instruments. Journal of Endodontics 2003;29:132–134.

33. Yared GM, Bou Dagher FE, Machtou P. Influence of rotational speed, torque and operator's proficiency on Profile failures. International Endodontic Journal 2001;34:47–53.

34. Gambarini G. Rationale for the use of low-torque endodontic motors in root canal instrumentation. Endodontics and Dental Traumatology 2000;16:95–100.

35. Gambarini G. Cyclic fatigue of ProFile rotary instruments after prolonged clinical use. International Endodontic Journal 2001;34:386–389.

36. Haïkel Y, Serfaty R, Bateman G, et al. Dynamic and cyclic fatigue of engine-driven rotary nickel-titanium endodontic instruments. Journal of Endodontics 1999;25: 434–440.

37. Li UM, Lee BS, Shih CT, et al. Cyclic fatigue on endodontic nickel titanium rotary instruments: static and dynamic tests. Journal of Endodontics 2002;28:448–451.

38. Sattapan B, Palamara JE, Messer HH. Torque during canal instrumentation using rotary nickel-titanium files. Journal of Endodontics 2000;26:156–160.

39. Martin B, Zelada G, Varela P, et al. Factors influencing the fracture of nickel-titanium rotary instruments. International Endodontic Journal 2003;36: 262–266.

40. Zelada G, Varela P, Martin B, et al. The effect of rotational speed and the curvature of root canals on the breakage of rotary endodontic instruments. Journal of Endodontics 2002;28:40–542.

41. Alapati SB, Brantley WA, Svec TA, et al. SEM observations of nickel-titanium rotary endodontic instruments that fractured during clinical use. Journal of Endodontics 2005;31:40–43.

42. Svec T, Powers JM. The deterioration of rotary nickel-titanium files under controlled conditions. Journal of Endodontics 2002;28:105–107.

43. Yared G. In vitro study of the torsional properties of new and used ProFile nickel titanium rotary files. Journal of Endodontics 2004;30:410–412.

44. Sattapan B, Nervo GJ, Palamara JE, Messer HH. Defects in rotary nickel-titanium files after clinical use. Journal of Endodontics 2000;26:161–165.

45. Yao JH, Schwartz SA, Beeson TJ. Cyclic fatigue of three types of rotary nickel-titanium files in a dynamic model. Journal of Endodontics 2006;32:55–57.

46. Shen Y, Haapasalo M, Cheung GS, Peng B. Defects in nickel-titanium instruments after clinical use. Part 1: Relationship between observed imperfections and factors leading to such defects in a cohort study. Journal of Endodontics 2009;35:129–132.

47. Shen Y, Cheung GS, Peng B, Haapasalo M. Defects in nickel-titanium instruments after clinical use. Part 2: Fractographic analysis of fractured surface in a cohort study. Journal of Endodontics 2009;35: 133–136.

48. Shen Y, Winestock E, Cheung GS, Haapasalo M. Defects in nickel-titanium instruments after clinical use. Part 4: an electropolished instrument. Journal of Endodontics 2009;35: 197–201.

49. Shen Y, Coil JM, Haapasalo M. Defects in nickel-titanium instruments after clinical use. Part 3: a 4-year retrospective study from an undergraduate clinic. Journal of Endodontics 2009; 35:193–196.

50. Di Fiore PM, Genov KA, Komaroff E, et al. Nickel-titanium rotary instrument fracture: a clinical practice assessment. International Endodontic Journal 2006;39:700–708.

51. Parashos P, Messer HH. Rotary NiTi instrument fracture and its consequences. Journal of Endodontics 2006;32: 1031–1043.

52. Di Fiore PM. A dozen ways to prevent nickel-titanium rotary instrument fracture. Journal of the American Dental Association 2007;138:196–201.

53. Bergmans L, Van Cleynenbreugel J, Wevers M, Lambrechts P. Mechanical root canal preparation with NiTi rotary instruments: rationale, performance and safety. Status report for the American Journal of Dentistry. American Journal of Dentistry 2001;14:324–333.

54. Guelzow A, Stamm O, Martus P, Kielbassa AM. Comparative study of six rotary nickel-titanium systems and hand instrumentation for root canal preparation. International Endodontic Journal 2005;38: 743–752.

55. Schirrmeister JF, Strohl C, Altenburger MJ, et al. Shaping ability and safety of five different rotary nickel-titanium instruments compared with stainless steel hand instrumentation in simulated curved root canals. Oral Surgery Oral Medicine, Oral Pathology, Oral Radiology, Endodontics 2006;101:807–813.

56. Vaudt J, Bitter K, Kielbassa AM. Evaluation of rotary root canal instruments *in vitro*: a review. ENDO (London, England) 2007;1:189–203.

57. Gambarini G, Gerosa R, De Luca M, et al. Mechanical properties of a new and improved nickel-titanium alloy for endodontic use: an evaluation of file flexibility. Oral Surgery, Oral Medicine, Oral Pathology, Oral Radiology, Endodontics 2008; 105:798–800.

58. Gambarini G, Grande NM, Plotino G, et al. Fatigue resistance

of engine-driven rotary nickel-titanium instruments produced by new manufacturing methods. Journal of Endodontics 2008;34: 1003–1005.

59. Larsen CM, Watanabe I, Glickman G. Cyclic fatigue analysis of a new generation of nickel titanium rotary instruments. Journal of Endodontics 2009;35:401–403.

60. Suzuki K. Experimental study on iontophoresis. Japanese Journal of Stomatology 1942;16: 411–417.

61. Sunada I. New method of measuring the length of the root canal. Journal of Dental Research 1962;41:375–387.

62. Kobayashi C. Electronic canal length measurement. Oral Surgery, Oral Medicine, Oral Pathology, Oral Radiology, Endodontics 1995;79:226–231.

63. Nekoofar MH, Ghandi MM, Hayes SJ, Dummer PM. The fundamental operating principles of electronic root canal length measurement devices. International Endodontic Journal 2006;39:595–609.

64. Gordon MPJ, Chandler NP. Electronic apex locators. International Endodontic Journal 2004;37:425–437.

65. Ebrahim AK, Wadachi R, Suda H. Electronic Apex Locators – A Review. Journal of Medical and Dental Sciences 2007;54: 125–136.

66. Chong BS, Pitt Ford TR. Apex locators in endodontics: which, when and how? Dental Update 1994;21:328–330.

67. Jenkins JA, Walker WA, Schindler WG, Flores CM. An in vitro evaluation of the accuracy of the Root ZX in the presence of various irrigants. Journal of Endodontics 2001;27:209–211.

68. Plotino G, Grande NM, Brigante L, et al. Ex vivo accuracy of three electronic apex locators: Root ZX, Elements Diagnostic Unit and Apex Locator and ProPex. International Endodontic Journal 2006;39:408–414.

69. Fouad AF, Reid LC. Effect of using electronic apex locators on selected endodontic treatment parameters. Journal of Endodontics 2000;26: 364–367.

70. Kobayashi C, Yoshioka T, Suda H. A new engine-driven canal preparation system with electronic canal measuring capability. Journal of Endodontics 1997;23:751–754.

71. Ebrahim AK, Wadachi R, Suda H. An in vitro evaluation of the accuracy of Dentaport ZX apex locator in enlarged root canals. Australian Dental Journal 2007;52:193–197.

72. Boutsioukis C, Lambrianidis T, Vasiliadis L. Clinical relevance of standardization of endodontic irrigation needle dimensions according to the ISO 9626:1991 and 9626:1991/Amd 1:2001 specification. International Endodontic Journal 2007;40: 700–706.

73. Ahmad M, Pitt Ford TR, Crum LA. Ultrasonic debridement of root canals: acoustic streaming and its possible role. Journal of Endodontics 1987;13:490–499.

74. van der Sluis LWM, Versluis M, Wu MK, Wesselink PR. Passive ultrasonic irrigation of the root canal: a review of the literature. International Endodontic Journal 2007;40:415–426.

75. Plotino G, Pameijer CH, Grande NM, Somma F. Ultrasonics in endodontics: a review of the literature. Journal of Endodontics 2007;33:81–95.

76. van der Sluis LWM. Ultrasound in endodontics. ENDO (London, England) 2007;1:29–36.

77. Hauser V, Braun A, Frentzen M. Penetration depth of a dye marker into dentine using a novel hydrodynamic system (RinsEndo®). International Endodontic Journal 2007;40: 644–652.

78. McGill S, Gulabivala K, Mordan N, Ng Y-L. The efficacy of dynamic irrigation using a commercially available system (RinsEndo®) determined by removal of a collagen 'bio-molecular film' from an ex vivo model. International Endodontic Journal 2008;41:602–608.

79. Fukumoto Y, Kikuchi I, Yoshioka T, et al. An ex vivo evaluation of a new root canal irrigation technique with intracanal aspiration. International Endodontic Journal 2006;39: 93–99.

80. Nielsen BA, Baumgartner JC. Comparison of the EndoVac system to needle irrigation of root canals. Journal of Endodontics 2007;33:611–615.

81. Chong BS. Managing Endodontic Failure in Practice. London, England: Quintessence Publishing Co. Ltd; 2004.

82. Masserann J. Entfernen metallischer Fragmente aus Wurzelkanälen. Journal of the British Endodontic Society 1979;5:55–59.

83. Williams VD, Bjorndal AM. The Masserann technique for the removal of fractured posts in endodontically treated teeth. Journal of Prosthetic Dentistry 1983;49:46–48.

84. Warren SR, Gutmann JL. Simplified method for removing intraradicular posts. Journal of Prosthetic Dentistry 1979;42: 353–356.

85. Stamos DE, Gutmann JL. Revisiting the Post Puller. Journal of Endodontics 1991;17:466–468.

86. Machtou P, Sarfati P, Cohen AG. Post removal prior to retreatment. Journal of Endodontics 1989; 15:552–554.

87. Berry KA, Loushine RJ, Primack RD, Runyan DA. Nickel-titanium versus stainless-steel finger spreaders in curved canals. Journal of Endodontics 1998;24: 752–754.

88. Schmidt KJ, Walker TL, Johnson JD, Nicoll BK. Comparison of nickel-titanium and stainless-steel spreader penetration and accessory cone fit in curved canals. Journal of Endodontics 2000;26:42–44.

89. Briseno Marroquin B, Wolter D, Willershausen-Zönnchen B. Dimensional variability of nonstandardized greater taper finger spreaders with matching gutta-percha-points. International Endodontic Journal 2001;34: 23–28.

90. Zmener O, Hilu R, Scavo R. Compatibility between standardized endodontic finger spreaders and accessory gutta-percha cones. Endodontics and Dental Traumatology 1996;12: 237–239.

91. Lee FS, Van Cura JE, BeGole E. A comparison of root surface temperatures using different obturation heat sources. Journal of Endodontics 1998;24: 617–620.

92. Silver GK, Love RM, Purton DG. Comparison of two vertical condensation obturation techniques: Touch 'n Heat modified and System B. International Endodontic Journal 1999;32:287–295.

93. McCullagh JJ, Biagioni PA, Lamey PJ, Hussey DL. Thermographic assessment of root canal obturation using thermomechanical compaction. International Endodontic Journal 1997;30:191–195.

94. Zmener O, Gimenes Frias J. Thermomechanical compaction of gutta-percha: a scanning electron microscope study. Endodontics and Dental Traumatology 1991;7:153–157.

95. Tagger M, Tamse A, Katz A, Korzen BH. Evaluation of the apical seal produced by a hybrid root canal filling method, combining lateral condensation and thermatic compaction. Journal of Endodontics 1984;10: 299–303.

96. Yee FS, Marlin J, Krakow AA, Gron P. Three-dimensional obturation of the root canal using injection molded thermoplasticized dental gutta-percha. Journal of Endodontics 1977;3:168–174.

97. Weller RN, Kimborough WF, Anderson RW. A comparison of thermoplastic obturation techniques: adaptation to the canal walls. Journal of Endodontics 1997;23:703–706.

98. Johnson WB. A new gutta-percha technique. Journal of Endodontics 1978;4:184–188.

99. Chu CH, Lo EC, Cheung GS. Outcome of root canal treatment using Thermafil and cold lateral condensation filling techniques. International Endodontic Journal 2005;38:179–185.

100. Royzenblat A, Goodell GG. Comparison of removal times of Thermafil plastic obturators using ProFile rotary instruments at different rotational speeds in moderately curved canals. Journal of Endodontics 2007;33: 256–258.

101. Department of Health. Health Technical Memorandum 01-05: Decontamination in primary care dental practices. London: Department of Health, England; 2008.

102. Burns H, Watkins R. Advice for dentists on re-use of endodontic instruments and variant Creutzfeldt-Jakob Disease (vCJD). Letter from the Chief Dental Officer & Chief Medical Officer, 19 April 2007. Scottish Executive; 2007.

103. Cockcroft B. Advice for dentists on re-use of endodontic instruments and variant Creutzfeldt-Jakob Disease (vCJD). Letter from the Chief Dental Officer England, 19 April 2007. Department of Health, England; 2007.

104. O'Carolan D, McBride M. Advice for dentists on re-use of endodontic instruments and variant Creutzfeldt-Jakob Disease (vCJD). Letter from the Acting Chief Dental Officer & Chief Medical Officer, 18 April 2007. The Department of Health, Social Services and Public Safety, Northern Ireland Executive; 2007.

105. Langmaid P. Advice for dentists on re-use of endodontic instruments and variant Creutzfeldt-Jakob Disease (vCJD). Letter from the Chief Dental Officer Wales, 19 April 2007. Welsh Assembly Government; 2007.

106. Azarpazhooh A, Fillery ED. Prion disease: The implications for dentistry. Journal of Endodontics 2008;34: 1158–1166.

107. Kim S. Principles of endodontic microsurgery. Dental Clinics of North America 1997;41:481–497.

108. Bahcall JK, Barss JT. Fiberoptic endoscope usage for intracanal visualization. Journal of Endodontics 2001;27:128–129.

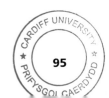

Chapter | 7 |

Preparation of the root canal system

J.S. Rhodes

SUMMARY

A major goal of root canal treatment is the removal of microorganisms from the root canal system. This chapter on preparation of the root canal system will cover gaining access to the root canals, determining working length, preparation techniques including with rotary nickel-titanium instruments, root canal irrigation and controversies associated with cleaning and shaping.

INTRODUCTION

It is widely accepted that microorganisms and their byproducts are the main aetiological factors in the initiation and progression of pulpal inflammation and periapical disease.[1,2,3] The central focus of root canal treatment is, therefore, to eliminate microbes and their substrates from the root canal system.[4] This may involve the removal of necrotic pulp and tissue debris, removal of an inflamed pulp or, in elective treatment, the removal of healthy pulp tissue. Retreatment of failing cases is addressed in Chapter 14.

Historically, a mechanistic approach to root canal treatment was frequently adopted. However, there is now a greater awareness of the microbiota and pattern of colonisation within the complexities of an infected root canal system (Fig. 7.1). This has led to the development of newer techniques, instruments and materials and a biologically-based rationale for root canal treatment:

1. Removal of all tissues, microorganisms, their byproducts and substrates from the root canal system.

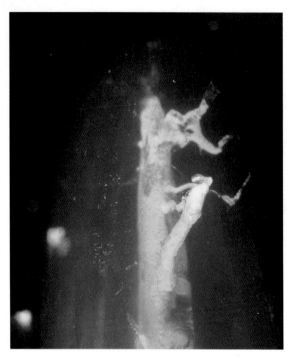

Figure 7.1 A root end which has been made transparent by clearing showing two lateral canals.

2. Shaping of the root canal system to facilitate placement of irrigants, medicaments and a root canal filling.
3. Filling of the shaped canal system coupled with an adequate and timely coronal restoration.

The traditional 'endodontic triad' concept of cleaning, shaping and filling may be modified. Considering that a major goal of root canal treatment is the removal of microorganisms from the complex root canal system 'shaping to facilitate cleaning and filling' might be a more appropriately modified concept. Nevertheless, these three objectives must be achieved while ensuring conservation of tooth structure and maintaining canal shape.

GAINING ACCESS TO THE ROOT CANAL SYSTEM

The main function of an access cavity is to create an unimpeded pathway to the pulp space and the apical foramen of the tooth. Good access cavity design and preparation is imperative for quality treatment results, prevention of iatrogenic problems and avoidance of technical failure of root canal treatment. Conservation of coronal tooth struc-

ture should never preclude the proper design and fulfilment of the requirements of the access opening.[5,6] On the other hand, injudicious tooth removal should be avoided. Pulp space anatomy and access cavities are covered in Chapter 4.

Pretreatment assessment

The dimensions of the pulp chamber and the location of the root canal orifice(s) will be influenced by the amount and position of tertiary 'irritation' dentine that has been deposited during the life of the tooth and in response to 'insults' that the tooth had suffered since eruption. Canal orifices may also become obstructed by pulp stones and/or dystrophic calcifications. Such calcifications and increased amounts of fibrotic tissue in the pulp chamber will make identifying and negotiating the root canals more challenging.

Preparation of the tooth

Caries and failing restorations must be completely removed prior to preparing the access cavity to prevent infected dentine and restorative material being inadvertently introduced into the root canal system, and to prevent microleakage or reinfection. If there is any doubt regarding the restorability of the tooth, the existing restoration should be completely removed[7,8] to confirm that there is sufficient tooth substance remaining. Removal of existing restorations and crowns may reveal caries, additional canals or hairline cracks on one or more axial walls, which may influence the prognosis and/or the design of the postendodontic restoration (Fig. 7.2).

Unsupported cusps should be removed or protected by, for example, placing an orthodontic band around the tooth to prevent cusp fracture during and after treatment. In some cases, following dismantling of the coronal restoration it may be necessary to place a provisional restoration to prevent microleakage, aid rubber dam isolation and create a reservoir for the irrigant solution in the access cavity.

Rubber dam

Isolation of the tooth with rubber dam is a necessary prerequisite for endodontic treatment. This topic is covered in Chapter 6. In addition, excellent reviews on the application of rubber dam have also been published.[8,9,10]

Removal of the pulp chamber roof and coronal pulp tissue

The number of canals and their approximate positions can be predicted from a sound knowledge of dentinogenesis

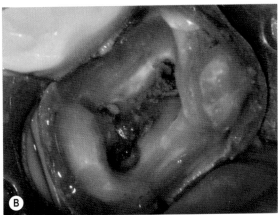

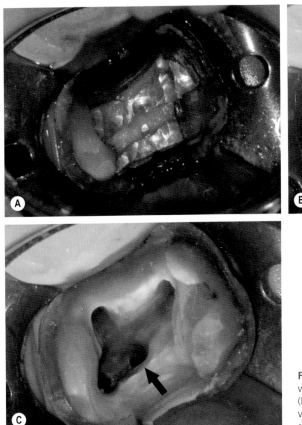

Figure 7.2 Retreatment case. (A) The cast restoration was removed to reveal caries around the core material. (B) Following caries removal the root filling material is visible. (C) Exploration of the pulp floor revealed the second mesiobuccal canal (arrowed).

and the nature of root formation. The pulp chamber and root canal space are always located in the cross-sectional centre of the crown and root respectively.[5] The location of canal orifices is best achieved with good illumination and carefully drying the pulp floor. Magnification with either loupes or an operating microscope is beneficial and the latter is better for detecting canal orifices.[11]

The design of the access cavity should reflect the anticipated position of the underlying root canal orifices. The relationship between the pulp chamber and the external anatomical outline is assessed from preoperative radiographs. Careful alignment of the bur will reduce the possibility of perforation either vertically, through the floor of the chamber into the furcation, or laterally (Fig. 7.3). Occasionally, where an extracoronal restoration is severely tilted relative to the root, or in cases with sclerosed root canal systems, initial access may best be made prior to rubber dam placement to permit more accurate orientation of instruments. When using instruments such as long-shank round burs or tungsten-carbide LN burs (Dentsply

Maillefer, Ballaigues, Switzerland), frequent re-evaluation of the alignment visually and/or radiographically will help reduce the risk of procedural errors. The direction of the search can then be adjusted if necessary (Fig 7.4).

The roof of the pulp chamber should be penetrated at a point where the roof and floor of the pulp chamber is the widest, this commonly occurs at the point where the pulp horn relating to the largest canal is situated, for example, the palatal root in maxillary molars. Tungsten carbide burs are ideal for cutting through metal. However, a diamond bur should be used to map out the access in porcelain fused to metal crowns, before using a tungsten carbide bur, to reduce the likelihood of porcelain fracture. For this reason, it is wise to warn the patient beforehand that a restoration may be irreversibly damaged and may need replacing following root canal treatment. Once the roof of the pulp chamber has been breached, the bur will suddenly drop into the pulp chamber space. To prevent damage to the floor of the pulp chamber a non-end-cutting bur is then used to remove the entire roof of the pulp chamber. The walls of the access cavity should be

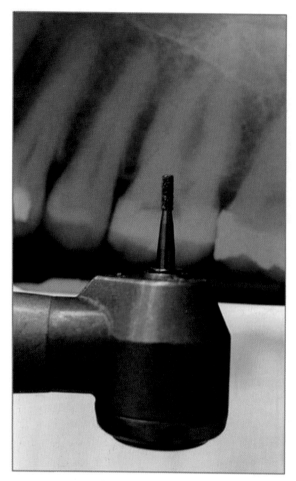

Figure 7.3 Alignment of the bur on the preoperative radiograph will help indicate the position and depth of the restoration and pulp chamber.

probed to ensure that the roof of the pulp chamber has been completely removed, i.e. no dentine ledges/lips are present (Fig 7.5).

Careful inspection of the pulp chamber floor will reveal subtle changes in the colour of the dentine, which aids identification of the canal orifices. Dark developmental lines may be visible linking canal orifices, which will appear as a small area of opaque dentine against a background of yellow/grey secondary dentine. A canal orifice will feel sticky when probed with a DG16 endodontic explorer or Micro-Opener (Dentsply Maillefer). In extensively calcified canals, transillumination or the use of dyes may provide some guidance for canal orifice identification.

The pulp chamber is irrigated with sodium hypochlorite during access cavity preparation to dissolve tissue and aid debridement. This will also reduce the inadvertent inoculation of microorganisms from the pulp chamber into the root canal system. Ultrasonically energized tips (Fig. 7.6) are useful for breaking up calcific masses and aid removal of gross debris.

Creating straight-line access

Once the canal orifice(s) have been identified it may be necessary to refine or modify the outline of the access cavity to allow endodontic files unimpeded, straight-line access into the coronal third of the root canal system. Straight-line access will reduce the likelihood of iatrogenic problems such as zips, elbows and ledges being created by large, and therefore, less flexible files as they attempt to straighten, particularly, in curved canals. Straight-line access will also allow unimpeded penetration of files for root canal preparation.

Although nickel-titanium (NiTi) rotary files are very flexible, poor straight-line access can still result in instrument separation.

A well-designed access cavity permits:

- complete debridement of the pulp chamber
- visualization of the pulp floor
- unimpeded placement of instruments into the root canals
- conservation of tooth tissue.

WORKING LENGTH DETERMINATION

Regardless of treatment philosophy on the desired final end point of preparation, it is always necessary to ascertain the length of the root canal accurately.[2,12,13,14] The most widely accepted method of establishing working length has been with radiography. In this method,[15] the working length is initially estimated by taking a measurement from an undistorted, preoperative radiograph. A file, preferably ISO size 15 or larger, so that it is easily discernible radiologically, is inserted into the canal to the estimated working length and a working length radiograph exposed. If the tip of the file is within 1 mm of the ideal location, then the radiograph can be accepted as an accurate representation of the tooth length. If adjustments of 2 mm or more are needed, the working length should be reconfirmed with an additional working length radiograph.[16] This method usually provides acceptable results but radiographs are, frequently difficult to interpret especially with posterior teeth. More importantly, the apical foramen may be distant from the radiographic apex further confusing interpretation. In such circumstances, additional methods of working length determination should be utilized.

Modern electronic apex locators measure the impedance of the root canal at different frequencies and have been reported to be accurate to within 0.5 mm in >90% of cases.[17,18,19] Consequently, an apex locator can be more reliable than a radiograph for determining working

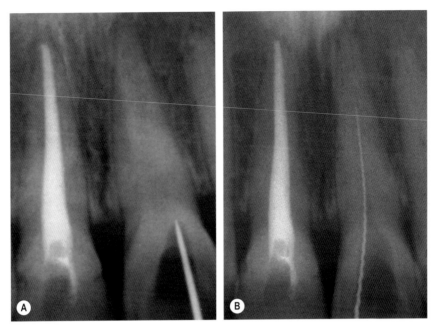

Figure 7.4 In a tooth with an extensively calcified canal (A) a check radiograph with a probe in the base of the cavity will provide guidance for instrument progression. (B) A later radiograph confirms that the file is in the root canal.

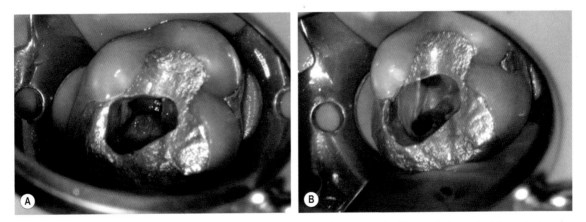

Figure 7.5 Inadequate access: (A) the pulp horns have been mistaken for the canal orifices and the roof of the pulp chamber is still in situ; (B) removal of the roof of the pulp chamber allows good visualization of the pulp floor.

length.[20] The use of an apex locator allows for a reduction in the number of radiographs required during root canal treatment. In a long-term retrospective study in which an apex locator was used solely to determine working length in infected root canals with periapical lesions, a high success rate was achieved[21] confirming its benefit. Not just one method but the combination of the radiographic method and the use of electronic apex locators will enhance the accuracy of working length determination.

ROOT CANAL IRRIGATION

Root canal treatment involves a chemomechanical approach; microorganisms are removed mechanically during canal preparation and eradicated chemically using irrigants. Microorganisms are present in the lumen of the root canal in a planktonic form and as a biofilm adhering to the canal walls. Regardless of the instrumentation tech-

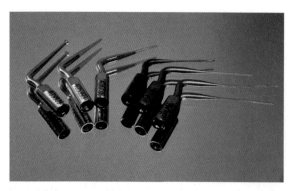

Figure 7.6 A selection of ultrasonic tips that can be used to break up calcific masses in the canal orifice.

nique or system chosen, the use of irrigants is essential for thorough debridement of the root canal system.[22]

The actions of an irrigant include:

- rinsing of debris
- lubrication of the canal system which facilitates instrumentation
- dissolution of remaining organic matter
- antibacterial properties
- softening and removing the smear layer
- penetrating into areas inaccessible to instruments, thereby extending the cleaning process.

Ideally, the irrigant should be non-toxic and have a low surface tension, in addition to being stable, inexpensive and easy to use. A plethora of irrigants have been used. Currently, the most widely used irrigant is sodium hypochlorite. It is highly effective at killing bacteria and breaking down organic material; various concentrations of sodium hypochlorite, varying from 0.5% to 5.25%, have been recommended.[23] The effectiveness of sodium hypochlorite has been shown to depend on the concentration and time of exposure. Higher concentrations of sodium hypochlorite have greater tissue-dissolving properties[24] but the higher the concentration, the more severe the potential reaction if it is inadvertently forced into the tissues. Accidental extrusion of sodium hypochlorite into the periapical tissues may result in tissue damage accompanied by varying degrees of pain, swelling and bruising. This topic is discussed in Chapter 14.

The use of calcium hydroxide as an intracanal medicament between visits has been shown to enhance disinfection following the use of sodium hypochlorite. Other irrigants used in root canal chemomechanical preparation include chlorhexidine,[25] iodine potassium iodide[26] and electrolytically-activated water.[27] Irrigants such as chlorhexidine and iodine potassium iodide have antibacterial properties but no tissue-dissolving properties. Apart from the rinsing effect, local anaesthetic solution or saline have none of the desired properties of a root canal irrigant and their use is not recommended. Photoactivated disinfec-

tion, involving a dye and a diode light, and lasers have also been advocated for disinfection of the root canal system[28] but its superiority over sodium hypochlorite is yet to be proven.

During root canal preparation a layer of 'sludge' is formed by the action of the instruments against the canal walls. This material is deposited on the canal wall and is called the 'smear layer'. It has both organic and inorganic components and exists as a superficial, loosely bound layer and a deeper adherent layer.[29] Considerable debate has taken place as to whether or not the smear layer should be removed. Complete removal of the smear layer may open up dentinal tubules to the passage of microorganisms from the root canal into the dentine. On the other hand, failure to remove the smear layer will, possibly allow bacteria to remain in the canal system and impair the adaptation of the root filling to the dentine wall and tubules.[30,31] A very close adaptation of thermoplasticized gutta-percha to the dentine wall has been shown following smear layer removal.[32,33] Removal of the smear layer is best achieved by irrigating the root canal system with sodium hypochlorite throughout the preparation procedure to flush out and prevent accumulation of debris on the canal walls. A final rinse with 17.5% ethylenediaminetetraacetic acid (EDTA), a chelating agent, is recommended for removal of the inorganic component.[34] The effects of chelating agents such as EDTA are self-limiting.

The irrigant is commonly delivered using specially designed endodontic needles and syringes. The needle is inserted into the canal to the level of the apical third. However, during initial canal preparation, the needle may not reach this depth so it should be inserted to the binding point, pulled out slightly so that it is loose in the canal and then the irrigant delivered gently and passively. As canal preparation proceeds, the needle will gradually reach deeper into the canal but at all times, the needle must not be jammed into the canal and the irrigant delivered with unnecessary force. Irrigants may also be delivered using ultrasonic devices. The effectiveness of ultrasonic irrigation is due to the creation of acoustic microstreaming and allows more effective delivery of irrigant to the apical part of the root canal system.[35,36] A passively vibrating ultrasonic instrument is more effective than one that is being dampened by the canal wall.[37,38] For this reason, modern tips designed for this purpose are fine in size (ISO size 15) or even smooth, without cutting flutes. There is limited evidence to specify the ideal length of time that passive ultrasonic irrigation should be activated within the canal.

INSTRUMENTATION TECHNIQUES

All root canal systems are curved in one or more planes with the degree and extent of curvature varying from root to root. Irrespective of the instrumentation technique used, the apical part of the root canal system is usually the least well-cleaned and prepared. The morphology of the apical root canal system is complex and highly variable. This has been clearly demonstrated from clearing techniques and micro-computed tomography.[39]

Preparation of the root canal system requires considerable skill, particularly in cases with more severely curved canals or other complex anatomical features. Despite advances in instrument design, the experience and tactile skills of the operator remains important.[40] There is no replacement for practical instructions on root canal preparation in order to acquire the necessary skills and competency. Regardless of the instrumentation technique or type of instrument used, the goals of shaping and cleaning of the root canal systems are:

- thorough debridement of the root canal system
- development of a continuously tapering preparation
- avoidance of procedural errors.

Maintaining the anatomy of the apical constriction (Fig. 7.7) during canal shaping is essential for predictable healing of the periapical tissues. Long-term studies have shown improved success rates when instrumentation and filling procedures are maintained within the canal system, at approximately the level of the cemento-dentinal junction.[41]

Historical methods of canal preparation that encompassed a mechanistic approach have largely been superseded. Canal preparation techniques can be broadly divided into those that adopt an 'apical-to-coronal' approach or those that adopt a 'coronal-to-apical' approach. Most endodontists would now advocate using a crown-down (coronal-to-apical) approach to preparation with hand files manipulated in a balanced-force action or nickel titanium rotary instruments in a handpiece. Numerous protocols have detailed the crown-down approach, these include: the Crown-down pressureless technique,[42] the Roane or Balanced-force technique,[43] the 'Double-flare' technique,[44] and the Modified double-flare technique.[45] In the Balanced-force technique, hand files of a triangular cross-section are rotated a quarter-turn clockwise to engage dentine of the root canal wall. Whilst applying apical pressure, this is followed by a half turn of the file in the counter-clockwise direction, which effectively 'cuts' the dentine that was engaged. The process can be repeated for two or three times before removing the instrument to clean the flutes and irrigate the canal. Unlike many other techniques, files are not pre-curved when used in this manner.

Crown-down rationale

There are several advantages with the crown-down approach:

- elimination of debris and microorganisms from the more coronal parts of the root canal system thereby

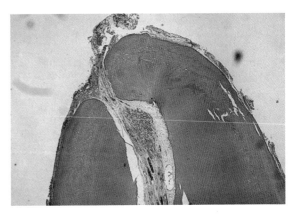

Figure 7.7 The anatomy of the apical constriction must be maintained during canal preparation.

preventing inoculation of periapical tissues with contaminated debris
- elimination of coronally-placed interferences that might adversely influence instrumentation
- early movement of large volumes of irrigant and lubricant to the apical part of the canal
- facilitating accurate working length determination as coronal curvature is eliminated early in the preparation.

The essentials of the coronal-to-apical approach to root canal cleaning and shaping are as follows:

- development of straight-line access from the occlusal or lingual surface into the pulp chamber
- removal of all overhanging ledges from the pulp chamber roof
- removal of lingual ledges or cervical bulges formed due to the deposition of dentine in the cervical part of the tooth
- development of divergent walls in the pulp chamber from the cavosurface margin to the chamber floor
- cutting of a funnel-shaped preparation, with its narrowest part located in the tooth apically.

The clinical benefits of the crown-down technique are:

- ease of removal of pulp stones
- enhanced tactile feedback with instruments by removal of coronal interferences
- enhanced apical movement of instruments into the canal
- enhanced working length determination due to minimal tooth contact in the coronal third
- increased space for irrigant penetration and debridement
- rapid removal of pulp tissue located in the coronal third
- straight-line access to root curves and canal junctions
- enhanced movement of debris coronally

- decreased deviation of instruments in canal curvatures by reducing root wall contact
- decreased canal blockages
- minimize instrument separation by reducing contact with canal walls
- improved quality of canal shaping
- improved quality of canal cleaning
- faster preparation, which may allow one-visit root canal treatment.

The biological benefits of the crown-down technique are:

- more rapid removal of contaminated, infected tissue from the root canal system
- removal of tissue debris coronally, thereby minimizing pushing debris apically
- reduction in postoperative pain that may occur with apical extrusion of debris
- better dissolution of tissue with increased irrigant penetration
- easier smear layer removal because of better contact with chelating agents
- enhanced disinfection of canal irregularities due to irrigant penetration.

Nickel-titanium instruments

Following the introduction of nickel-titanium (NiTi) alloy to endodontic instrument design,[46] many new NiTi hand and rotary instruments have become available. The clinical and mechanical properties of these NiTi instruments have been compared with those of stainless steel instruments; these include the efficacy of canal preparation, cleanliness of the canals after preparation, the shaping ability of the instruments and fracture properties of the instruments.[32,47–56] There is a general acceptance that rotary NiTi instruments produce well-shaped canals in an efficient manner with the creation of relatively fewer iatrogenic problems than stainless steel files. However, direct comparison between stainless steel and NiTi instruments is difficult unless the instrument design is identical.[57]

In addition, most testing procedures were carried out in vitro, frequently in plastic blocks with simulated canals, and long-term clinical evidence of the superiority of one instrument type is unproven. Since NiTi is more flexible than stainless steel, instruments can be manufactured with greater tapers whilst retaining flexibility. A canal of pre-determined, desired taper can be created using the corresponding tapered instrument instead of relying on a series of standardized lesser tapered files. This also decreases the risk of iatrogenic problems during preparation as generally fewer instruments are required to prepare the canal.

Benefits of NiTi instrumentation

1. Files are superflexible and able to work round significant curvatures.

2. NiTi flexibility enables manufacturers to produce files with tapers greater than standard stainless steel hand files. Therefore, fewer instruments are generally required.
3. NiTi instruments will efficiently taper a preformed pilot channel, avoiding the need for stepping back.
4. The instruments tend not to deviate from the centre-point of the canal, and transportation of the canal is uncommon.

Disadvantages of NiTi instrumentation

1. Instrument fracture can still be unpredictable.
2. The instruments are flexible but are liable to fracture when worked around curvatures with a small radius. This risk increases with increasing file diameter.
3. Overuse will still result in zipping and transportation of the canal despite superflexibility.
4. NiTi instruments tend to be more expensive.

Crown-down technique

The basic steps common to all 'crown-to-apical' techniques involve early coronal and mid-root flaring and enlargement before proceeding to the apical part of the canal. Early coronal flaring significantly reduces the change in working length during canal preparation.[58] As an instrument initially moves into the coronal third of the canal and as the pathway is enlarged, this facilitates further movement of small instruments and allows passage of irrigants deeper into the root canal. This entire process is continued until the working length can be determined easily. Instrument placement into the middle and apical parts of the canal system is unimpeded. Irrigants and lubricants will penetrate more easily and will facilitate passage of instruments in an apical direction.

When using NiTi instruments, larger instruments will make space for smaller instruments. This may involve using an instrument with a greater taper before one with a smaller taper, or a series of instruments in decreasing tip sizes. Some systems have been designed with variable tapers and as long as the instruments are used in sequence, dentine will be selectively removed in a coronal-to-apical direction.

As a general rule, most systems consist of a series of shorter, more tapered instruments that are used for coronal flaring followed by another series of longer, more flexible instruments meant to be used more apically. The final taper of the preparation is usually decided by the operator depending on the dimensions and the degree of curvature of the original canal. Using micro-computed tomography it has been possible to see the changes to the internal anatomy of the root canal as a sequence of instruments is used during preparation and it is interesting to see that the files rarely contact the entire wall of the root canal and actually remove relatively little dentine, especially in the

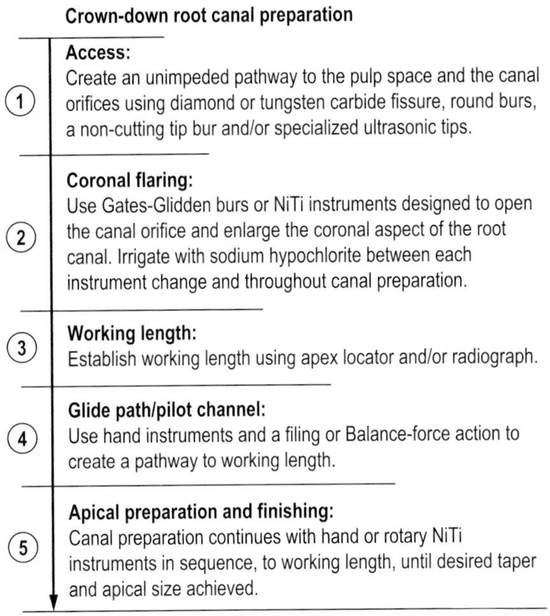

Crown-down root canal preparation

(1) **Access:**
Create an unimpeded pathway to the pulp space and the canal orifices using diamond or tungsten carbide fissure, round burs, a non-cutting tip bur and/or specialized ultrasonic tips.

(2) **Coronal flaring:**
Use Gates-Glidden burs or NiTi instruments designed to open the canal orifice and enlarge the coronal aspect of the root canal. Irrigate with sodium hypochlorite between each instrument change and throughout canal preparation.

(3) **Working length:**
Establish working length using apex locator and/or radiograph.

(4) **Glide path/pilot channel:**
Use hand instruments and a filing or Balance-force action to create a pathway to working length.

(5) **Apical preparation and finishing:**
Canal preparation continues with hand or rotary NiTi instruments in sequence, to working length, until desired taper and apical size achieved.

Figure 7.8 A composite protocol for use with a 'coronal-to-apical' root canal preparation concept.

apical region.[39,59] An example of a composite protocol for use with a 'coronal-to-apical' preparation concept is shown in Figure 7.8.

Calcified canals

The same basic principles apply to preparation of calcified canals. However, the operator should proceed with caution, irrigate frequently to keep dentine chips in suspension, flush them away and check for patency with a small file between instruments. Ultrasound can be used to loosen debris in the sclerosed canal orifice. The tip of the ultrasonic instrument can be used either to activate the solution in the chamber or it can be placed into the calcified orifice in an attempt to provide some initial patency. A small K-file, or a specific file designed for canal penetration (e.g. Pathfinder, SybronEndo or C-file, Dentsply Maillefer), can be used to begin canal penetration. At this point, a small NiTi rotary instrument designed for coronal flaring can be used to taper the orifice and remove any constriction. The clinician can return to a small ultrasonic tip to penetrate further into the canal. Gates-Glidden burs will not be beneficial as they have a non-cutting tip. This procedure will take time and patience, and the temptation to try to drill a canal into the root should be resisted as this invariably leads to deviation and potential root perforation.

CONTROVERSIES IN ROOT CANAL CLEANING AND SHAPING

A number of issues remain unresolved concerning endodontic treatment procedures.

Where should the preparation end?

This question was addressed succinctly in a short paper entitled 'Where shall the root filling end?'.[13] Current treatment protocols used by many clinicians are frequently based on opinion rather than fact, for example, there is little or no evidence to support the belief that the presence of sealer 'puffs' on a postoperative radiograph indicates better quality of treatment. In fact, there is considerable evidence for maintaining all instrumentation procedures and filling material within the root canal system.[4,60,61,62,63,64] There should be differentiation between vital teeth, those with infected canals, and retreatment cases, when deciding where to terminate the instrumentation and filling.[41] Based on biological principles and experimental evidence, instrumentation should terminate 2–3 mm from the radiographic apex in vital cases. In cases where canals are infected, the position should be 0–2 mm from the apex, while in retreatment cases the ideal termination should be at the apical foramen. However, irrespective of the preoperative condition of the canal system, it is recommended that all instrumentation and filling procedures should not extend beyond the apical foramen.

Discussion on the ideal termination of the preparation and filling procedures presupposes the existence of the 'ideal' root apex as described by Kuttler.[14] However, it has been found that this ideal apical terminus exists in less than half of teeth.[65] Instead, a number of apical anatomical configurations have been described (Fig. 7.9). No apical constriction may be present especially in the presence of any resorptive process.[66] Consequently, it is often very difficult or even impossible to locate either the apical constriction or the apical foramen.

When should the preparation end?

Removal of all microorganisms, tissue and debris is the aim of root canal treatment and hence this can be taken to be the end point of preparation. However, determining when this has been achieved remains difficult clinically.[22] Historically, instrumentation procedures have taken little account of canal anatomy, such as fins, webs, anastomoses or apical ramifications. Outdated standardized preparation techniques in which the presence of white dentine chips was used as a sign of canal cleanliness have been shown to be unreliable.[67]

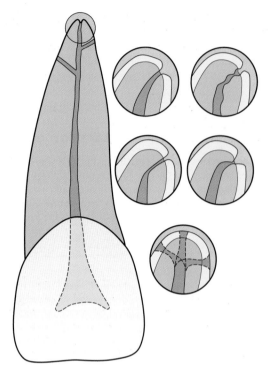

Figure 7.9 Five major apical morphological forms.

Due to the complexities of canal anatomy, the emphasis has shifted to chemomechanical preparation of the root canal system.[22,68,69] Removal of the smear layer also improves disinfection.[22] The importance of an intracanal dressing such as calcium hydroxide has been demonstrated as canals can be more reliably rendered bacteria-free.[69] An unanswered question is how long, ideally, should the irrigant be left in the canal system to achieve 'adequate' disinfection of the canal? This concern has fuelled a further controversy; namely can root canal treatment be completed in one visit or should it be carried out in multiple visits?

What about the apical size of preparation?

There is controversy concerning the ideal diameter of the apical preparation. Some authorities consider that dentine should be removed apically to eliminate contamination whilst others consider that a narrow preparation, combined with a suitable flare to allow irrigant penetration is satisfactory.[70,71,72]

Increasing the apical size of the preparation to allow better debridement, irrigant penetration and making a defined stop were discussed as the 'apical clearing' concept.[73] This involved sequentially rotating files, two to four sizes larger than the initial apical file at working length, then rotating the largest apical file again after final irrigation and drying. Apical clearing is recommended in canals which have been prepared with an apical stop. However, apical clearing in teeth without an apical stop would increase the chances of overpreparation and overfilling.

Preparation should be carried out to produce sufficient space for irrigants to be effective. This was achieved, historically, by using files with a greater tip size. However, modern NiTi instruments provide space by creating larger tapers for a minimal apical size.

Should apical patency filing be performed?

'Apical patency' is described as the placement of small files to and through the apical constriction during preparation.[36,73] The aim is to allow for creation of a preparation and filling extending fully to the periodontal ligament. Evidence to support this concept is unavailable. It is, however, important to make sure that the canal does not become blocked apically with infected dentine chips during preparation and, therefore, there is merit in recapitulating with a small instrument to keep the canal patent. Inoculating infected material beyond the apical constriction could result in postoperative discomfort or flare-ups.

Should treatment be completed in one or multiple visits?

One-visit root canal treatment has assumed a position of controversy for many reasons. Clinical studies have addressed the advantages and disadvantages.

The advantages of one-visit treatment are:

- reduced number of appointments
- no risk of intra-appointment microbial recontamination
- use of canal space for immediate post-retention restorations.

The disadvantages are:

- longer appointments may cause patient fatigue
- inability to control exudates may prevent completion of the procedure.

Whether completed in one or multiple visits, studies concerning postoperative pain[74–82] as well as effective healing rates[82,83,84] have shown that outcomes are similar. However, many of these studies have used older preparation techniques, which have the potential for less effective canal cleaning. There are some indications and contraindications that should be considered when contemplating one-visit treatment.

The indications include:

- uncomplicated teeth with vital pulps
- fractured teeth where aesthetics is important and extensive restoration is indicated immediately
- patient unable to return for additional appointments
- patient requires antibiotic prophylaxis or sedation.

Contraindications include:

- patients with acute apical periodontitis
- teeth with severe anatomical anomalies
- molars with necrotic pulps and periapical radiolucencies
- root canal retreatment.[62]

One-visit treatment does not sit easily with evidence on effective and predictable canal disinfection in infected cases[22,68] so cases should be selected carefully.

LEARNING OUTCOMES

Following completion of this chapter, the reader should be able to:

- appreciate the steps to undertake when gaining access to the root canals
- explain the methods of determining working length
- understand the role of root canal irrigants
- explain the concepts of root canal preparation including the crown-down approach and use of NiTi rotary instruments
- tackle calcified canals
- discuss controversies associated with root canal preparation.

REFERENCES

1. Bergenholtz G. Pathogenic mechanisms in pulpal disease. Journal of Endodontics 1990;16: 98–101.

2. Blaney JR. The biologic aspect of root canal therapy. Dental Items of Interest 1927;49:681–708.

3. Kakehashi S, Stanley HR, Fitzgerald RJ. The effects of surgical exposures of dental pulps in germ-free and conventional laboratory rats. Oral Surgery, Oral Medicine, Oral Pathology 1965;20:340–349.

4. Ng YR, Mann V, Rahbaran S, et al. Outcome of primary root canal treatment: systematic review of the literature. International Endodontic Journal 2008;41:6–31.

5. Gutmann JL, Dumsha TC, Lovdahl PE, Hovland EJ. Problem Solving in Endodontics. Prevention, Identification and Management. 3rd edn. St Louis, MO, USA: Mosby-Year Book; 1997. p. 47.

6. Patel S, Rhodes JS. A practical guide to endodontic access cavity preparation in molar teeth. British Dental Journal 2007;203:133–140.

7. Abou-Rass M. Evaluation and clinical management of previous endodontic therapy. Journal of Prosthetic Dentistry 1982;47: 528–534.

8. Reuter JE. The isolation of teeth and the protection of the patient during endodontic treatment. International Endodontic Journal 1983;16;173–181.

9. Bhuva B, Chong BS, Patel S. Rubber dam in clinical practice ENDO (London, England) 2008;2:131–141.

10. Marshall K. Rubber dam. British Dental Journal 1990;184:218–219.

11. Yoshioka T, Kobayashi C, Suda H. Detection rate of root canal orifices with a microscope. Journal of Endodontics 2002;28:452–453.

12. Bramante CM, Berbert A. A critical evaluation of some methods of determining tooth length. Oral Surgery, Oral Medicine, Oral Pathology 1974;37:463–473.

13. Hasselgren G. Where shall the root filling end? New York State Dental Journal 1994;60:34–35.

14. Kuttler Y. Microscopic investigation of root apexes. Journal of the American Dental Association 1955;50:544–552.

15. Ingle JI. Endodontic instruments and instrumentation. Dental Clinics of North America 1957;1:805–822.

16. Cox VS, Brown CE, Bricker SL, Newton CW. Radiographic interpretation of endodontic file length. Oral Surgery, Oral Medicine, Oral Pathology 1991;72:340–344.

17. Czerw RJ, Fulkerson MS, Donnelly JC, Walmann JO. In vitro evaluation of the accuracy of several electronic apex locators. Journal of Endodontics 1995;21: 572–575.

18. Gordon MP, Chandler NP. Electronic Apex Locators. International Endodontic Journal 2004;37:425–437.

19. Shabahang S, Goon WW, Gluskin AH. An in vivo evaluation of Root ZX electronic apex locator. Journal of Endodontics 1996;22:616–618.

20. Pratten DH, McDonald NJ. Comparison of radiographic and electronic working lengths. Journal of Endodontics 1996;22:173–176.

21. Murakami M, Inoue S, Inoue N. Clinical evaluation of audiometric control root canal treatment: a retrospective study. Quintessence International 2002;33:465–474.

22. Byström A, Sundqvist G. The antibacterial action of sodium hypochlorite and EDTA in 60 cases of endodontic therapy. International Endodontic Journal 1985;18:35–40.

23. Moorer WR, Wesselink PR. Factors promoting the tissue dissolving capability of sodium hypochlorite. International Endodontic Journal 1982;15:187–196.

24. Hand RE, Smith ML, Harrison JW. Analysis of the effect of dilution on the necrotic tissue dissolution property of sodium hypochlorite.

Journal of Endodontics 1978;4: 60–64.

25. Leonardo MR, Tanomaru Filho M, Silva LA, et al. In vivo antimicrobial activity of 2% chlorhexidine used as a root canal irrigating solution. Journal of Endodontics 1999;25:167–171.

26. Safavi KE, Spangberg LS, Langeland K. Root canal dentinal tubule disinfection. Journal of Endodontics 1990;16:207–210.

27. Marais JT, Williams WP. Antimicrobial effectiveness of electro-chemically activated water as an endodontic irrigation solution. International Endodontic Journal 2001;34:237–243.

28. Koba K, Kimura Y, Matsumoto K, et al. Post-operative symptoms and healing after endodontic treatment of infected teeth using pulsed Nd:YAG laser. Endodontics and Dental Traumatology. 1999;15: 68–72.

29. McComb D, Smith DC. A preliminary scanning electron microscopic study of root canals after endodontic procedures. Journal of Endodontics 1975;1:238–242.

30. Gutmann JL. Adaptation of injected thermoplasticized gutta-percha in the absence of the dentinal smear layer. International Endodontic Journal 1993;26: 87–92.

31. Karagöz-Kücükay I, Bayirli G. An apical leakage study in the presence and absence of the smear layer. International Endodontic Journal 1994;27:87–93.

32. Shuping GB, Ørstavik D, Sigurdsson A, Trope M. Reduction of intracanal bacteria using nickel-titanium rotary instrumentation and various medications. Journal of Endodontics 2000;26:751–755.

33. von Fraunhofer JA, Fagundes DK, McDonald NJ, Dumsha TC. The effect of root canal preparation on microleakage within endodontically treated teeth: an in vitro study. International Endodontic Journal 2000;33: 355–360.

34. Behrend GD, Cutler CW, Gutmann JL. An in-vitro study of smear layer removal and microbial leakage along root-canal fillings. International Endodontic Journal 1996;29:99–107.

35. Ahmad M. Effect of ultrasonic instrumentation on Bacteroides intermedius. Endodontics and Dental Traumatology 1989;5:83–86.

36. Ahmad M, Pitt Ford TR, Crum LA. Ultrasonic debridement of root canals: an insight into the mechanisms involved. Journal of Endodontics 1987;13:93–101.

37. Carver K, Nusstein J, Reader A, Beck M. In vivo antibacterial efficacy of ultrasound after hand and rotary instrumentation in human mandibular molars. Journal of Endodontics 2007;33: 1038–1043.

38. van de Sluis LW, Versluis M, Wu MK, Wesselink PR. Passive ultrasonic irrigation of the root canal a review of the literature. International Endodontic Journal 2007;40:415–426.

39. Peters OA, Schonenberger K, Laib A. Effects of four Ni-Ti preparation techniques on root canal geometry assessed by micro computed tomography. International Endodontic Journal 2001;34:221–230.

40. Gulabivala K, Abdo S, Sherriff M, Regan JD. The influence of interfacial forces and duration of filing on root canal shaping. Endodontics and Dental Traumatology 2000;16: 166–174.

41. Wu MK, Wesselink PR, Walton RE. Apical terminus location of root canal treatment procedures. Oral Surgery, Oral Medicine, Oral Pathology, Oral Radiology and Endodontics 2000;89:99–103.

42. Marshall FJ, Pappin J. A crown-down pressureless preparation root canal enlargement technique. Portland, USA: Technique manual, University of Oregon Health Sciences University; 1988.

43. Roane J, Sabala CL, Duncanson MG. The 'balanced force' concept for instrumentation of curved canals. Journal of Endodontics 1985;11:203–211.

44. Fava LR. The double-flared technique: an alternative for biomechanical preparation. Journal of Endodontics 1983;9:76–80.

45. Saunders WP, Saunders EM. Effect of noncutting tipped instruments on the quality of root canal preparation using a modified double-flared technique. Journal of Endodontics 1992;18:32–36.

46. Walia HM, Brantley WA, Gerstein H. An initial investigation of the bending and torsional properties of Nitinol root canal files. Journal of Endodontics 1988;14:346–351.

47. Ahlquist M, Henningsson O, Hultenby K, Ohlin J. The effectiveness of manual and rotary techniques in the cleaning of root canals: a scanning electron microscopy study. International Endodontic Journal 2001;34: 533–537.

48. Bishop K, Dummer PM. A comparison of stainless steel Flexofiles and nickel-titanium NiTiFlex files during the shaping of simulated canals. International Endodontic Journal 1997;30: 25–34.

49. Fabra-Campos H. Rodriguez-Vallejo J. Digitization, analysis and processing of dental images during root canal preparation with Quantec Series 2000 instruments. International Endodontic Journal 2001;34:29–39.

50. Gambarini G. Rationale for the use of low-torque endodontic motors in root canal instrumentation. Endodontics and Dental Traumatology 2000;16: 95–100.

51. Jardine SJ, Gulabivala K. An in vitro comparison of canal preparation using two automated rotary nickel-titanium instrumentation techniques. International Endodontic Journal 2000;33:381–391.

52. Kavanagh D, Lumley PJ. An in-vitro evaluation of canal preparation using Profile .04 and .06 taper instruments. Endodontics and Dental Traumatology 1998;14:16–20.

53. Pruett JP, Clement DJ, Carnes DL. Cyclic fatigue testing of nickel-titanium endodontic instruments. Journal of Endodontics 1997;23:77–85.

54. Short JA, Morgan LA, Baumgartner JC. A comparison of canal centering ability of four instrumentation techniques. Journal of Endodontics 1997;23: 503–507.

55. Tepel J, Schafer E, Hoppe W. Properties of endodontic hand instruments used in rotary motion. Part 1. Cutting efficiency. Journal of Endodontics 1995;21:418–421.

56. Tepel J, Schafer E, Hoppe W. Properties of endodontic hand instruments used in rotary motion. Part 3. Resistance to bending and fracture. Journal of Endodontics 1997;23:141–145.

57. Kazemi RB, Stenman E, Spangberg L. A comparison of stainless steel and nickel-titanium H-type instruments of identical design: torsional and bending tests. Oral Surgery, Oral Medicine, Oral Pathology, Oral Radiology and Endodontics 2000;90:500–506.

58. Davis RD, Marshall JG, Baumgartner JC. Effect of early coronal flaring on working length change in curved canals using rotary nickel-titanium versus stainless steel instruments. Journal of Endodontics 2002;28:438–442.

59. Paque F, Barbakow F, Peters OA. Root canal preparation with Endo-Eze AET: changes in root canal shape assessed by micro-computed tomography. International Endodontic Journal 2005;38:456–464.

60. Grahnen H, Hansson L. The prognosis of pulp and root canal therapy. A clinical and radiographic follow-up examination. Odontolgisk Revy 1961;12: 146–165.

61. Molven O. The frequency, technical standard and results of endodontic therapy. Bergen, Norway: Dr Odont thesis, University of Bergen; 1974.

62. Sjögren U, Hägglund B, Sundqvist G, Wing K. Factors affecting the long-term results of endodontic treatment. Journal of Endodontics 1990;16:498–504.

63. Smith CS, Setchell DT, Harty FJ. Factors affecting the success of root canal therapy – a five year retrospective study. International Endodontic Journal 1993;26: 321–333.

64. Strindberg LZ. The dependence of the results of pulp therapy on certain factors. An analytic study based on radiographic and clinical follow-up examinations. Acta Odontologica Scandinavica 1956;14(Suppl. 21):1–175.

65. Dummer PM, McGinn JH, Rees DG. The position and topography of the apical canal constriction and apical foramen. International Endodontic Journal 1984;17:192–198.

66. Simon JH. The apex: how critical is it? General Dentistry 1994;42: 330–334.

67. Walton RE. Current concepts of canal preparation. Dental Clinics of North America 1992;36: 309–326.

68. Byström A, Claesson R, Sundqvist G. The antibacterial effect of camphorated paramonochlorophenol, camphorated phenol and calcium hydroxide in the treatment of infected root canals. Endodontics and Dental Traumatology 1985;1:170–175.

69. Byström A, Sundqvist G. Bacteriologic evaluation of the efficacy of mechanical root canal instrumentation in endodontic therapy. Scandinavian Journal of Dental Research 1981;89: 321–328.

70. Card SJ, Sigurdsson A, Ørstavik D, Trope M. The effectiveness of increased enlargement in reducing intracanal bacteria. Journal of Endodontics 2002;28: 779–783.

71. Coldero LG, McHugh S, MacKenzie D, Saunders WP. Reduction in intracanal bacteria during root canal preparation with and without apical enlargement. International Endodontic Journal 2002;35: 437–446.

72. Siqueira JF Jnr, Lima KC, Magalhães FA, et al. Mechanical reduction of the bacterial population in the root canal by three instrumentation techniques. Journal of Endodontics 1999;25: 332–335.

73. Mullaney TP. Instrumentation of finely curved canals. Dental Clinics of North America 1979;23: 575–592.

74. Alaçam T. Incidence of postoperative pain following the use of different sealers in immediate root canal filling. Journal of Endodontics 1985;11: 135–137.

75. Eleazer PD, Eleazer KR. Flare-up rate in pulpally necrotic molars in one-visit versus two-visit endodontic treatment. Journal of Endodontics 1998;24:614–616.

76. Fava LR. A clinical evaluation of one and two-appointment root canal therapy using calcium hydroxide. International Endodontic Journal 1994;27: 47–51.

77. Figini L, Lodi G, Gorni F, Gagliani M. Single versus multiple visits for endodontic treatment of permanent teeth. Evidence based dentistry 2008;34: 1041–1047.

78. Fox J, Atkinson JS, Dinin AP, et al. Incidence of pain following one-visit endodontic treatment. Oral Surgery, Oral Medicine, Oral Pathology 1970;30:123–130.

79. Mulhern JM, Patterson SS, Newton CW, Ringel AM. Incidence of postoperative pain after one-appointment endodontic treatment of asymptomatic pulpal necrosis in single-rooted teeth. Journal of Endodontics 1982;8:370–375.

80. Oliet S. Single-visit endodontics: a clinical study. Journal of Endodontics 1983;9:147–152.

81. Pekruhn RB. Single-visit endodontic therapy: a preliminary clinical study. Journal of the American Dental Association 1981;103:875–877.

82. Pekruhn RB. The incidence of failure following single-visit endodontic therapy. Journal of Endodontics 1986;12:68–72.

83. Soltanoff W. A comparative study of the single-visit and the multiple-visit endodontic procedure. Journal of Endodontics 1978;4:278–281.

84. Weiger R, Rosendahl R, Löst C. Influence of calcium hydroxide intracanal dressings on the prognosis of teeth with endodontically induced periapical lesions. International Endodontic Journal 2000;33:219–226.

Chapter | 8 |

Intracanal medication

D. Ørstavik

SUMMARY

Endodontics may be considered the treatment or prevention of apical periodontitis, which translates into the elimination or control of root canal infection. Over the years, medicaments used for this purpose have changed from strong and toxic chemicals to more selective and effective, yet tissue tolerant agents. Antibiotics have found limited use in root canal treatment, but may be useful in the treatment of immature teeth. The bacterial flora of different types of root canal infections is variable, and so is their susceptibility to conventional medicaments; this has led to alternatives, or combinations of, medicaments

© 2009 Elsevier Ltd, Inc, BV
DOI: 10.1016/B978-0-7020-3156-4.00011-5

that show promise in managing persistent and recurrent infections. A better understanding of factors influencing the local availability and potency of medicaments has helped facilitate improved means of application. Medicaments are also used with the intention of controlling pain and supporting the tissue healing process; however, they are always secondary to their main, antimicrobial function. While irrigation with sodium hypochlorite and dressing with calcium hydroxide remain standard treatment protocol, chlorhexidine and iodine compounds are emerging as alternatives or supplements to these classical medicaments.

INTRODUCTION

Endodontic success or failure is related to the absence or presence of signs and symptoms of apical periodontitis.[1] Root canal treatment can, therefore, be considered the prevention or cure of this disease.[2] Apical periodontitis includes periapical granuloma and radicular cyst as well as acute manifestations of inflammation. The aetiology of apical periodontitis is, primarily, a bacterial infection of the root canal system;[3,4,5,6] consequently, the technical and pharmacological aspects of prevention and treatment are mainly aimed at controlling infection. Thus, preventive endodontics entails treatment of a tooth without previous signs of apical periodontitis by aseptic pulp extirpation. Curative endodontics is the chemomechanical elimination of infection in the root canal system of a tooth with signs of apical periodontitis. Both procedures are completed by the placement of a bacteria-tight filling to prevent new infection.

The use of intracanal medicaments is an adjunct to the prevention, and essential for, the treatment of apical periodontitis. The primary function is to prevent root canal infection where none is present, and/or to inactivate bacteria already infecting the root canal space. Intracanal medicaments would include any agent with intended pharmacological action introduced into the root canal space. Antibacterial and other active compounds currently used as irrigating solutions during instrumentation rightly belong in this category. Intracanal dressings more concisely describe medicaments left in the root canal space to exert their effects over a longer time period.

HISTORY

The role of microorganisms in pulpless teeth was recognized more than a century ago,[7] and strong, caustic antiseptics were popular as intracanal medicaments at the turn of the twentieth century. Formaldehyde-containing materials, e.g. formocresol,[8] and iodoform pastes[9] belong

to this category and remained popular for decades. Formulations with sulphonamides[10] and later antibiotics were tried as intracanal medicaments; Grossman's polyantibiotic paste[11] and Ledermix®[12] (Haupt Pharma GmbH, Wolfratshausen, Germany) are examples of these types of dressings.

The reduction of pain through pharmacological control of the inflammatory process has also been attempted in endodontics by the application of eugenol,[13] and later corticosteroids and other anti-inflammatory drugs,[14] as dressings. The focus on the possible adverse toxic effects of medicaments[15,16] led to a more systematic selection from the list of disinfectants available for use. Phenol derivatives and iodine formulations gained popularity as medicaments in endodontics; sodium hypochlorite was confirmed as a suitable irrigant.

Calcium hydroxide, while advocated since 1930,[17] has gained popularity in endodontics in the last three decades. Calcium hydroxide has had success in a variety of clinical situations including pulpotomy, root resorption, root-end closure, control of exudation and root canal infection.[18]

RATIONALE AND OVERVIEW OF APPLICATIONS

The primary function of endodontic medicaments is to provide antimicrobial activity. In a few instances, other, secondary functions are desirable (Table 8.1). The rationale for applying intracanal medicaments in various clinical situations has been reviewed.[19]

Asepsis, antisepsis and disinfection

Asepsis is the assurance that no pathogenic microorganisms are present in the field of operation. It entails the use, not only of clean, but also of sterile or disinfected instruments and utensils, liquids, etc. In the course of treating teeth with no signs of root canal infection, maintaining asepsis is the primary means of preserving a bacteria-free

Table 8.1 Functions of intracanal medicaments

Primary function: antimicrobial activity
Antisepsis
Disinfection
Secondary functions
Hard tissue formation
Pain control
Exudation control
Resorption control

canal. Antisepsis is the endeavour to prevent or arrest the growth of microorganisms on living tissue. In vital pulp extirpation, antiseptic measures are necessary to prevent infection in case there is a breach in the chain of asepsis. Irrigating solutions and interappointment dressings need to be antibacterial in action to prevent any microorganisms, which may contaminate the root canal system, from multiplying and establishing themselves.

Disinfection is the elimination of pathogenic microorganisms, usually by chemical or physical means. Disinfection by antiseptic agents is what is attempted in the treatment of infected teeth. Sterilization, on the other hand, implies the use of irradiation or heat to reach a state of complete freedom from live microbes and cannot be applied to root canal treatment. Disinfection entails mechanical removal of tissue and debris containing microbes, irrigation and dressing with antiseptic agents; also, surgical removal of an infected apex contributes to the antiseptic efforts of treatment. The presence of radiologically discernible apical periodontitis is a sign that the root canal system is infected.[6] This state of pre-existing infection also has a negative influence on prognosis.[20] In these cases, bacterial reduction, and effective disinfection, of the root canal system is a prerequisite for successful treatment.

Secondary functions of medicaments

Root canal treatment is sometimes associated with clinical features only indirectly related to infection of the root canal system. Pain during and after treatment may occur, and the associated tissue reactions include exudation, transudation, swelling and resorption. Each of these phenomena, either singularly or in conjunction with infection, has been a target for attempts at medication during, between and after treatment sessions.

Pain control

Pain is mostly associated with infection, and the primary means of pain control in endodontic treatment is infection control. Pharmacological agents that result in pain reduction through a decrease in the tissue responses to inflammation may have a role in further alleviating clinical pain from both infectious and aseptic pulpal-periodontal inflammation.

Control of exudation or bleeding

Persistent exudation in the root canal may occur, despite apparently successful technical treatment. Exudation reflects inflammation, however, and residual infection should be suspected. Therefore, treatment is aimed at dealing with potential infection as well as drying, or coagulating the exudating site.

Control of inflammatory root resorption

Trauma to the teeth may result in various forms of resorptive damage; inflammatory root resorption being the most aggressive and destructive. Inflammatory root resorption is normally associated with infection of the root canal combined with physical damage to the cementum; again, a primary function of treatment is to eliminate infection in the root canal system. Secondarily, medicaments may influence the resorption process itself.

Induction of hard tissue formation

It is often considered desirable to allow hard tissue to form, to continue apical root development, to close a wide foramen, or to create a mechanical barrier at a fracture line. Although the mechanism of action is largely unknown, dressings are available with claims of inducing hard tissue formation (see later).

MICROBIOLOGY OF ENDODONTIC INFECTIONS

Following pulpal necrosis, sooner or later, the entire root canal system will become infected. A long-standing infection will have bacteria not only in the main, but also in accessory canals, and for a distance into the dentinal tubules.[21] If apical periodontitis has progressed to the point where resorption of the cementum occurs, bacteria may be found throughout the length of the dentinal tubules.[22]

The source of the infecting bacteria may be dental caries, salivary contamination through fractures, cracks or leaking fillings, or contamination of the pulp space during dental, including endodontic, treatment. The microbial flora will vary with the clinical condition, and endodontic infection may be one of three types: primary, secondary, or persistent infection. Infected canals typically contain 2–10 different cultivable species; the total number of microorganism ranging from 10^3 to 10^7.[23] The exact number of microorganisms is not known as they vary from tooth to tooth, and because of a lack of established quantitative methods of determination.

Primary root canal infection

With increasing time and depth, a primary root canal infection, i.e. one in existence prior to any intervention, the microbial flora changes from a predominantly facultative, Gram-positive flora to an almost completely anaerobic and mainly Gram-negative set of microorganisms.[24] Strains belonging to the genera *Tannerella, Dialister, Fusobacterium, Prevotella, Porphyromonas, Peptostreptococcus,* and *Treponema* are frequently found in teeth with apical periodontitis.[25] Other microorganisms not found by normal culturing techniques may be present. Facultative streptococci are also common. These same types of microorganisms are found in exacerbations or periapical abscesses.[26] In addition, infections involving other microorganisms, e.g. *streptococci, Eubacterium, Veillonella*[27] and *Actinomyces/Arachnia*[28] frequently occur.[29]

In most infected teeth, several species are recovered from the root canals.[25] Many of the dominating species, e.g. *Fusobacterium, Prevotella* and *Porphyromonas*, may require the presence of some other synergistic species for their survival and propagation. It may be noteworthy in this context that these same species have not been found in dentinal tubules, which when infected harbour less fastidious microorganisms, such as lactobacilli and streptococci.[30]

Secondary root canal infection

The microbial flora in retreatment cases, a secondary root canal infection, occurring during or after treatment, has been shown to differ significantly from microorganism in primary apical periodontitis. Typically, retreatment cases show enterococci, streptococci, and anaerobic cocci in high frequencies;[31,32] enteric rods and *Candida* are also relatively more frequent than in primary apical periodontitis.[33,34,35,36]

Persistent root canal infection

A similar flora is found in persistent root canal infection. Here, a pre-existing infection has withstood the antimicrobial effects of treatment, and a selection of species survived, having adapted to the new environment in the root canal system. In these cases, dependent on the healing response after non-surgical root canal treatment, follow-up surgery may be necessary.

Extraradicular infection

Some organisms, notably *Actinomyces* and *Propionibacterium* species, but also others, are known to survive and propagate in soft tissues and also at the periapex as extraradicular infection.[37] These infections may be one of the causes of what has been termed 'treatment-resistant cases'. Intracanal medicaments are of little use in extraradicular infections; surgery is indicated.

ANTIMICROBIAL AGENTS

Antibiotics

The successful use of various antibiotics, both systemically and topically, in other areas of medicine made them likely candidates for antibacterial action in the root canal system.

There are three main concerns about the local use of antibiotics in the root canal:

- Sensitization. Topical application of an antibiotic increases the risk of the patient becoming allergic to it.[38] Life-threatening anaphylactic reactions may occur from the administration of antibiotics to sensitized individuals. Induced allergy to an antibiotic may limit the options for treatment of more severe infections, which would, otherwise, be curable with that particular drug.
- Development of bacterial drug resistance. The drug kinetics of antibiotics applied in the root canal is not well known.[39] Conditions may become favourable for the development of antibiotic-resistant microbial strains, causing an infection, which in turn is more difficult to treat.[40] Moreover, beyond the scope of treatment of the individual patient, the widespread use of antibiotics causes a general increase in pathogenic and indigenous microorganisms that are resistant to a variety of antibiotics.[41]
- Limited spectrum. No one antibiotic is efficacious against all endodontic microorganisms.[42] Given that most endodontic infections are caused by a combination of species, the chance of one antibiotic achieving effective bacterial inhibition or elimination is small.

Sulpha preparations

Sulphathiazole as part of a dressing was advocated in the 1950s and 1960s.[10] While irrefutably antibacterial, variable results were shown in comparative clinical studies.[43,44] Moreover, although effective against many Gram-negative and Gram-positive microorganisms, sulpha drugs are ineffective against enterococci and *Pseudomonas aeruginosa*.

Penicillin

Grossman's polyantibiotic paste contained penicillin as an important ingredient. Beta-lactamase produced by several microbial species found in the root canal makes them resistant to penicillin. This includes *P. aeruginosa* and several anaerobic Gram-negative rods.

Metronidazole

Metronidazole has good effect against several Gram-negative anaerobic microorganisms.[45] It has been suggested for use in irrigating solutions,[46] as an intracanal dressing[47] and for parenteral applications in combination with other antibiotics, particularly penicillin.[37] It has limited activity against enterococci.[48]

Tetracycline

Tetracycline shows affinity for hard tissues and may be retained on tooth surfaces.[49] It is used locally in periodontics with good clinical and bacteriological results,[50] and the derivative, doxycycline, forms the antibiotic ingredient in Ledermix.[51] However, its antimicrobial spectrum is quite narrow, and it may be ineffective against several oral and endodontic pathogens. The fact that resistance to tetracycline occurs through the formation of transferable R factors also suggests caution in its application.

MTAD (BioPure MTAD, Dentsply Tulsa Dental, Tulsa, OK, USA) is an irrigant containing a mixture of tetracycline, an acid and a detergent. The tetracycline component, doxycycline is retained in the dentine after application. Apart from the criticism that doxycyline is bacteriostatic and not bacteriocidal, another disadvantage is the potential iatrogenic staining of teeth when sodium hypochlorite reacts with MTAD with alternating usage.[52]

Clindamycin

One study has reported on the use of clindamycin as an inter-appointment dressing, but only limited antibacterial efficacy could be demonstrated.[53] An experimental delivery device for clindamycin in the root canal has been reported,[54] and in vitro experiments suggest that clindamycin may penetrate deep into dentinal tubules.[55]

Antibiotic combinations

While the traditional polyantibiotic pastes[11] have been largely discontinued, a new combination of three or four antibiotic compounds has received interest,[56,57] Successful revascularization, with hard tissue formation in the pulp and complete root formation, has been observed in immature, permanent teeth with pulp necrosis and apical periodontitis after application of this mixture.[58,59,60]

Disinfectants

While antibiotics work through biological interference with essential biochemical processes, disinfectants (Table 8.2) are a group of chemicals that act by direct toxicity to the microbes. Their action is thus quicker and more general, and they usually have a broader antibacterial spectrum than antibiotics. On the other hand, they may be more toxic to host tissues, and their action is generally more dose dependent.

Aldehydes

Formaldehyde, paraformaldehyde and glutaraldehyde have been widely used in dentistry including endodontics. They are water-soluble, protein-denaturing agents and are among the most potent disinfectants. Aldehydes have applications in the disinfection of surfaces and medical equipment that cannot be sterilized, but they are quite toxic and allergenic, and some may be carcinogenic.

Formocresol is an aqueous solution containing cresol, formaldehyde, and glycerine, used for pulpotomy proce-

Table 8.2 Root canal disinfectants

HALOGENS
Chlorine Irrigating solution: sodium hypochlorite 0.5% in 1% sodium bicarbonate as Dakin's solution; or 0.5–5.25% in aqueous solution.
Iodine Irrigating solution and short-term dressing: 2% iodine in 5% potassium iodide aqueous solution; iodophors. Field disinfection: 5% iodine in tincture of alcohol.
CHLORHEXIDINE
Chlorhexidine gluconate Field disinfection and irrigating solution: 0.12–2.0% aqueous solution. Irrigation and dressing: 1–5% gel.
CALCIUM HYDROXIDE
Dressing: aqueous, viscous or oily suspension/paste with varying amounts of salts added. Other antibacterial agents (iodine, chlorophenols, chlorhexidine) may be added.
ALDEHYDES
Formocresol Dressing: 19% formaldehyde, 35% cresol, 46% water and glycerine.

dures in primary teeth,[61] but its toxic and mutagenic properties are of concern. It is no longer favoured and it has been suggested that its use should be discontinued.[62]

Paraformaldehyde is the polymeric form of formaldehyde, best known for its inclusion in some root canal filling materials, e.g. N2 and Endométhasone. It slowly decomposes to release its monomer, formaldehyde; its toxic, allergenic, and genotoxic properties are as for formaldehyde.

Halogens

Halogens include chlorine and iodine, which are both used in various formulations in endodontics. They are potent oxidizing agents with rapid bactericidal effects. Chlorine is released from sodium hypochlorite and from chloramine. The latter releases active chlorine at a lower rate, and has been used for short-term dressing of the root canal. Sodium hypochlorite is currently the irrigating solution of choice. It is used clinically in concentrations from 0.5–5.25%. Both in vitro and in vivo bacteriological studies support its application. Necrotic tissue and debris are dissolved by sodium hypochlorite,[63] a property exploited in biomechanical cleansing of root canals.[64,65] Its toxicity is low; however, its bleaching properties can be a nuisance if spilled onto a patient's clothes, its smell is objectionable to some patients, and it may cause severe symptoms if accidentally injected beyond the apex.[66]

Iodine is used mainly as iodine potassium iodide and in iodophors, which are organic iodine-containing compounds that release iodine over time. Iodine is also a very potent antibacterial agent of low toxicity, but may stain clothing if spilled. As iodoform (triiodomethane), it was used in a paste formulation as a permanent root canal filling.[9] Iodine compounds are used as an irrigating solution and short-term dressing as 2% solution of iodine in 4% aqueous potassium iodide. It has also been added to gutta-percha points for root canal filling.[67,68] Some patients may be allergic to iodine compounds, and their use in these patients is contraindicated.

Phenol derivatives

Phenol itself is no longer used in endodontics because of its high toxicity, but the derivative paramonochlorophenol has been a very popular component of interappointment dressings. It has been used both in aqueous solution[69] and in combination with camphor (as camphorated monochlorophenol); it was long recognized as the dressing of choice for infected teeth. Thymol, similarly, enjoyed widespread popularity, but is less antibacterial than the chlorophenol compounds.

Eugenol is frequently used as a dressing for temporary control of pain after vital pulp exposure.[70] It has a well-documented, but limited, antimicrobial effect and is applied primarily for its pain-relieving effect.[71]

Chlorhexidine

Chlorhexidine has been widely used in periodontology.[72] Its substantivity (persistence in the area of interest), its relatively broad spectrum of activity, and its low toxicity may make it well suited for irrigation and as dressings in endodontics. Results of in vitro studies pointed to the suitability of chlorhexidine in endodontics[73-77] and some in vivo bacteriological data are emerging.[36,78] Effective concentrations are in the 0.2–2% range. Innovative attempts to utilize the disinfecting properties of chlorhexidine include its inclusion in gutta-percha points for root canal filling.[68]

Calcium hydroxide

Calcium hydroxide has reached a unique position as a dressing in endodontics.[79] After its successful clinical application for a variety of indications,[18,80] multiple biological functions have been ascribed to calcium hydroxide.[81] Its primary function is probably antibacterial in most clinical situations, with the added benefits of cauterizing activity and high pH; also in the consistency

of a paste, it physically restricts bacterial colonization of the canal space. Calcium hydroxide is applied as a thick, creamy suspension in sterile water, saline, and a variety of other, viscous or oily vehicles.[82,83]

Calcium hydroxide with antimicrobial additives

Complete disinfection by calcium hydroxide cannot be expected in all cases.[84] Moreover, in root filled teeth the flora may contain microorganisms relatively resistant to its action. Numerous attempts have been made to mix calcium hydroxide with other aqueous and non-aqueous disinfectants.[85] Parachlorophenol, camphorated parachlorophenol,[82] metacresol,[86] and iodoform[87] have all been added to calcium hydroxide suspensions. Combinations of calcium hydroxide with chlorhexidine have also been tested in vitro.[88,89,90]

RESISTANCE OF ORAL MICROBES TO MEDICAMENTS

In some cases, bacteria persist and produce symptoms of inflammation despite apparently optimal cleansing and disinfection procedures.[91] They may either be inaccessible to the cleaning instruments or to the medicaments, or they may be resistant to the medicaments used.[57] Special interest has recently focussed on streptococci, enterococci and yeasts in persistent infections; these have been shown to be relatively resistant to calcium hydroxide[84,90,92,93] and occur in high frequency in retreatment cases.[27,33,94] Organic and inorganic debris in the root canal system will also affect and limit the antimicrobial activity of irrigating solutions and interappointment dressings.[95]

CONCEPT OF PREDICTABLE DISINFECTION IN ENDODONTICS

Given the infectious nature of apical periodontitis, any clinical procedure should be based on the ability of each step to prevent contamination and to eliminate infection. A standard procedure should, furthermore, be based on a worst-case scenario, which would be the infected root canal with associated chronic apical periodontitis. Individual treatment steps have been assessed for their efficacy in eliminating bacteria from infected root canals[23,91,96,97,98,99,100] (Fig. 8.1).

Mechanical instrumentation

Even in the absence of an antibacterial irrigating solution and subsequent dressing, there is still a dramatic decrease

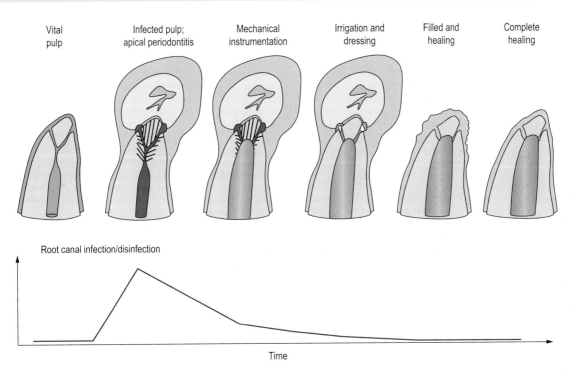

Figure 8.1 Apical periodontitis develops when the root canal system becomes infected. Treatment entails the reduction of bacteria by mechanical instrumentation and antibacterial irrigation. The antibacterial dressing, if effective, eliminates infection. Total disinfection allows for complete healing of the tooth with apical periodontitis following root canal filling.

in bacterial numbers in a root canal from mechanical cleansing alone.[23,101,102,103] However, in the majority of cases, bacteria, which are left in the canal, have the potential to multiply between appointments[23] and after root canal filling.[94]

Antibacterial effect of irrigation

The addition of sodium hypochlorite as an antibacterial irrigating solution increases the number of bacteria-free canals substantially.[96] The use of 5% rather than 0.5% sodium hypochlorite appears slightly more effective, and the reduction in the number of infected teeth has been shown to be even greater, when ethylenediaminetetraacetic acid (EDTA) was alternated with sodium hypochlorite,[96,97] and when ultrasonic instrumentation of the canal was performed.[100] Increasing the temperature of sodium hypochlorite also increases its efficacy.[104] Chlorhexidine (applied as a 2% gel) has been shown to be similarly or even more effective than sodium hypochlorite in reducing intracanal bacteria during instrumentation.[105]

Effect of antibacterial dressing

The number of bacteria-free canals may be further increased when a dressing of calcium hydroxide is placed in fully instrumented canals between visits.[84,102,106,107] Calcium hydroxide has been found to be more effective than camphorated monochlorophenol in comparative experiments,[84] but the added effect on the reduction from instrumentation and irrigation is variable.[79] Attempts at potentiating the antimicrobial effect of calcium hydroxide by the addition of other medicaments in the dressing has met with some,[108] but limited success.[109]

Follow-up studies

Teeth treated as described above have been followed for periods of up to 7 years, a successful outcome (definite signs of healing of apical periodontitis) shown in more than 90% of the cases.[91] While success rates from different studies may be difficult to compare, it would appear that these clinical results are better than most, if not all, previous reports.[110]

Adequate disinfection in single-visit endodontics

Single-visit ('one-step') endodontics implies shaping, cleaning and disinfection of the root canal in the course of one treatment session. This is followed by permanent root canal filling at the same appointment. Immediate root canal filling of teeth that are not infected is not controversial and, in principle, probably preferable to treatment in multiple appointments; if asepsis is maintained, there is no need for a disinfecting dressing between appointments and the risk of leakage. The debatable issue is whether the time duration and the type of medicament that can be applied during one appointment endodontics will provide predictable disinfection and, subsequently, healing of infected teeth with apical periodontitis. It is highly desirable to achieve effective disinfection quickly, and data from clinical studies have shown that treatment in one visit may be as effective, and as predictable, as procedures utilizing an interim dressing.[111,112] However, some clinical follow-up studies suggest better treatment outcome after dressing-based disinfection compared with single-visit procedures.[113,114] Human and animal histological studies have also reported the presence of residual bacteria and inflammation in teeth treated in one visit.[115,116]

From controlled to predictable disinfection

Scientific data from clinical studies should be the basis for a rational, evidence-based approach to treatment of infected teeth.[117]Clinical experiments have documented controlled disinfection by advanced bacteriological techniques. When applied to clinical practice, adherence to the principles of mechanical instrumentation, irrigation with sodium hypochlorite and EDTA, and dressing with calcium hydroxide, would be expected to produce predictable disinfection (bacteria-free canals) in a very high percentage of cases (Fig. 8.2), and in turn, a very high rate of clinical and radiological evidence of healing of apical periodontitis. Indeed, large series of follow-up studies using this treatment regimen for infected teeth have borne out the high success rate.[118] A need for routine chairside bacteriological control of procedures is not implied in clinical practice.

Treatment of non-infected teeth

None of the steps advocated for the treatment of the infected tooth place in jeopardy the success of treatment of a tooth with an initially non-infected pulp. Vital pulp extirpation followed by instrumentation with sodium hypochlorite and a dressing of calcium hydroxide give a clean pulp wound with minimal or no inflammation (Fig. 8.3). Therefore, as a means of securing the absence of microbes in these cases, the same treatment principles should apply. One exception is when permanent root canal filling is possible at the first appointment; then there is no need for a period of canal dressing for the purpose of disinfection. Also, it may be questioned whether EDTA

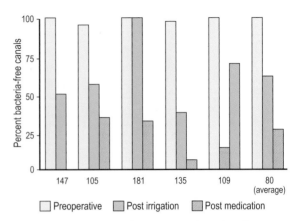

Figure 8.2 Percentage reduction in canals positive for bacterial growth after instrumentation/irrigation and dressing of initially infected root canals. Numbers beneath bars refer to the articles cited.

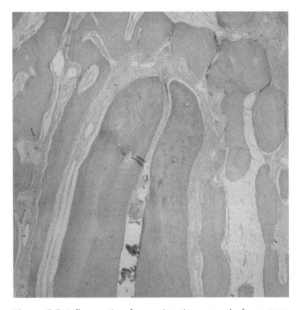

Figure 8.3 Inflammation-free extirpation wound of a mature central incisor (monkey) after two weeks of dressing with calcium hydroxide.

serves any purpose in the treatment of teeth with non-infected pulps.

Other principles of treatment may have the potential for equal or better efficacy and success rates. However, the extensive literature with clinical and bacteriological controls, and clinical and radiological follow-ups makes the above guidelines a standard of reference. Alternative methods and medicaments should be tested and compared similarly prior to receiving general clinical acceptance.

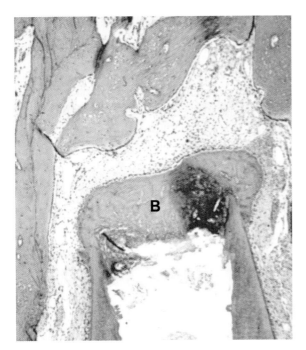

B

Figure 8.4 Formation of a hard tissue barrier (B) at the apex of an immature central incisor (monkey). The pulp was extirpated and a dressing of calcium hydroxide placed for three weeks.

INDUCTION OF HARD TISSUE FORMATION

The process of creating a hard tissue barrier at an open apex or at a grossly over-instrumented apex is termed root end closure or apexification.[119,120] When calcium hydroxide is used in long-term treatment of traumatized young permanent incisors and infection is controlled, a barrier of bone/cementum-like tissue at the apex is formed with a high degree of predictability[120,121] (Fig. 8.4). This barrier allows mechanical compression of the root filling, and any toxic responses of the tissues to the filling materials are minimized by this intervening barrier. While it may not be essential that calcium hydroxide be used as a dressing for this purpose, its clinical application is the most extensively documented. Similar principles apply in the formation of a hard tissue barrier more coronally, e.g. at the line of a horizontal root fracture or at a pulpotomy or pulp-capping wound surface.[122] Mineral trioxide aggregate (MTA) is now the material of choice for these purposes; it is a filling or sealant material rather than a medicament, and thus falls outside the scope of this chapter[123] but is covered elsewhere in this book (see Chs 9 & 12).

PAIN OF ENDODONTIC ORIGIN

Endodontic pain is mainly associated with both inflammation and infection.[124–129] The inflammatory responses to the trauma of pulp extirpation and instrumentation may elicit pain of lesser magnitude and duration than pain following bacterial activity.[29,130] The rationale behind pain control by interappointment dressings is thus, primarily, to combat infection. This is reflected also in the finding that interappointment pain is significantly more frequent in infected, necrotic teeth than in vital cases.[131,132] There are strong psychological components to the clinical expression of pain of endodontic origin.[133,134] Clinical pain is further confounded by the concomitant presence of microbial and iatrogenic and other factors. The quantification of pain clinically is also very difficult to standardize for comparative purposes.

The incidence of interappointment or post-treatment pain seems to be very much dependent on the criteria defining pain.[135,136,137] As an operating definition, the incidence of patients requiring an extra, non-scheduled visit following self-reported pain may have some merit. It would not include the discomfort sometimes associated with, the practical necessities of the treatment itself (local anaesthetic injection, rubber dam clamp placement, severance and laceration of the pulp). By such criteria, no significant advantage of one medicament over another has been reported.[138,139,140,141]

Due to the lack of precise knowledge of the source of pain in individual cases, the introduction of medicaments in dressings to alleviate inter- and post-treatment pain has been by theoretical considerations, and by trial and error, rather than by clinical research. Most interest has focused on the use of corticosteroids in the interappointment dressing; particularly, the use of Ledermix containing triamcinolone, has been popular.[12,51,142,143] It is doubtful whether initial concerns about the systemic effects of locally administered corticosteroids are justified; there is no indication that harmful side-effects are associated with its use in dentistry, and the doses applied are rather small compared with other medical indications.[144] However, while concerns for side-effects may have been exaggerated, the clinical benefits, if any, over calcium hydroxide medication remain questionable.[143] Non-steroidal anti-inflammatory drugs have also been tested clinically as intracanal dressings,[14] but any clinical advantages again remain obscure.

For the control of pain, little seems to be gained either by the prophylactic addition to dressings or by the routine prescription of parenteral drugs.[137] It seems that endodontic pain may be better dealt with on a case-by-case approach, providing relief with pain control medication and by treatment appropriate for the individual patient.

EXUDATION AND BLEEDING

Purulent exudate is a clear sign of infection. A serous exudate ('the weeping canal') is a more elusive clinical condition. It may also be associated with a relatively large apical foramen or an over-instrumented, patent foramen. Both conditions are usually controlled by instrumentation and dressing with calcium hydroxide. The application for a few minutes of dry calcium hydroxide packed against the exuding surface may succeed in desiccating or necrotizing the site to the point where seepage is controlled and treatment may continue. However, an interim dressing with calcium hydroxide may be necessary to control the exudation more effectively.

To the extent that exudation is associated with inflammation, and it may be reduced by local corticosteroids, it would be rational in these cases to include steroid-containing dressings.[142] Given the limited nature of this problem, clinical studies are hard to design and carry out, and data are lacking to support this suggested mode of treatment.

Bleeding from the canal is usually easily controlled by simple occlusion of the bleeding site with paper points, dry or moistened with 3% hydrogen peroxide. Calcium hydroxide packed onto the bleeding site is also effective in stopping bleeding within a few minutes.

ROOT RESORPTION

Root resorption is a complication of root canal infection and trauma, in some instances with deleterious consequences to the tooth.[145] The external apical root resorption associated with chronic apical periodontitis is self-limiting and stops when the root canal infection is adequately controlled. It is likely that this resorption occurs to eliminate necrotic and/or infected cementum and dentine at the apex.

Traumatic tooth injuries, particularly luxations and avulsions followed by replantation, frequently lead to resorptive processes. Surface resorption is self-limiting and followed by repair of cemental damage induced by the trauma. Ankylosis or replacement resorption, however, may be progressive in nature. Inflammatory resorption of the root surface occurs in response to a necrotic and infected root canal system, and may be extremely rapid causing tooth loss in months if left untreated.[146] Root canal treatment is essential when inflammatory root resorption is evident or imminent, and calcium hydroxide is currently the medicament of choice for this purpose.[147,148] Prolonged use of calcium hydroxide with multiple changes of the dressing may lead to necrosis of cells trying to recolonize the cementum surface. While this finding may suggest that the duration of treatment with calcium hydroxide in these cases should be kept short (1–2

weeks),[149] longer-term placement of calcium hydroxide remains a clinically proven procedure in the treatment of resorption.[150]

It has been suggested that because Ledermix inhibits the spread of dentinoclasts,[151] it may provide added benefits in the control of inflammatory root resorption,[152,153] particularly when mixed with calcium hydroxide.[39] More experimental is the use of calcitonin, a hormone that inhibits osteoclastic bone resorption, in canal dressings for inflammatory root resorption.[154]

TISSUE DISTRIBUTION OF MEDICAMENTS

There is limited knowledge of the actual distribution, in hard and soft tissues, of medicaments applied to the root canal.[155,156,157] Several barriers limit the penetration of chemical agents from the pulp canal space through tooth structures and into the periapical tissues.[92,158] There is also limited knowledge on the localization of microorganisms, inflamed tissues and cells targeted by the medicaments.[159,160]

Diffusion and solubility

The ability of a medicament to dissolve and diffuse in the predominantly aqueous periapical environment may be essential for its action. Lipid soluble substances may have difficulty reaching targets at a distance in the tissues. Amphipathic drugs may have particular benefits; it may not be coincidental that aldehydes and phenol derivatives have had clinical success.[161] Thus, aqueous solutions of paramonochlorophenol may penetrate further and have greater antimicrobial activity than the more concentrated lipid solute.[25] The low but significant solubility in water of calcium hydroxide has the dual advantage of limiting its toxic effects while the depot of the compound in suspension at the same time provides continuous release of the agent.

Penetration of dentine

Studies in vivo have found the raised pH effect of calcium hydroxide to pervade the width of dentine,[157] but to decrease rapidly in the tissues beyond. However, precise measurements of dentinal pH following application of calcium hydroxide in the root canal ex vivo show that the pH in apical dentine is only moderately elevated.[162] The application of calcium hydroxide on a dentine surface in turn significantly reduces its permeability.[163] Nevertheless, calcium hydroxide is slower than many other medicaments in killing bacteria in experimentally infected dentinal tubules.[92] Similarly, the active ingredients in Ledermix show a gradient in dentine decreasing from the site of application to the cementum surface.[39] Eugenol, a constituent in several root canal sealer formulations, decreases in concentration 100-fold over 1 mm of dentine.[71] Moreover, intact cementum appears to be an effective, if not complete, barrier to medicament penetration.[158] Both the organic and the inorganic components of dentine may also interact with medicaments and reduce their antibacterial properties.[164]

Effect of the smear layer

Bacteriological data, both in vitro[76,165] as well as in vivo,[84] indicate that medicaments penetrate and act more effectively, when applied in a root canal that has been treated to remove the smear layer. In infected teeth with chronic apical periodontitis, it may be assumed that bacteria are lodged peripheral to the main canal where the medicaments are applied.[21,22] The removal of the smear layer through the use of EDTA seems prudent in these cases. Following complete disinfection, however, or in the treatment of a non-infected tooth, retention or recreation of the smear layer may be advantageous in adding to the sealing off of the canal by the final root canal filling, although there are conflicting reports on the effects of the smear layer on root canal fillings.[166]

TISSUE TOXICITY AND BIOLOGICAL CONSIDERATIONS

Endodontic medicaments can cause tissue damage, which will lead to inflammatory responses in soft tissues. These responses may interfere with the healing of apical periodontitis or serve as a locus for colonization by microorganisms, to create a lesion where none existed. Any antiseptic will have a concentration gradient in the tissues with bactericidal and then bacteriostatic activity, but the cytotoxic effects will always be wider-ranging (Fig. 8.5). Experiments with cell-culture techniques and toxicity tests in animals have aided the selection of chemicals and medicaments for endodontic use.[15] Moreover, the allergenic and genotoxic properties of medicaments must form part of the selection criteria.[167,168]

The very strong tissue toxicity, as well as the allergenicity and mutagenicity of aldehydes, have been part of the reason why these agents are no longer recommended for routine use. Similarly, phenols are strongly cytotoxic and can hardly be recommended for use by current standards.[15] Although toxicity is reduced by the addition of camphor, the toxicity/efficacy ratio is still very high. In recommended concentrations, halogen compounds have high antibacterial activity combined with low tissue toxicity. This forms part of the reason why sodium hypochlorite is the irrigating solution of choice and why iodine potassium iodide has been an attractive alternative for short-term intracanal dressing.[107] Cases have been

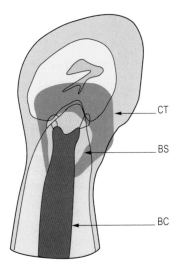

Figure 8.5 Theoretical zones of bactericidal (BC), bacteriostatic (BS) and cytotoxic (CT) activity from an antiseptic in the root canal.

reported, however, of patients experiencing extremely painful reactions to sodium hypochlorite inadvertently placed or injected into the periapical tissues.[66,169]

Calcium hydroxide is, by virtue of its extremely high pH, potentially quite toxic. However, applied on vital tissue, the damage is limited to a narrow zone of superficial necrosis with the potential for complete regeneration.[170] Misplaced or placed in areas where diffusion of the ions may reach soft tissues in high concentrations, calcium hydroxide may cause necrosis.[171]

SUGGESTED CLINICAL PROCEDURES

Mechanical reduction of bacteria

Mechanical instrumentation is the main factor in reducing most bacteria infecting the root canal system. Rubber dam is essential in preventing the root canal system from salivary infection. All efforts should be made to complete the mechanical phases of cleaning and shaping early in treatment, preferably at the first appointment. Any caries must be completely excavated, defective restorations removed, and the tooth and surrounding rubber dam surface thoroughly disinfected. All instrumentation should be carried out in the presence of an irrigating solution. The clinical studies with bacteriological control have employed master apical file sizes of ISO 40 or larger, which exceed the general recommendations in many current treatment protocols. Clinical experiments indicate that more bacteria are removed when canals were prepared to larger files sizes,[102,172] while other studies did not find an effect,[173] and the type of file or instrumentation technique may not be relevant.[174,175,176]

Primary root canal infection

Irrigation: Sodium hypochlorite has the best clinical and laboratory documentation. It may be applied, as a 1–5% aqueous solution, in a sterile syringe with a short 12–25 mm needle with an outer diameter as low as practical (0.25 mm). Care should be taken to prevent the needle from being wedged in the canal so as to prevent the accidental injection of sodium hypochlorite into the periapical tissues. Fresh solution is introduced and the exhausted suctioned off between each change of files. Syringes of 10 mL capacity are practical for this purpose. Sodium hypochlorite may also be used with ultrasonic equipment, and the alternate use of sodium hypochlorite and EDTA will further reduce the number of bacteria. EDTA should be the final rinse if adhesive root filling materials are used.

Dressing: Prior to the application of a dressing to disinfect an infected root canal, the canal is flushed with a 15–17% neutral aqueous solution of EDTA. After allowing the chelating agent to act for 1–2 minutes, it is suctioned off and the canal is dried with paper points.

Calcium hydroxide has clearly the best record and fulfils most, if not all, indications. It may be applied with a Lentulo spiral filler or a syringe. Care must be taken to avoid overfilling. Paper points may be used to suck up excess fluid, and root canal pluggers of suitable dimensions may be used to ensure that the suspension or paste reaches the apical part of the canal. More material may be added if needed and the packing procedure repeated until a homogeneous filling is obtained (Fig. 8.6).

There are many commercially available calcium hydroxide products; some are in injection syringes for ease of application. In teeth with large root canals, as in very young maxillary incisors, the syringe may suffice for placement.

Secondary and persistent root canal infections

Irrigation: The microbial flora may be resistant to conventional medicaments, and an even greater antimicrobial effort may be warranted. Following removal of the previous root canal filling by mechanical and/or chemical (e.g. chloroform) means, the root canal system is irrigated with sodium hypochlorite and EDTA as in primary cases. Towards the end of each appointment and as instrumentation is nearing completion, chlorhexidine (0.2–2% in aqueous solution or as a gel) is applied during the final stages. EDTA should precede the chlorhexidine application, as mixing sodium hypochlorite with chlorhexidine may lead to the precipitation of a brown-coloured flocculate, suspected of being an aniline.[177,178] EDTA should be the final rinse if adhesive root filling materials are used.

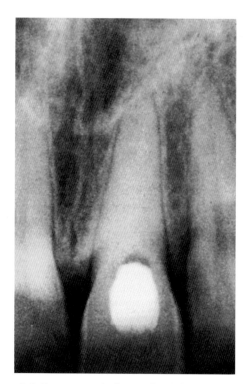

Figure 8.6 The root canal of a maxillary left central incisor filled with calcium hydroxide. The radiopacity of the thick suspension of calcium hydroxide is close to that of dentine and an effective dressing gives the appearance of a completely filled canal.

Dressing: A mixture of calcium hydroxide with aqueous chlorhexidine has been tested in vitro[88,89] and in vivo.[179] Chlorhexidine may also be used in a gel form in concentrations of 2–5%. Given the predominance of streptococci and enterococci in secondary and persistent root canal infections, chlorhexidine preparations may be indicated in these cases.

Temporary filling

A bacteria-tight temporary filling is of paramount importance in preventing secondary contamination and infection of the root canal system. There are increasing numbers of complex endodontic cases as more and more people seek conservative restorative treatment rather than extractions. In these cases, treatment in two or several appointments is usually the rule rather than the exception. It may, reasonably, be assumed that a significant proportion of apical periodontitis developing after pulp extirpation are caused by reinfection through coronal leakage and, therefore, the quality of the seal afforded by the temporary filling should be given careful attention.

The pulp chamber should be free of medicament and cleaned to receive the temporary filling. The dressing should be protected from saliva by a 3–4 mm thick layer of sealing material. When the temporary filling is at particular risk of fracture or dislodgement, extra precautions should be considered. A dual filling ('the double seal') is then advisable: one internal, sealing the dressing and designed to remain even if the external part breaks off, and one external, designed to withstand occlusal function and/or for aesthetic reasons. Should the temporary filling fail, the root canal system is at risk of recontamination, so defeating the purpose of placing a medicament.

Materials for temporary sealing of endodontic access cavities include reinforced zinc oxide-eugenol and calcium sulphate-based materials. There is very limited data on the true clinical efficacy of these materials, and the results are very variable, with one product type being superior in one experiment, while falling short in another study.[180,181] In a clinical study of bacterial penetration along temporary fillings placed in vivo, calcium sulphate and reinforced zinc oxide-eugenol cements performed equally well and better than a resin-based material.[182] Given the greater strength and resistance to dissolution and disintegration, reinforced zinc oxide-eugenol cements combine optimum

leakage resistance and good physical properties making it the temporary filling material of choice in most clinical situations.

LEARNING OUTCOMES

Having read and understood this chapter, the reader should be able to:

- distinguish and know the mode of action of the different types of disinfectants and antibiotics used in endodontics;
- recognize the most important species of microorganisms associated with different types of root canal infection, their differential susceptibility to medicaments and intracanal factors that may limit the efficacy of medicaments;
- assess the overall importance of medicaments in root canal treatment;
- critically evaluate the efficacy of newer medicaments as root canal dressings and irrigants.

REFERENCES

1. Strindberg LZ. The dependence of the results of pulp therapy on certain factors. An analytic study based on radiographic and clinical follow-up examinations. Acta Odontologica Scandinavica 14, Supplement 1956;21:99–101.

2. Ørstavik D. Antibacterial properties of endodontic materials. International Endodontic Journal 1988;21:161–169.

3. Kakehashi S, Stanley HR, Fitzgerald RJ. The effects of surgical exposures of dental pulp in germ-free and conventional laboratory rats. Oral Surgery, Oral Medicine, Oral Pathology 1965;20:340–349.

4. Möller ÅJR, Fabricius L, Dahlén G, et al. Influence on periapical tissues of indigenous oral bacteria and necrotic pulp tissue in monkeys. Scandinavian Journal of Dental Research 1981;89: 475–484.

5. Ricucci D, Siqueira JF Jr, Bate AL, Pitt Ford TR. Histologic investigation of root canal-treated teeth with apical periodontitis: a retrospective study from twenty-four patients. Journal of Endodontics 2009;35: 493–502.

6. Sundqvist G. Bacteriological studies of necrotic dental pulps. Sweden: Thesis no. 7 Umeå University, Umeå; 1976.

7. Miller WD. Micro-organisms of the Human Mouth. Philadelphia, PA, USA: SS White Dental Mfg Co.; 1890.

8. Buckley JP. The rational treatment of putrescent pulps and their sequelae. Dental Cosmos 1906; 48:537–544.

9. Walkhoff O. Mein System der Medikamentösen Behandlung Schwerer Erkrankungen der Zahnpulpa und des Periodontiums. Berlin, Germany: Hermann Meusser; 1928.

10. Nygaard-Östby B. Introduction to endodontics. Norway: Universitetsforlaget Oslo; 1971.

11. Grossman LI. Polyantibiotic treatment of pulpless teeth. Journal of the American Dental Association 1951;43:265–278.

12. Schroeder A. Cortisone in dental surgery. International Dental Journal 1962;12:356–373.

13. Markowitz K, Moynihan M, Liu M, Kim S. Biologic properties of eugenol and zinc oxide-eugenol. A clinically oriented review. Oral Surgery, Oral Medicine, Oral Pathology 1992;73:729–737.

14. Negm MM. Effect of intracanal use of nonsteroidal anti-inflammatory agents on posttreatment endodontic pain. Oral Surgery, Oral Medicine, Oral Pathology 1994;77:507–513.

15. Spångberg L. Intracanal medication. In: Ingle JI, Bakland LK, editors. Endodontics. 4th edn. USA: Williams and Wilkins, Malvern, PA; 1994. p. 627–640.

16. Wennberg A. Biological evaluation of root canal antiseptics using in vitro and in vivo methods. Scandinavian Journal of Dental Research 1980;88:46–52.

17. Hermann BW. Dentinobliteration der Wurzelkanäle nach Behandlung mit Calcium.

Zahnärztliche Rundschau 1930;39:888–899.

18. Heithersay GS. Calcium hydroxide in the treatment of pulpless teeth with associated pathology. Journal of the British Endodontic Society 1975;8: 74–93.

19. Chong BS, Pitt Ford TR. The role of intracanal medication in root canal treatment. International Endodontic Journal 1992;25: 97–106.

20. Ørstavik D, Kerekes K, Eriksen HM. Clinical performance of three endodontic sealers. Endodontics and Dental Traumatology 1987;3:178–186.

21. Shovelton DS. The presence and distribution of micro-organisms within non-vital teeth. British Dental Journal 1964;117: 101–107.

22. Valderhaug J. A histologic study of experimentally induced periapical inflammation in primary teeth in monkeys. International Journal of Oral Surgery 1974;3:111–123.

23. Byström A, Sundqvist G. Bacteriologic evaluation of the efficacy of mechanical root canal instrumentation in endodontic therapy. Scandinavian Journal of Dental Research 1981;89: 321–328.

24. Fabricius L, Dahlén G, Öhman AE, Möller ÅJR. Predominant indigenous oral bacteria isolated from infected root canals after varied times of closure. Scandinavian Journal of Dental Research 1982;90:134–144.

25. Sundqvist G. Taxonomy, ecology, and pathogenicity of the root canal flora. Oral Surgery, Oral Medicine, Oral Pathology 1994;78:522–530.

26. Brook I, Frazier EH, Gher ME. Aerobic and anaerobic microbiology of periapical abscess. Oral Microbiology and Immunology 1991;6:123–125.

27. Molander A, Reit C, Dahlen G, Kvist T. Microbiological status of root-filled teeth with apical periodontitis. International Endodontic Journal 1999;31:1–7.

28. Sjögren U, Happonen RP, Kahnberg KE, Sundqvist G.

Survival of Arachnia propionica in periapical tissue. International Endodontic Journal 1988;21: 277–282.

29. Siqueira JF Jr. Microbial causes of endodontic flare-ups. International Endodontic Journal 2003;36:453–463.

30. Ando N, Hoshino E. Predominant obligate anaerobes invading the deep layers of root canal dentine. International Endodontic Journal 1990;23: 20–27.

31. Engström B. The significance of enterococci in root canal treatment. Odontologisk Revy 1964;15:87–106.

32. Möller ÅJR. Microbiological examination of root canals and periapical tissues of human teeth. Methodological studies. Odontologisk Tidskrift 1966;74: 1–380.

33. Peciuliene V, Reynaud AH, Balciuniene I, Haapasalo M. Isolation of yeasts and enteric bacteria in root-filled teeth with chronic apical periodontitis. International Endodontic Journal 2001;34:429–434.

34. Siren EK, Haapasalo MP, Ranta K et al. Microbiological findings and clinical treatment procedures in endodontic cases selected for microbiological investigation. International Endodontic Journal 1997;30:91–95.

35. Waltimo TM, Siren EK, Torkko HL et al. Fungi in therapy-resistant apical periodontitis. International Endodontic Journal 1997;30:96–101.

36. Zamany A, Safavi K, Spångberg LS. The effect of chlorhexidine as an endodontic disinfectant. Oral Surgery, Oral Medicine, Oral Pathology, Oral Radiology, Endodontics 2003;96: 578–581.

37. Tronstad L, Kreshtool D, Barnett F. Microbiological monitoring and results of treatment of extraradicular endodontic infection. Endodontics and Dental Traumatology 1990;6: 129–136.

38. Van Joost T, Dikland W, Stolz E, Prens E. Sensitization to chloramphenicol; a persistent

problem. Contact Dermatitis 1986;14:176–178.

39. Abbott PV, Hume WR, Heithersay GS. Effects of combining Ledermix and calcium hydroxide pastes on the diffusion of corticosteroid and tetracycline through human tooth roots in vitro. Endodontics and Dental Traumatology 1989;5: 188–192.

40. Wade WG, Moran J, Morgan JR, et al. The effects of antimicrobial acrylic strips on the subgingival microflora in chronic periodontitis. Journal of Clinical Periodontology 1992;19: 127–134.

41. Cohen ML. Antimicrobial resistance: prognosis for public health. Trends in Microbiology 1984;2:422–425.

42. Abbott PV, Hume WR, Pearman JW. Antibiotics and endodontics. Australian Dental Journal 1990;35:50–60.

43. Frank AL, Glick DH, Weichman JA, Harvey H. The intracanal use of sulfathiazole in endodontics to reduce pain. Journal of the American Dental Association 1968;77:102–106.

44. Seltzer S, Bender IB, Ehrenreich J. Incidence and duration of pain following endodontic therapy: relationship to treatment with sulfonamides and to other factors. Oral Surgery, Oral Medicine, Oral Pathology 1961;14:74–82.

45. Slots J, Rams TE. Antibiotics in periodontal therapy: advantages and disadvantages. Journal of Clinical Periodontology 1990;17:479–493.

46. Sanjiwan R, Chandra S, Jaiswal JN, Mats AN. The effect of metronidazole on the anaerobic micro-organisms of the root canal—a clinical study. Federation of Operative Dentistry 1990;1:30–36.

47. Hess JC. Germes anaérobies et gangrènes pulpaires. Experience clinique du traitement local au métronidazole. Journal Dentaire du Quebec 1986;23:15–18.

48. Dahlen G, Samuelsson W, Molander A, Reit C. Identification and antimicrobial susceptibility

of enterococci isolated from the root canal. Oral Microbiology and Immunology 2000;15: 309–312.

49. Bjorvatn K. Scanning electron-microscopic study of pellicle and plaque formation on tetracycline-impregnated dentin. Scandinavian Journal of Dental Research 1986;94:89–94.

50. Genco RJ. Using antimicrobial agents to manage periodontal diseases. Journal of the American Dental Association 1991;122: 31–38.

51. Ehrmann EH. The effect of triamcinolone with tetracycline on the dental pulp and apical periodontium. Journal of Prosthetic Dentistry 1965;15: 144–152.

52. Tay FR, Mazzoni A, Pashley DH, et al. Potential iatrogenic tetracycline staining of endodontically treated teeth via NaOCl/MTAD irrigation: a preliminary report. Journal of Endodontics 2006;32:354–358.

53. Molander A, Reit C, Dahlen G. Microbiological evaluation of clindamycin as a root canal dressing in teeth with apical periodontitis. International Endodontic Journal 1990;23: 113–118.

54. Gilad JZ, Teles R, Goodson M, et al. Development of a clindamycin-impregnated fiber as an intracanal medication in endodontic therapy. Journal of Endodontics 1999;25:722–727.

55. Lin S, Levin L, Peled M, et al. Reduction of viable bacteria in dentinal tubules treated with clindamycin or tetracycline. Oral Surgery, Oral Medicine, Oral Pathology, Oral Radiology, Endodontics 2003;96:751–756.

56. Sato I, Ando-Kurihara N, Kota K, et al. Sterilization of infected root-canal dentine by topical application of a mixture of ciprofloxacin, metronidazole and minocycline in situ. International Endodontic Journal 1996;29: 118–124.

57. Sato T, Hoshino E, Uematsu H, Noda T. In vitro antimicrobial susceptibility to combinations of drugs on bacteria from carious

and endodontic lesions of human deciduous teeth. Oral Microbiology and Immunology 1993;8:172–176.

58. Banchs F, Trope M. Revascularization of immature permanent teeth with apical periodontitis: new treatment protocol? Journal of Endodontics 2004;30:196–200.

59. Huang GT. A paradigm shift in endodontic management of immature teeth: conservation of stem cells for regeneration. Journal of Dentistry 2008;36: 379–386.

60. Windley W 3rd, Teixeira F, Levin L, et al. Disinfection of immature teeth with a triple antibiotic paste. Journal of Endodontics 2005;31:439–443.

61. Strange DM, Seale NS, Nunn ME, Strange M. Outcome of formocresol/ZOE sub-base pulpotomies utilizing alternative radiographic success criteria. Pediatric Dentistry 2001;23: 331–336.

62. Casas MJ, Kenny DJ, Judd PL, Johnston DHl. Do we still need formocresol in pediatric dentistry? Journal of the Canadian Dental Association 2005;71:749–751.

63. Hand RE, Smith ML, Harrison JW. Analysis of the effect of dilution on the necrotic tissue dissolution property of sodium hypochlorite. Journal of Endodontics 1978;4:60–64.

64. Moorer WR, Wesselink PR. Factors promoting the tissue dissolving capability of sodium hypochlorite. International Endodontic Journal 1982;15: 187–196.

65. Rubin LM, Skobe Z, Krakow AA, Gron P. The effect of instrumentation and flushing of freshly extracted teeth in endodontic therapy: a scanning electron microscope study. Journal of Endodontics 1979;5: 328–335.

66. Becker GL, Cohen S, Borer R. The sequelae of accidentally injecting sodium hypochlorite beyond the root apex. Oral Surgery, Oral Medicine, Oral Pathology 1974;38:633–638.

67. Melker KB, Vertucci FJ, Rojas MF, Progulske-Fox A, Bélanger M. Antimicrobial efficacy of medicated root canal filling materials. Journal of Endodontics 2006;32:148–151.

68. Podbielski A, Boeckh C, Haller B. Growth inhibitory activity of gutta-percha points containing root canal medications on common endodontic bacterial pathogens as determined by an optimized quantitative in vitro assay. Journal of Endodontics 2000;26:398–403.

69. Taylor GN, Madonia JV, Wood NK, Heuer MA. In vivo autoradiographic study of relative penetrating abilities of aqueous 2% parachlorophenol and camphorated 35% parachlorophenol. Journal of Endodontics 1977;2:81–86.

70. Hasselgren G, Reit C. Emergency pulpotomy: pain relieving effect with and without the use of sedative dressings. Journal of Endodontics 1989;15:254–256.

71. Hume WR. The pharmacologic and toxicological properties of zinc oxide-eugenol. Journal of the American Dental Association 1986;113:789–791.

72. Jolkovsky DL, Waki MY, Newman MG, et al. Clinical and microbiological effects of subgingival and gingival marginal irrigation with chlorhexidine gluconate. Journal of Periodontology 1990;61: 663–669.

73. Heling I, Sommer M, Steinberg D, et al. Microbiological evaluation of the efficacy of chlorhexidine in a sustained-release device for dentine sterilization. International Endodontic Journal 1992;25: 15–19.

74. Heling I, Steinberg D, Kenig S, et al. Efficacy of a sustained-release device containing chlorhexidine and Ca(OH)2 in preventing secondary infection of dentinal tubules. International Endodontic Journal 1992;25: 20–24.

75. Jeansonne MJ, White RR. A comparison of 2.0% chlorhexidine gluconate and

5.25% sodium hypochlorite as antimicrobial endodontic irrigants. Journal of Endodontics 1994;20:276–278.

76. Ørstavik D, Haapasalo M. Disinfection by endodontic irrigants and dressings of experimentally infected dentinal tubules. Endodontics and Dental Traumatology 1990;6:142–149.

77. Vahdaty A, Pitt Ford TR, Wilson RF. Efficacy of chlorhexidine in disinfecting dentinal tubules in vitro. Endodontics and Dental Traumatology 1993;9:243–248.

78. Kuruvilla JR, Kamath MP. Antimicrobial activity of 2.5% sodium hypochlorite and 0.2% chlorhexidine gluconate separately and combined, as endodontic irrigants. Journal of Endodontics 1998;24: 472–476.

79. Sathorn C, Parashos P, Messer H. Antibacterial efficacy of calcium hydroxide intracanal dressing: a systematic review and meta-analysis. International Endodontic Journal 2007;40: 2–10.

80. Athanassiadis B, Abbott PV, Walsh LJ. The use of calcium hydroxide, antibiotics and biocides as antimicrobial medicaments in endodontics. Australian Dental Journal 2007;52(Suppl. 1):S64–S82.

81. Foreman PC, Barnes IE. Review of calcium hydroxide. International Endodontic Journal 1990;23:283–297.

82. Fava LR, Saunders WP. Calcium hydroxide pastes: classification and clinical indications. International Endodontic Journal 1999;32:257–282.

83. Siqueira JF Jr, De Uzeda M. Intracanal medicaments: evaluation of the antibacterial effects of chlorhexidine, metronidazole, and calcium hydroxide associated with three vehicles. Journal of Endodontics 1997;23:167–169.

84. Byström A, Claesson R, Sundqvist G. The antibacterial effect of camphorated paramonochlorophenol, camphorated phenol and calcium hydroxide in the treatment of infected root canals. Endodontics and Dental Traumatology 1985;1:170–175.

85. de Souza-Filho FJ, Soares Ade J, Vianna ME, et al. Antimicrobial effect and pH of chlorhexidine gel and calcium hydroxide alone and associated with other materials. Brazilian Dental Journal 2008;19:28–33.

86. Weiss M. Pulp capping in older patients. New York State Dental Journal 1966;32:451–457.

87. Eda S, Kawakami T, Hasegawa H et al. Clinico-pathological studies on the healing of periapical tissues in aged patients by root canal filling using pastes of calcium hydroxide added iodoform. Gerodontics 1985;1: 98–104.

88. Gomes BP, Vianna ME, Sena NT et al. In vitro evaluation of the antimicrobial activity of calcium hydroxide combined with chlorhexidine gel used as intracanal medicament. Oral Surgery, Oral Medicine, Oral Pathology, Oral Radiology, Endodontics 2006;102:44–50.

89. Sirén EK, Haapasalo MP, Waltimo TM, Ørstavik D. In vitro antibacterial effect of calcium hydroxide combined with chlorhexidine or iodine potassium iodide on Enterococcus faecalis. European Journal of Oral Sciences 2004;112:326–331.

90. Waltimo TM, Ørstavik D, Sirén EK, Haapasalo MP. In vitro susceptibility of Candida albicans to four disinfectants and their combinations. International Endodontic Journal 1999;32: 421–429.

91. Byström A, Sundqvist G. Bacteriological evaluation of the effect of 0.5 percent sodium hypochlorite in endodontic therapy. Oral Surgery, Oral Medicine, Oral Pathology 1983;55:307–312.

92. Byström A, Happonen RP, Sjögren U, Sundqvist G. Healing of periapical lesions of pulpless teeth after endodontic treatment with controlled asepsis. Endodontics and Dental Traumatology 1987;3:58–63.

93. Haapasalo M, Ørstavik D. In vitro infection and disinfection of dentinal tubules. Journal of Dental Research 1987;66: 1375–1379.

94. Waltimo TM, Siren EK, Ørstavik D, Haapasalo MP. Susceptibility of oral Candida species to calcium hydroxide in vitro. International Endodontic Journal 1999;32:94–98.

95. Pitt Ford TR. The effects on the periapical tissues of bacterial contamination of the filled root canal. International Endodontic Journal 1982;15:16–22.

96. Haapasalo M, Qian W, Portenier I, Waltimo T. Effects of dentin on the antimicrobial properties of endodontic medicaments. Journal of Endodontics 2007;33: 917–925.

97. Byström A, Sundqvist G. The antibacterial action of sodium hypochlorite and EDTA in 60 cases of endodontic therapy. International Endodontic Journal 1985;18:35–40.

98. Siqueira JF Jr, Guimarães-Pinto T, Rôças IN. Effects of chemomechanical preparation with 2.5% sodium hypochlorite and intracanal medication with calcium hydroxide on cultivable bacteria in infected root canals. Journal of Endodontics 2007;33: 800–805.

99. Sjögren U, Figdor D, Spångberg L, Sundqvist G. The antimicrobial effect of calcium hydroxide as a short-term intracanal dressing. International Endodontic Journal 1991;24:119–125.

100. Sjögren U, Sundqvist G. Bacteriologic evaluation of ultrasonic root canal instrumentation. Oral Surgery, Oral Medicine, Oral Pathology 1987;63:366–370.

101. Garcez AS, Nunez SC, Lage-Marques JL, et al. Photonic real-time monitoring of bacterial reduction in root canals by genetically engineered bacteria after chemomechanical endodontic therapy. Brazilian Dental Journal 2007;18:202–207.

102. Ørstavik D, Kerekes K, Molven O. Effects of extensive apical

reaming and calcium hydroxide dressing on bacterial infection during treatment of apical periodontitis: a pilot study. International Endodontic Journal 1991;24:1–7.

103. Peters LB, van Winkelhoff AJ, Buijs JF, Wesselink PR. Effects of instrumentation, irrigation and dressing with calcium hydroxide on infection in pulpless teeth with periapical bone lesions. International Endodontic Journal 2002;35:13–21.

104. Sirtes G, Waltimo T, Schaetzle M, Zehnder M. The effects of temperature on sodium hypochlorite short-term stability, pulp dissolution capacity, and antimicrobial efficacy. Journal of Endodontics 2005;31:669–671.

105. Wang CS, Arnold RR, Trope M, Teixeira FB. Clinical efficiency of 2% chlorhexidine gel in reducing intracanal bacteria. Journal of Endodontics 2007;33: 1283–1289.

106. Cvek M, Hollender L, Nord CE. Treatment of non-vital permanent incisors with calcium hydroxide. Odontologisk Revy 1976;27: 93–108.

107. Safavi KE, Dowden WE, Introcaso JH, Langeland K. A comparison of antimicrobial effects of calcium hydroxide and iodine-potassium iodide. Journal of Endodontics 1985;11:454–456.

108. Barthel CR, Zimmer S, Zilliges S, et al. In situ antimicrobial effectiveness of chlorhexidine and calcium hydroxide: gel and paste versus gutta-percha points. Journal of Endodontics 2002;28: 427–430.

109. Siqueira JF Jr, Magalhães KM, Rôças IN. Bacterial reduction in infected root canals treated with 2.5% NaOCl as an irrigant and calcium hydroxide/camphorated paramonochlorophenol paste as an intracanal dressing. Journal of Endodontics 2007;33:667–672.

110. Friedman S. Expected Outcomes in the Prevention and Treatment of Apical Periodontitis. In: Ørstavik D, Pitt Ford TR, editors. Essential Endodontology. 2nd edn. Oxford, UK: Blackwell Munksgaard; 2008. p. 402–463.

111. Penesis VA, Fitzgerald PI, Fayad MI, et al. Outcome of one-visit and two-visit endodontic treatment of necrotic teeth with apical periodontitis: a randomized controlled trial with one-year evaluation. Journal of Endodontics 2008;34: 251–257.

112. Sathorn C, Parashos P, Messer HH. Effectiveness of single-versus multiple-visit endodontic treatment of teeth with apical periodontitis: a systematic review and meta-analysis. International Endodontic Journal 2005;38: 347–355.

113. Sjögren U, Figdor D, Persson S, Sundqvist G. Influence of infection at the time of root filling on the outcome of endodontic treatment of teeth with apical periodontitis. International Endodontic Journal 1997;30:297–306.

114. Trope M, Delano EO, Ørstavik D. Endodontic treatment of teeth with apical periodontitis: single vs. multivisit treatment. Journal of Endodontics 1999;25: 345–350.

115. Nair PN, Henry S, Cano V, Vera J. Microbial status of apical root canal system of human mandibular first molars with primary apical periodontitis after 'one-visit' endodontic treatment. Oral Surgery, Oral Medicine, Oral Pathology, Oral Radiology, Endodontics 2005;99:231–252.

116. Silveira AM, Lopes HP, Siqueira JF Jr, et al. Periradicular repair after two-visit endodontic treatment using two different intracanal medications compared to single-visit endodontic treatment. Brazilian Dental Journal 2007;18:299–304.

117. Law A, Messer H. An evidence-based analysis of the antibacterial effectiveness of intracanal medicaments. Journal of Endodontics 2004;30:689–694.

118. Eriksen HM, Ørstavik D, Kerekes K. Healing of apical periodontitis after endodontic treatment using three different root canal sealers. Endodontics and Dental Traumatology 1988;4:114–117.

119. Dylewski JJ. Apical closure of nonvital teeth. Oral Surgery, Oral Medicine, Oral Pathology 1971;32:82–89.

120. Cvek M, Sundström B. Treatment of non-vital permanent incisors with calcium hydroxide. V. Histologic appearance of roentgenographically demonstrable apical closure of immature roots. Odontologisk Revy 1974;25:379–391.

121. Sheehy EC, Roberts GJ. Use of calcium hydroxide for apical barrier formation and healing in non-vital immature permanent teeth: a review. British Dental Journal 1997;183:241–246.

122. Kirk EE, Lim KC, Khan MO. A comparison of dentinogenesis on pulp capping with calcium hydroxide in paste and cement form. Oral Surgery, Oral Medicine, Oral Pathology 1989;68:210–219.

123. Roberts HW, Toth JM, Berzins DW, Charlton DG. Mineral trioxide aggregate material use in endodontic treatment: a review of the literature. Dental Materials 2008;24:149–164.

124. Hahn CL, Falkler WA, Minah GE. Correlation between thermal sensitivity and micro-organisms isolated from deep carious dentin. Journal of Endodontics 1993;19:26–30.

125. Hashioka K, Suzuki K, Yoshida T, et al. Relationship between clinical symptoms and enzyme-producing bacteria isolated from infected root canals. Journal of Endodontics 1994;20:75–77.

126. Hashioka K, Yamasaki M, Nakane A, et al. The relationship between clinical symptoms and anaerobic bacteria from infected root canals. Journal of Endodontics 1992;18:558–561.

127. Sassone LM, Fidel RA, Faveri M, et al. A microbiological profile of symptomatic teeth with primary endodontic infections. Journal of Endodontics 2008;34:541–545.

128. Siqueira JF Jr, Rôças IN, Rosado AS. Investigation of bacterial communities associated with asymptomatic and symptomatic endodontic infections by denaturing gradient gel

electrophoresis fingerprinting approach. Oral Microbiology and Immunology 2004;19: 363–370.

129. Skidmore AE. Pain of dental origin. Clinical Journal of Pain 1991;7:192–204.

130. Chávez de Paz Villanueva LE. Fusobacterium nucleatum in endodontic flare-ups. Oral Surgery, Oral Medicine, Oral Pathology, Oral Radiology, Endodontics 2002;93:179–183.

131. Mor C, Rotstein I, Friedman S. Incidence of interappointment emergency associated with endodontic therapy. Journal of Endodontics 1992;18:509–511.

132. Sim CK. Endodontic interappointment emergencies in a Singapore private practice setting: a retrospective study of incidence and cause-related factors. Singapore Dental Journal 1997;22:22–27.

133. Mohorn S, Maixner W, Fillingim R, et al. Effect of psychological factors on preoperative and postoperative endodontic pain. Journal of Dental Research 1995;74:43 (Abstract 254).

134. Schweinhardt P, Loggia ML, Villemure C, Bushnell MC. Psychological State and Pain Perception. In: Sessle BJ, Lavigne GJ, Lund JP, Dubner R, editors. Orofacial Pain: From Basic Science to Clinical Management. 2nd edn. Chicago, Il, USA: Quintessence; 2008.

135. Oguntebi BR, DeSchepper EJ, Taylor TS, et al. Postoperative pain incidence related to the type of emergency treatment of symptomatic pulpitis. Oral Surgery, Oral Medicine, Oral Pathology 1992;73:479–483.

136. Tammaro S, Berggren U, Bergenholtz G. Representation of verbal pain descriptors on a visual analogue scale by dental patients and dental students. European Journal of Oral Sciences 1997;105:207–212.

137. Torabinejad M, Cymerman JJ, Frankson M, et al. Effectiveness of various medications on postoperative pain following complete instrumentation.

Journal of Endodontics 1994;20:345–354.

138. Fava LR. Human pulpectomy: incidence of postoperative pain using two different intracanal dressings. International Endodontic Journal 1992;25:257–260.

139. Rogers MJ, Johnson BR, Remeikis NA, BeGole EA. Comparison of effect of intracanal use of ketorolac tromethamine and dexamethasone with oral ibuprofen on post treatment endodontic pain. Journal of Endodontics 1999;25:381–384.

140. Sathorn C, Parashos P, Messer H. The prevalence of postoperative pain and flare-up in single- and multiple-visit endodontic treatment: a systematic review. International Endodontic Journal 2008;41:91–99.

141. Trope M. Relationship of intracanal medicaments to endodontic flare-ups. Endodontics and Dental Traumatology 1990;6:226–229.

142. Abbott PV. Medicaments: aids to success in endodontics. Part 2. Clinical recommendations. Australian Dental Journal 1990;35:491–496.

143. Ehrmann EH, Messer HH, Clark RM. Flare-ups in endodontics and their relationship to various medicaments. Australian Endodontic Journal 2007;33:119–130.

144. Abbott PV. Systemic release of corticosteroids following intra-dental use. International Endodontic Journal 1992;25:189–191.

145. Andreasen JO, Andreasen F. Root resorption following traumatic dental injuries. Proceedings of the Finnish Dental Society 1992;88:95–114.

146. Donaldson M, Kinirons MJ. Factors affecting the time of onset of resorption in avulsed and replanted incisor teeth in children. Dental Traumatology 2001;17:205–209.

147. Flores MT, Andersson L, Andreasen JO, et al. International Association of Dental Traumatology. Guidelines for the management of traumatic dental

injuries. I. Fractures and luxations of permanent teeth. Dental Traumatology 2007;23:66–71.

148. Flores MT, Andersson L, Andreasen JO, et al. International Association of Dental Traumatology. Guidelines for the management of traumatic dental injuries. II. Avulsion of permanent teeth. Dental Traumatology 2007;23:130–136.

149. Lengheden A, Blomlöf L, Lindskog S. Effect of delayed calcium hydroxide treatment on periodontal healing in contaminated replanted teeth. Scandinavian Journal of Dental Research 1991;99:147–153.

150. Trope M. Clinical management of the avulsed tooth. Dental Clinics of North America 1995;39:93–112.

151. Pierce A, Heithersay G, Lindskog S. Evidence for direct inhibition of dentinoclasts by a corticosteroid/antibiotic endodontic paste. Endodontics and Dental Traumatology 1988;4:44–45.

152. Chen H, Teixeira FB, Ritter AL et al. The effect of intracanal anti-inflammatory medicaments on external root resorption of replanted dog teeth after extended extra-oral dry time. Dental Traumatology 2008;24:74–78.

153. Pierce A, Lindskog S. The effect of an antibiotic/corticosteroid paste on inflammatory root resorption in vivo. Oral Surgery, Oral Medicine, Oral Pathology 1987;64:216–220.

154. Pierce A, Berg JO, Lindskog S. Calcitonin as an alternative therapy in the treatment of root resorption. Journal of Endodontics 1988;14:459–464.

155. Abbott PV, Hume WR, Heithersay GS. The release and diffusion through human coronal dentine in vitro of triamcinolone and demeclocycline from Ledermix paste. Endodontics and Dental Traumatology 1989;5:92–97.

156. Ciarlone AE, Pashley DH. Medication of the dental pulp: a review and proposals. Endodontics and Dental Traumatology 1992;8:1–5.

157. Tronstad L, Andreasen JO, Hasselgren G, et al. pH changes in dental tissues after root canal filling with calcium hydroxide. Journal of Endodontics 1981;7: 17–21.

158. Abbott PV, Hume WR, Heithersay GS. Barriers to diffusion of Ledermix paste in radicular dentine. Endodontics and Dental Traumatology 1989;5:98–104.

159. Molven O, Olsen I, Kerekes K. Scanning electron microscopy of bacteria in the apical part of root canals in permanent teeth with periapical lesions. Endodontics and Dental Traumatology 1991;7:226–229.

160. Nair PN, Luder HU. Wurzelkanal und periapikale Flora: eine licht- und elektronenmikroskopische Untersuchung. Schweizerische Monatsschrift fur Zahnmedizin 1985;95:992–1003.

161. Wesley DJ, Marshall FJ, Rosen S. The quantitation of formocresol as a root canal medicament. Oral Surgery, Oral Medicine, Oral Pathology 1970;29:603–612.

162. Teixeira FB, Levin LG, Trope M. Investigation of pH at different dentinal sites after placement of calcium hydroxide dressing by two methods. Oral Surgery, Oral Medicine, Oral Pathology, Oral Radiology, Endodontics 2005;99:511–516.

163. Pashley DH, Kalathoor S, Burnham D. The effects of calcium hydroxide on dentin permeability. Journal of Dental Research 1986;65:417–420.

164. Haapasalo HK, Siren EK, Waltimo TM, et al. Inactivation of local root canal medicaments by dentine: an in vitro study. International Endodontic Journal 2000;33:126–131.

165. Guignes P, Faure J, Maurette A. Relationship between endodontic preparations and human dentin permeability measured in situ. Journal of Endodontics 1996;22: 60–67.

166. Saleh IM, Ruyter IE, Haapasalo M, Ørstavik D. Bacterial penetration along different root canal filling materials in the presence or absence of smear layer. International Endodontic Journal 2008;41:32–40.

167. Nunn JH, Smeaton I, Gilroy J. The development of formocresol as a medicament for primary molar pulpotomy procedures. ASDC Journal of Dentistry for Children 1996;63:51–53.

168. Ørstavik D. Endodontic materials. Advances in Dental Research 1988;2:12–24.

169. Hülsmann M, Hahn W. Complications during root canal irrigation—literature review and case reports. International Endodontic Journal 2000;33: 186–193.

170. Schröder U, Granath LE. Early reaction of intact human teeth to calcium hydroxide following experimental pulpotomy and its significance to the development of hard tissue barrier. Odontologisk Revy 1971;22: 379–396.

171. Bramante CM, Luna-Cruz SM, Sipert CR, et al. Alveolar mucosa necrosis induced by utilisation of calcium hydroxide as root canal dressing. International Dental Journal 2008;58:81–85.

172. Yared GM, Dagher FE. Influence of apical enlargement on bacterial infection during treatment of apical periodontitis. Journal of Endodontics 1994;20: 535–537.

173. Coldero LG, McHugh S, MacKenzie D, Saunders WP. Reduction in intracanal bacteria during root canal preparation with and without apical enlargement. International Endodontic Journal 2002;35: 437–446.

174. Aydin C, Tunca YM, Senses Z, et al. Bacterial reduction by extensive versus conservative root canal instrumentation in vitro.

Acta Odontologica Scandinavica 2007;65:167–170.

175. Dalton BC, Ørstavik D, Phillips C, et al. Bacterial reduction with nickel-titanium rotary instrumentation. Journal of Endodontics 1998;24:763–767.

176. Shuping GB, Ørstavik D, Sigurdsson A, Trope M. Reduction of intracanal bacteria using nickel-titanium rotary instrumentation and various medications. Journal of Endodontics 2000;26:751–755.

177. Basrani BR, Manek S, Sodhi RN, et al. Interaction between sodium hypochlorite and chlorhexidine gluconate. Journal of Endodontics 2007;33:966–969.

178. Bui TB, Baumgartner JC, Mitchell JC. Evaluation of the interaction between sodium hypochlorite and chlorhexidine gluconate and its effect on root dentin. Journal of Endodontics 2008;34: 181–185.

179. Zerella JA, Fouad AF, Spångberg LS. Effectiveness of a calcium hydroxide and chlorhexidine digluconate mixture as disinfectant during retreatment of failed endodontic cases. Oral Surgery, Oral Medicine, Oral Pathology, Oral Radiology, Endodontics 2005;100:756–761.

180. Mayer T, Eickholz P. Microleakage of temporary restorations after thermocycling and mechanical loading. Journal of Endodontics 1977;23: 320–322.

181. Scotti R, Ciocca L, Baldissara P. Microleakage of temporary endodontic restorations in overdenture tooth abutments. International Journal of Prosthodontics 2002;15:479–482.

182. Beach CW, Calhoun JC, Bramwell JD, et al. Clinical evaluation of bacterial leakage of endodontic temporary filling materials. Journal of Endodontics 1996;22: 459–462.

Chapter | 9 |

Root canal filling

N.P. Chandler

SUMMARY

Over the past decade several newer root canal filling materials have been introduced, the focus being to improve on the perceived deficiencies of gutta-percha and to achieve savings in both time and cost. Most of these developments aimed to replace gutta-percha with a variety of new resins as the core filling material. Newer root canal sealers have also been introduced to complement these systems. Gutta-percha and the newer core materials are now made to match the size and taper of modern root canal preparation instruments. Single-cone, matched root fillings may provide an acceptable result in carefully selected cases. Mineral Trioxide Aggregate is finding an increasing role as a root canal filling material, following its successful application in immature teeth. The ideal root canal filling material is yet to be developed and some root canal shapes remain challenging to fill irrespective of the method used. The aim of this chapter is to describe the fundamental principles of canal filling using gutta-percha and to provide a brief overview of relevant alternative methods.

INTRODUCTION

The entire root canal system should be filled following cleaning and shaping. The objectives of root canal filling are:

© 2009 Elsevier Ltd, Inc, BV
DOI: 10.1016/B978-0-7020-3156-4.00012-7

1. To prevent microorganisms which remain in the root canal system after preparation from proliferating and passing into the periapical tissues via the apical foramen and other pathways.
2. To seal the pulp chamber and root canal system from leakage via the coronal restoration in order to prevent passage of microorganisms and/or toxins along the root canal and into the periapical tissues via the apical foramen and other pathways.
3. To prevent percolation of periapical exudate and possibly microorganisms into the pulp space via the apical foramen and other pathways.
4. To prevent percolation of gingival exudate and microorganisms into the pulp space via lateral/furcation canals opening into the gingival sulcus or through exposed, patent dentinal tubules around the neck of the tooth.

The quality of the root canal filling depends on the complexity of the root canal system, the efficacy of canal preparation, the materials and techniques employed, and the skill and experience of the operator. Filling of the canal does not represent the end of root canal treatment, as restoration of the clinical crown to prevent leakage of fluids and oral microorganisms into the pulp space is critical to long-term success.[1] There is mounting evidence that the quality of the coronal seal affects the prognosis of root canal treatment.[2]

Many materials and techniques have been used to fill root canals.[3] The current material of choice is gutta-percha combined with a sealer, because it is versatile and can be used in a variety of techniques.

CANAL ANATOMY

Pulp anatomy is complex with many root canals having apical deltas, lateral canals and other aberrations; accessory canals, fins, and anastomoses are not uncommon, especially in posterior teeth. These, together with the consequences of physiological and pathological dentine deposition and procedural problems during canal preparation, present challenges. The inherent anatomy of the root canal system has a major influence on the techniques used to fill canals and on the quality of the final result.

ACCESS AND CANAL PREPARATION

The aims of preparation are to clean and shape the root canal system. Access and preparation have been discussed in Chapters 4 and 7 respectively. It should be emphasized that time and care spent during access and canal preparation will facilitate root canal filling. As well as removing microorganisms and debris from the root canal system, preparation produces the desired canal shape to receive the root filling. Cleaning of the canal may be achieved

with irrigants and minimal removal of dentine from canal walls. However, achieving the correct canal shape invariably requires additional effort to create the flowing, flared preparation demanded by most root canal filling techniques. Inappropriate access and root canal preparation can leave microorganisms, pulpal remnants and dentine debris within the root canal system. These will, invariably, affect proper adaptation of the root filling to the canal walls, and the physical properties of the sealer will determine the effectiveness of the seal produced. Furthermore, creation of an inappropriate canal shape will make it difficult to introduce root filling materials along the length of the canal, resulting in a poorly condensed filling with voids. Thus, the ability to fill canals predictably is, significantly, dependent on the adequacy of access and the quality of the root canal preparation.

The method of root canal filling will be dictated by the preparation technique and the shaping objectives. Some operators prefer to create an apical stop at the dentine-cementum junction where a natural apical constriction is believed to exist; in this way instrumentation does not extend beyond the apical foramen.[4] With this shape of canal, the filling technique of choice is cold lateral condensation of gutta-percha. Other operators create a continuously tapering canal shape where the smallest diameter is at the foramen.[5] With this shape, a variety of warm gutta-percha techniques are more appropriate; the lack of an apical stop will predispose the master gutta-percha cone, used in lateral condensation, to being distorted and pushed beyond the foramen when a spreader is introduced.

CRITERIA FOR FILLING

Root canal filling is often delayed for one or more visits following preparation to allow interappointment medicaments placed in the canal to act on the microbial flora and for signs and symptoms to resolve.[6,7] Unfortunately, delaying root canal filling may lead to loss of, or microleakage, through provisional restorations. Also, all medicaments have limited antimicrobial activity[7] and duration of effectiveness. Under the right circumstances, modern root canal preparation techniques are effective in eliminating microorganisms so in selected cases root canal preparation and filling may be completed in one visit.

The decision as to when to fill root canals is controversial and debatable. Advocates for immediate filling of canals following preparation believe that their regimen for eliminating microorganisms by preparing a continuously tapering canal shape[5] and the extensive use of sodium hypochlorite and ethylenediaminetetraacetic acid (EDTA) or alternative irrigation is effective. It was argued that the root canal system is likely to be sufficiently cleared of microorganisms and substrate to allow filling to proceed immediately.[8] Meanwhile, there is strong evidence that delaying root canal filling and the use of an intracanal medicament will reduce the microbial population further[9] and enhance the long-term outcome, particularly if the root canal is infected. It will encourage more rapid resolution of apical periodontitis and an improved prognosis.[10,11] To further confuse the issue, there is research reporting no difference between the outcome of one-visit or two-visit root canal treatment incorporating calcium hydroxide medication.[12]

Logically, teeth with non-infected pulps and no sign of apical periodontitis can be prepared and filled in one visit, whereas infected cases with apical periodontitis should be treated cautiously, with additional appointments to allow an intracanal medicament to further reduce the microbial population. Unfortunately, research in this area is difficult and time-consuming and so far, a definitive answer is lacking.[13] Irrespective of the number of treatment visits, it is essential that the root canal can be thoroughly dried prior to filling, otherwise it will influence the effectiveness of the seal.

MATERIALS USED TO FILL ROOT CANALS

Many materials have been used to fill root canals. Historically, these range from feathers and wood sticks through a range of precious metals to amalgam and dental cements. The requirements for a root canal filling material have been specified for many years.[14] A large number of materials have proved to be inadequate, impractical or biologically unacceptable.

SEALERS

A root canal sealer (cement) is used in combination with the core root canal filling material, e.g. gutta-percha. The primary role of the sealer is to obliterate the irregularities between the root canal wall and the core material. Almost all of today's root canal filling techniques use a sealer to enhance the seal of the root canal filling.[15]

Root canal sealers are used for the following purposes:

- cementing (luting, binding) the core material to the canal
- filling the discrepancies between the root canal walls and core material
- acting as a lubricant
- acting as an antimicrobial agent
- acting as a marker for accessory canals, resorptive defects, root fractures and other spaces into which the main core material may not penetrate.

The requirements and characteristics of an ideal sealer are:[16]

- non-irritating to periapical tissues
- insoluble in tissue fluids
- dimensionally stable
- hermetic sealing ability
- radiopaque
- bacteriostatic
- sticky and good adhesion to canal wall when set
- easily mixed
- non-staining to dentine
- good working time
- readily removable if necessary.

No current material satisfies all these requirements but many work well in clinical practice. As well as providing a satisfactory seal, it must be well tolerated by the periapical tissues and be relatively easy to handle. Sealers are toxic when freshly prepared;[17] however, their toxicity is reduced substantially after setting.[18] Thus, although sealers produce varying degrees of periapical inflammation, it is normally only temporary and depending on composition, it does not appear to prevent tissue healing.[19]

Most sealers are absorbed to some extent when exposed to tissue fluid,[20] so the volume of sealer must be kept to a minimum with the core material forming the bulk of the root filling. The core material should force the sealer into inaccessible areas and into irregularities along the root canal walls. Excess sealer should ideally flow backwards and into the access cavity, but some gutta-percha techniques tend to force sealer apically and laterally via the foramen and accessory canals.[21,22] The passage of sealer into the periapical tissues is not encouraged. However, there is equivocal evidence that it will reduce the success rate of treatment provided that canal preparation and filling have been performed with care. Clinical experience suggests that most excess sealer in the periapical region is absorbed with time but large volumes of extruded sealer must be avoided.

Sealers in use today can be divided into five groups based on their constituents:

- zinc oxide–eugenol sealers
- calcium hydroxide sealers
- resin sealers
- glass ionomer sealers
- silicone-based sealers.

Zinc oxide-eugenol sealers

Most of the zinc oxide-eugenol sealers are based on Grossman's formula.[23] Commercial products include Tubli-Seal (SybronEndo, Orange, CA, USA), Pulp Canal Sealer (SybronEndo) and Roth Sealer (Roth International Ltd, Chicago, IL, USA). Modified formulations with extended working times are also available.

Once set, zinc oxide-eugenol sealers are relatively weak and porous, and are susceptible to decomposition in tissue fluids, particularly when extruded into the periapical tissues.[24] All zinc oxide-eugenol cements are cytotoxic and the cellular response may last longer than those produced by other materials.[18] However, these problems are not usually apparent clinically, and zinc oxide-eugenol materials are, probably, the most commonly used sealers. The various zinc oxide-eugenol sealers have a range of setting times and flow characteristics so the choice of formulation is dependent on the case. Difficult canals that need some time to fill require a sealer with an extended working time. If heat is applied during root canal filling, its influence on the setting time of sealers should also be taken into account.

Calcium hydroxide sealers

Calcium hydroxide-based sealers have been developed on the assumption that they preserve the vitality of the pulp stump and stimulate healing and hard tissue formation at the apical wound. Laboratory research has demonstrated their sealing ability to be similar to zinc oxide-eugenol sealers[25] although it remains to be seen whether during long-term exposure to tissue fluids they maintain their integrity, since calcium hydroxide is soluble and may leach out and weaken the remaining cement.[24]

Commercial products include Sealapex (SybronEndo), a calcium hydroxide-containing polymeric resin, Apexit Plus (Ivoclar Vivadent, Schaan, Liechtenstein) and epoxy-based Acroseal (Septodont, Saint-Maur Cedex, France).

Resin-based sealers

Resin-based materials have been available for many years but they remain less popular than zinc oxide-eugenol sealers. The first resin sealer, AH 26 (Dentsply DeTrey, Konstanz, Germany), a powder and a liquid, consisted of an epoxy resin base which set slowly when mixed with an activator. It has good sealing[26] and adhesive properties, and antibacterial activity. However, it produces an initial severe inflammatory reaction[18] which subsides after some weeks and the material is then well tolerated by the periapical tissues. The resin has a strong allergenic and mutagenic potential[27] and cases of contact allergy and paraesthesia[28] have been reported. The material releases formaldehyde[29] which may explain its strong antibacterial effect.[30] AH 26 has largely been superseded by AH Plus (Dentsply DeTrey), a two paste system formulated to polymerize without the release of formaldehyde; this sealer is also marketed as TopSeal (Dentsply Maillefer, Ballaigues, Switzerland). AH Plus is also less cytotoxic, with a thinner film thickness and lower solubility.

EndoREZ (Ultradent, South Jordan, UT, USA) is a urethane dimethacrylate (UDMA) based resin sealer. It is recommended for use with EndoREZ points (Ultradent), methacrylate resin coated gutta-percha points so that there is bonding between the root filling, sealer and the root canal dentine. Other resin sealers include Hybrid Root SEAL (Sun Medical Co. Ltd., Moriyama City, Shiga, Japan) or MetaSEAL (Parkell, Edgewood, NY, USA), both of the same chemical formulation and based on 4-methacryloethyl trimellitate anhydride(4-META).

Glass ionomer sealers

The ability of glass ionomer cement to adhere to dentine would appear to provide a number of potential advantages over conventional sealers. Its endodontic potential was recognized soon after its introduction as a restorative material[31] but it was many years before a product for endodontic use was formulated. The results of a multicentre clinical trial evaluating its performance[32] suggested that it was similar to traditional sealers, but this sealer is no longer available.

Activ GP glass ionomer sealer (Brasseler, Savannah, Georgia, USA) was recently introduced for use with Activ GP points (Brasseler). The surface of these gutta-percha points is coated with glass ionomer. The sealer is meant to adhere chemically and micromechanically to the Activ GP points and also bond to the root canal dentine.

Silicone-based sealers

RoekoSeal (Coltène/Whaledent, Cuyahoga Falls, OH, USA) is a polydimethylsiloxane-based sealer. The manufacturer stated that this silicone-based sealer expands slightly on setting (0.2%) and is highly radiopaque; the claimed advantages include good sealing ability[33] and excellent biocompatibility.[34] However, in a histopathological study on periapical healing in dog's teeth, no differences were noted between RoekoSeal and AH Plus.[35]

GuttaFlow (Coltène/Whaledent), introduced in 2004, is a modification of RoekoSeal. GuttaFlow contains particles of gutta-percha less than 30 μm in size and and also expands slightly (0.2%) on curing according to the manufacturer. The material is considered to be almost insoluble. It is used with a single master gutta-percha cone, without mechanical compaction, although lateral or vertical condensation are acceptable. Its flow is significantly better into lateral grooves and depressions in the apical regions of root canals than lateral condensation or warm compaction with AH 26 sealer.[36] Its sealing qualities are similar to lateral compaction or the System B technique with AH 26.[37] All traces of irrigants must be thoroughly rinsed from the canal with water or isopropyl alcohol prior to introducing the material. GuttaFlow has a working time of 15 minutes and a setting time of about 30 minutes; GuttaFlow FAST has a 5 minute working time and a 10 minute set. A potential concern is extrusion of material beyond the apex[36,37] although its cytotoxicity is lower than some other sealers.

Calcium silicate-based sealers

An advantage with these, newer types of sealer is their potential bioactive property. Similar to other tricalcium silicate and dicalcium silicate-containing biomaterials, calcium hydroxide is produced on reaction with water. It is anticipated that release of calcium and hydroxyl ions from the set sealer will result in the formation of apatites as it comes into contact with phosphate-containing fluids.

ProRoot Endo sealer (Dentsply Tulsa Dental, Tulsa, OK, USA) is a calcium silicate-based endodontic sealer that is designed to be used in conjunction with a root filling material in either the cold lateral, warm vertical or carrier-based filling techniques. The major components of the powder are tricalcium silicate and dicalcium silicate, with the inclusion of calcium sulphate as a setting retardant, bismuth oxide as a radiopacifier and a small amount of tricalcium aluminate. The liquid component consists of a viscous aqueous solution of a water-soluble polymer (polyvinyl-pyrrolidone homopolymer). Other calcium silicate-based sealers on the market include iRoot SP sealer (Innovative Bioceramix Inc., Vancouver, BC, Canada) and Endosequence BC sealer (Brasseler); the same product marketed under different names in different countries.

SMEAR LAYER

The smear layer, comprising both organic and inorganic components, is found on the root canal walls after endodontic instrumentation.[38,39,40] It is composed largely of particulate dentine debris created by endodontic instruments during root canal preparation but also contains pulpal remnants and microorganisms. With further instrumentation the material is forced against the canal walls forming a friable and loosely adherent layer. The smear layer is typically 1–2 μm thick, although it can also be found within the dentinal tubules for up to 40 μm.[38]

The smear layer has received much attention, not only because it may harbour microorganisms already in the canal but it may create an avenue for leakage of microorganisms and act as a substrate for microbial proliferation. It may also be broken down by bacterial action[41] to provide a pathway for leakage. In addition, the smear layer has the potential to interfere with the adaptation of sealer against the root canal walls and prevent tubular penetration of sealer, thereby increasing the likelihood of leakage.[1,42] Indeed, it has been shown that most leakage occurs between the sealer and the wall of the root canal.[43]

Smear layer removal prior to filling would appear to be desirable as it would eliminate microorganisms and allow for better adaptation of sealer. However, this procedure has been questioned since opening the tubules might increase the diffusion of potentially irritant root filling materials through the tubules to the root surface,[44] allow microorganisms trapped in the tubules to escape[45] or to proliferate within the tubules and, potentially, increase leakage.[46] Nevertheless, the present consensus is that the removal of the smear layer is beneficial and desirable, particularly when treating infected teeth.

In laboratory studies, a number of methods have been shown to be effective in removing the smear layer.[40] The key method involves 17% EDTA as a chelating agent together with sodium hypochlorite to dissolve the organic component.[42]

GUTTA-PERCHA

Gutta-percha has been used to fill root canals for over 130 years and is the most widely used and accepted root filling material. Gutta-percha is a form of rubber obtained from tropical trees of the *Sapotaceae* family. It is a trans isomer of polyisoprene, which exists in two crystalline forms, the α- and β-phases. The α-phase occurs naturally and the β-phase arises during refining; the two are interchangeable depending on temperature. Gutta-percha is mixed with other materials to produce a blend that can be used effectively within the root canal. Commercial gutta-percha cones contain gutta-percha (19–22%), zinc oxide (59–75%), various waxes, colouring agents, antioxidants, and metal salts to provide radiopacity. There is considerable variation in the stiffness, brittleness and tensile strength of commercially available gutta-percha cones and obturating products.[47]

Gutta-percha cones are:

- inert
- dimensionally stable
- non-allergenic to almost all individuals
- antibacterial
- non-staining to dentine
- radiopaque
- compactible
- softened by heat
- softened by organic solvents
- removable from the root canal when necessary.

However, the disadvantages are:

- lack of rigidity
- do not adhere to dentine.

Canal filling with gutta-percha

The objective of root canal filling is to completely fill the canal system in an attempt to seal the canal from leakage apically and coronally. Gutta-percha is versatile and can be used in a variety of techniques, but a sealer is always necessary to cement the material to the canal wall and to fill minor irregularities.

Over the years, a large number of newer filling techniques have been described, accompanied by claims of greater efficacy, reduced leakage or time and money saving. Unfortunately, new does not necessarily mean better, and sadly there is little evidence from clinical trials to suggest that there are significant differences between root canal filling techniques and treatment outcome. Caution is required when considering newer filling techniques and it is prudent to wait for the published results of laboratory and clinical studies before investing in and learning a newer technique.

Methods for filling canals using gutta-percha can, broadly, be divided into three main groups:

- cold gutta-percha
- heat-softened gutta-percha
- solvent-softened gutta-percha.

Cold gutta-percha techniques

Cold gutta-percha techniques are relatively simple to master as they are not complicated by the need to soften the material with heat or solvents, hence they do not require expensive devices or equipment. However, cold gutta-percha cannot be effectively compacted into all the irregularities in a root canal system so this is the role of the sealer. Lateral condensation is the most popular method of root filling with cold gutta-percha.

Lateral condensation

With the advent of the standardized preparation technique,[48] the method of filling root canals with a single, full length gutta-percha cone and sealer became popular. The concept was simple and attractive; the root canal was prepared to a round cross-sectional shape of a standard size with reamers and filled with a gutta-percha cone of the same diameter. Unfortunately, a round canal shape was rarely achieved, especially in curved roots,[49,50] and the single cone required large amounts of sealer to fill the intervening gaps resulting in increased leakage.[51] It was also clear that discrepancies in size[52] and taper between gutta-percha cones and equivalent numbered instruments were prevalent. While many clinicians appreciated these problems and adopted other filling techniques, others continued to fill canals using this method (Fig. 9.1).

Current canal preparation techniques produce a flared canal with a flowing conical shape and cannot be filled adequately with a single 0.02 taper gutta-percha cone. Gutta-percha cones with ISO standardized tip sizes but with varying tapers, e.g. 0.04 or 0.06 tapers are available (Fig. 9.2). These cones with increased taper can fill funnel-shaped canals more effectively because they are more likely to correspond to the canal shape created by instruments with similar taper. In a laboratory study on curved canals, a single tapered cone technique has been found to be comparable with lateral condensation in terms of the

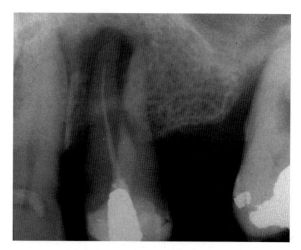

Figure 9.1 Maxillary left first premolar with a short, single cone filling in one canal and an untreated second canal.

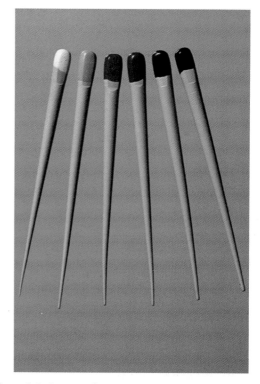

Figure 9.2 Gutta-percha cones, 0.06 taper with standardized 15–40 tip sizes.

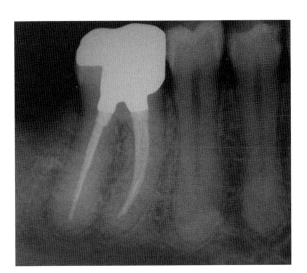

Figure 9.3 Mandibular right first molar. The mesial canals are filled with 0.04 taper, size 40 gutta-percha cones and the distal canal with a 0.06 taper, size 40 cone. Canal entrances covered with IRM and an amalgam intraradicular core for the coronal restoration. Reproduced courtesy of D Violich.

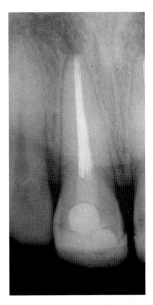

Figure 9.4 Maxillary central incisor filled with laterally condensed gutta-percha.

amount of gutta-percha occupying the root canal space; the technique is also faster than lateral condensation.[53] A clinical example shows radiographically acceptable results (Fig. 9.3).

Lateral condensation of cold gutta-percha is taught and practised throughout the world and is the technique of choice for many clinicians. It is simple and rapid to carry out. It can be used in virtually all cases where canal preparation results in an apical stop, and is the standard against which most newer techniques are compared (Fig. 9.4). Lateral condensation involves the placement of a master (primary) gutta-percha cone to the terminus of the preparation followed by placing additional (accessory) gutta-percha cones alongside (Fig. 9.5). The use of a standardized master cone provides the possibility of a predictable fit at the apex, while the accessory cones fill the intervening space, produced as a result of the flared canal shape. The root filling, therefore, consists of numerous cones cemented together and to the canal wall by sealer; there is no merging of the cones into a homogeneous mass of gutta-percha (Fig. 9.6). The technique is not recommended when the canal has no apical stop and files can easily pass through the foramen (when the canal has a continuous taper with the foramen being the narrowest).

A spreader is inserted alongside the master cone to improve its adaptation at the terminus of the preparation and to create the space for the accessory gutta-percha cones. When inserted to within 1 mm of the terminus to condense the master cone apically[54] and laterally, the

result will be considerably less leakage than if the spreader had only entered part of the way into the canal.[55] The need to advance the spreader well into the root canal is one of the main reasons why canals are flared. A narrow, parallel shape will not allow the spreader to influence the adaptation of the apical region of the master gutta-percha cone. Narrow canal preparations also risk removing the master gutta-percha cone when withdrawing the spreader, as it might pierce the cone instead of condensing the material.

The requirements for successful lateral condensation are:

- a flared canal preparation with an apical stop
- a well-fitting master gutta-percha cone
- speader/s of the appropriate size and shape
- accessory cones which match the dimensions of the spreader/s
- an appropriate sealer.

The master gutta-percha cone must fit to the full length of the preparation, be tight at the end-point of the canal preparation (ideally present some resistance to withdrawal or 'tug-back'), and it must not be able to pass through the foramen.

The size of the master gutta-percha cone should correspond to the master apical file used to prepare the apical stop. The selected gutta-percha cone is held with tweezers at the correct length, equivalent to the working distance and then inserted into the canal. Ideally, the gutta-percha cone should:

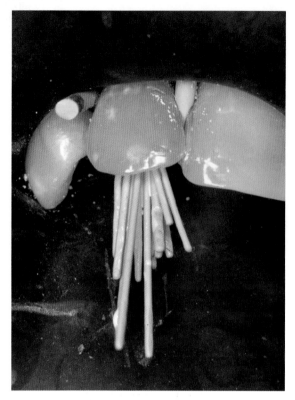

Figure 9.5 Maxillary lateral incisor with multiple gutta-percha cones in place during lateral condensation.

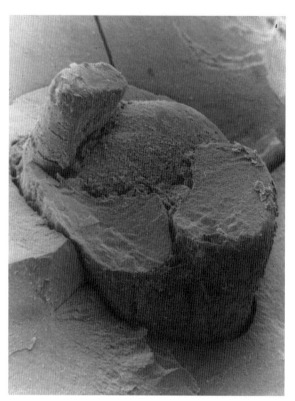

Figure 9.6 Scanning electron micrograph of a section of a root with laterally condensed gutta-percha in situ. Close adaptation of the cones to the wall of the canal and the limited space occupied by sealer or voids is evident. The circular cross section of the cones have been modified by spreader insertion.

- pass down to the full working distance
- be impossible to push beyond this depth or through the foramen
- fit tightly giving some resistance to withdrawal (tug-back).

The tweezers are squeezed slightly to mark the gutta-percha cone and the tweezers removed, leaving the cone in situ (Fig. 9.7). A radiograph may be taken to confirm the correct depth in relation to the terminus of the preparation and the radiographic apex. If the canal length is correctly estimated, the gutta-percha cone should be at the right depth and position, and the canal filling procedure can proceed. However, a number of problems can occur, either as a result of technical difficulties during canal preparation or because of size discrepancies in the gutta-percha cones and/or instruments. Most of these problems can be easily addressed but they require some thought to ensure that the exact problem is identified.

Gutta-percha cone reaches the working distance but is loose

This may occur for a number of reasons.

- The gutta-percha cone was smaller than expected. During manufacture, a tolerance of ±0.05 mm is allowed at d_1 so that it is possible for a gutta-percha cone with the correct nominal size to be smaller than the equivalent master apical file size and prepared canal width. The solution may be to remove 1 mm increments from the tip of the cone with a sharp scalpel blade to increase the tip diameter, or to select a larger gutta-percha cone.
- The end-point of preparation was wider than expected. Just as the size of cones may vary so can the size of files. The tolerance of files can be ±0.02 mm at d_1 so it is possible for the canal to be wider than anticipated. The solution to this problem is the same as that described above.

The canal can become wider than expected through inappropriate choice of instruments and/or preparation technique leading to the excessive removal of tooth tissue from the outer wall of the canal apically. If this is the problem, then either a selection of gutta-percha cones can be tried-in until one is found to fit or an alternative filling method chosen.

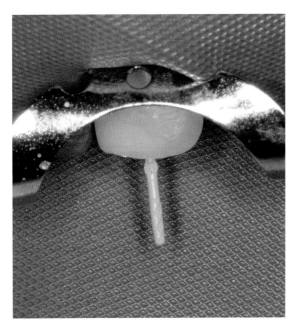

Figure 9.7 Master gutta-percha cone notched at working distance corresponding to the chosen incisal edge reference point.

- The canal was not widened sufficiently at the end-point or the canal taper was too narrow. This is a common problem and occurs when the master apical file is either smaller than its nominal size or, more likely, that it was not used sufficiently to widen the canal fully. In this way, either the apical dimensions of the canal are too small or the curved region of the canal is too narrow and causes the gutta-percha cone to bind. It is essential that the master apical file be manipulated until it can pass down freely to the termination of the preparation without the application of any undue force. With insufficient preparation it may be possible to force the master apical file to the working distance, but the gutta-percha cone will bind and buckle before reaching the expected length. The solution to this problem is to select a new file and reinstrument the canal to the working length until the file is loose. Increasing the taper along the length of the canal may also be necessary.
- Dentine debris is blocking the apical region of the canal, usually as a result of insufficient irrigation. Blockages are difficult to eliminate, so during canal preparation copious volumes of irrigant should be used and frequent recapitulation is necessary to ensure the canal is patent at the termination of the preparation. Passive ultrasonic irrigation may also be helpful to remove blockages.[56]

Gutta-percha cone passes beyond working distance or through foramen

This can occur when the apical stop is inadequate or when the gutta-percha cone is too small. If the stop is not sufficiently definite, then the cone will pass more deeply and through the foramen. The solution is either to reprepare the canal with larger instruments until a distinct stop is created at the end-point of preparation, or to remove 1 mm increments from the gutta-percha cone until its diameter is sufficient to bind in the canal at the working distance.

Gutta-percha cone does not reach the working distance

This is the most common problem with positioning of the master cone and there are a number of reasons:

- The gutta-percha cone was larger than expected. Just as gutta-percha cones can be smaller than the nominal size and appear loose, they can also be larger. Thus, if a cone is a short distance (<2 mm) away from the end-point of the preparation it may be possible to try a selection of cones of the same diameter to find one that fits.

Selection of spreaders and accessory gutta-percha cones

Once the master gutta-percha cone has been chosen, it is important to select and try-in the spreader to ensure that it can pass down the canal to within 1 mm of the termination of the preparation. Spreaders should be precurved in curved canals and a silicone stop used to mark the depth of insertion. Nickel-titanium spreaders, which are more flexible, are also available. To reduce the risk of root fracture due to excessive condensation pressures, finger rather than hand-held spreaders may be used.

Spreaders come in non-standardized or standardized 0.02 tapers, the same as for most hand files. Non-standardized spreaders have relatively small diameters at the tip but a range of tapers ranging from extra-fine through fine, medium to large; some manufacturers use letters rather than words to denote the degree of taper, e.g. A, B, C, D. Spreaders with a standardized taper are manufactured in a range of ISO diameters.

The choice of spreader design, that is, with non-standardized or standardized taper, and the type of accessory cones are determined by operator preference. When non-standardized spreaders are used the cones should also be non-standardized. However, standardized spreaders require standardized accessory gutta-percha cones. In this way, the cone will fill the space created by the corresponding spreader. The space created by a standardized spreader cannot be filled adequately with a non-standardized cone. It is also beneficial to use instruments and materials from the same manufacturer to ensure accurate sizing.

The size of the spreader, and thus cones, are determined by the size of the canal. Large canals with a substantial taper are more efficiently filled with larger taper cones, whilst smaller canals with narrower tapers should be filled with finer cones. On most occasions, an extra-fine or fine spreader is required along with matching accessory gutta-percha cones.

Completion of lateral condensation

1. The master gutta-percha cone, spreader, accessory gutta-percha cones and sealer should be organized to ensure they can be handled efficiently.
2. The canal should be dried thoroughly with paper points.
3. The sealer should be mixed and smeared onto the canal wall using either a hand file rotated anticlockwise, by coating a paper point and inserting it into the canal, or by coating the master cone itself. Large volumes of sealer introduced with motor driven devices are not necessary and may be hazardous.
4. The master cone should be 'buttered' lightly with sealer and then inserted immediately to the full working length.
5. The spreader is then placed alongside the gutta-percha cone and pushed apically with controlled force until it reaches the appropriate depth, 1 mm from the end-point of preparation. These forces can be considerable,[57] and the direction of force should be apical with no lateral action, which could risk root fracture. Apical pressure is applied in a constant manner for 10 to 20 seconds to compact the gutta-percha in an apical and lateral direction. In curved canals, the spreader may be precurved and applied either lateral to, or on the outer aspect of the master gutta-percha cone. It should not be applied along the inner aspect of the curve as it could pierce the cone and drag it out when the spreader is removed.
6. The first accessory gutta-percha cone is inserted into the space created by the spreader.
7. The spreader is then cleaned and reinserted immediately into the canal. It should not go down to the full working length.
8. The second accessory gutta-percha cone is inserted into the space created.
9. The sequence of spreader application and cone insertion continues until the canal is full, with the number of accessory cones required varying from canal to canal (Fig. 9.8). If a post-retained

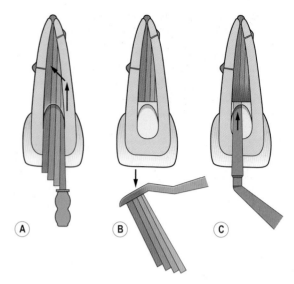

Figure 9.8 Cold lateral condensation. (A) After master gutta-percha cone fitted, accessory cones added and condensed until no longer space for spreader. (B) A heated instrument is used to sever the gutta percha cones and (C) vertically condensed (based on an original drawing by M Monteith).

restoration is planned, if desired, lateral condensation can cease when the apical 5–6 mm have been filled.

10. If the final coronal restoration is not post-retained, the excess gutta-percha emerging from the canal entrance should be removed with a hot instrument and condensed vertically with a plugger to promote a satisfactory seal. The gutta-percha should be reduced to below the gingival level, particularly in anterior teeth, in order to maintain the translucency of the crown and to prevent the possibility of sealer staining the dentine.[58] In all cases, having the root filling confined to well within the root and protected by suitable restorations will reduce the risk of microleakage.

When a post-retained restoration is planned gutta-percha can be removed immediately but carefully, leaving approximately 4–5 mm of apical root filling undisturbed.[59,60] Post space preparation at this stage is advantageous as the operator is very conscious of the anatomy and length of the canal. A rubber dam is already in place and the required length of post is easily assessed.

Lateral condensation is relatively simple to carry out, rapid, and has been used for many years with considerable success, even in quite demanding cases (Fig. 9.9). However, since it is impossible for cold gutta-percha to flow into all the irregularities in the root canal system, parts of the canal must either remain unfilled[61] or be filled only with

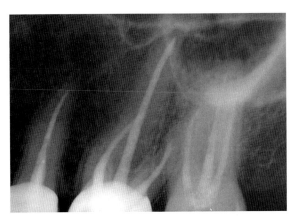

Figure 9.9 Three maxillary posterior teeth filled with laterally condensed gutta-percha. Condensation is insufficient in the palatal canal of the second molar.

sealer. The importance of cleaning anatomical irregularities in oval canals has been emphasized. Otherwise, they remain packed with debris and reduce the quality of the root filling;[61,62] canals which are this shape present a challenge for most obturation methods.[63]

Innovative means of obturation using gutta-percha aimed at reducing the time involved with lateral condensation include SimpliFill (Discus Dental, Culver City, CA, USA). A section of gutta-percha or Resilon (see later) is held at the end of the SimpliFill disposable delivery device, which is inserted into the canal to the desired depth. An apical plug of root filling is left inside the canal by twisting, to free the delivery device, which is then withdrawn; the remainder of the canal is then back-filled if required.

The perceived deficiencies of lateral condensation have resulted in the development of techniques in which gutta-percha is softened by heat or solvents so that the core material can be condensed into anatomical irregularities.[62] Some of these techniques are 'hybrids' which use the controllability and safety of cold lateral condensation in the apical region and heat-softening to fill the coronal two-thirds more quickly. Other techniques involve heat to soften the whole length of gutta-percha in the root canal.

Heat-softened gutta-percha techniques

For decades the only technique that used heat-softened gutta-percha was warm vertical condensation[64] but a number of innovative methods for warming and condensing gutta-percha are now available. In some, cold gutta-percha is placed in the canal and warmed in situ; these can be referred to as intracanal heating techniques. Others rely on warming gutta-percha outside and then delivering it into the canal, the extracanal heating techniques.

For canals prepared with an apical stop, lateral condensation of gutta-percha is an excellent and popular method of filling and the one best suited for most operators. The heat-softened techniques are technically more demanding for inexperienced and non-specialist operators, and caution is required. Practising on simulated canals in plastic blocks and on extracted teeth is very valuable and will aid familiarity.

Intracanal heating techniques

In these techniques, cold gutta-percha is placed in the canal and then heated to become soft and condensable. All the techniques involve the use of a sealer. The popularity of these methods was limited until Schilder[64] described his method for filling canals using warm vertical condensation.

Warm vertical condensation

The aim of the Schilder technique[64] is to fill the canal with heat-softened gutta-percha packed with sufficient vertical pressure to force it to flow into the entire root canal system, including accessory and lateral canals. The traditional technique requires a flared canal preparation with a definite apical stop. The flared nature of the canal is necessary to accommodate the pluggers used to condense the gutta-percha and facilitate the flow of the material apically. Excessive widening of the canal at the apical stop is counterproductive and actually results in more apical leakage[65] and an increased incidence of over-extensions.[66]

The traditional warm vertical condensation technique uses spreaders heated with an open flame, but electrically-heated devices (e.g. Touch 'n Heat, SybronEndo) are relatively inexpensive and more convenient. The method produces homogeneous, compact fillings with gutta-percha flowing into irregularities, apical deltas and lateral canals;[67] signs of sealer and gutta-percha extrusion into the apical and lateral periodontal ligament are not infrequent. However, no substantial improvement in apical[46] or coronal seal[68] has been demonstrated compared to cold lateral condensation. Despite the use of very hot instruments the actual rise in temperature within the mass of gutta-percha is minimal with no long-term adverse periodontal effects reported.[69] Intracanal heating of gutta-percha with ultrasonic devices has also been described[70,71] and is reported to save time.

Continuous wave of condensation technique

In recent years, the traditional warm vertical condensation technique has been simplified considerably through the use of electrically-heated spreaders and pluggers (Touch 'n Heat, System B Heat Source, Elements Obturation Unit, SybronEndo). With the introduction and evolution of these devices came a revival of interest in warm vertical condensation techniques.

The continuous wave of condensation technique[72] uses the System B type heat sources. There are two stages, down-packing and back-packing. In down-packing, heat is carried along the length of the master gutta-percha cone starting coronally and ending in apical 'corkage'. The apical and lateral movement of thermosoftened gutta-percha is referred to as a 'wave of condensation'. The temperature set at the tip of the plunger of a System B is controlled and maintained throughout down-packing. Thus, the technique is simpler and more rapid than other techniques because down-packing is completed in a single continuous vertical movement. Back-packing involves filling the middle and coronal portions of the canal and can be accomplished using thermoplasticized gutta-percha devices, e.g. injection delivery systems (see later) that can deposit increments of warm gutta-percha.

The continuous wave technique requires a smooth tapering canal shape with the smallest diameter at the foramen. A non-standardized gutta-percha cone of similar taper is then selected and tried in to ensure it achieves the correct length and fits snugly, with tug-back. This should allow the tip of the cone to fit into, but not protrude through, the foramen. This is essential to provide resistance during condensation and prevent extrusion of the gutta-percha cone. The tip of the cone can be adjusted to provide a snug fit by removing increments with a scalpel until tug-back is achieved; a radiograph should be taken to confirm the fit. Alternatively, instead of needing to modify a non-standardized gutta-percha point, one that corresponds to the taper and apical size of the prepared canal may be used; these variable taper gutta-percha cones are now available.

A System B plugger that matches the canal taper is chosen, attached to the heating device and then tried in the canal so that it stops between 4–5 mm from the termination of the preparation, a position termed the 'binding point'; this is marked with a silicone stop. It is important that the taper of the plugger matches the taper produced following canal preparation, and that it does not contact the canal walls at this point. The pluggers can be precurved if required.

Following sealer application, the selected gutta-percha cone is positioned into the canal and the excess protruding out of the canal entrance removed with the heated plugger. The plugger is then placed on the point, activated (maximum power, 200°C) and driven down (downpacked) through the gutta-percha to the level of the binding point as indicated by the silicone stop on the plugger (Fig. 9.10). After 1 second, the activating button is released and further vertical pressure applied on the cooling plugger for another 10 seconds to counteract shrinkage on cooling. Finally, the heat source is activated for a further second whilst apical pressure is maintained before the plugger is withdrawn. Most of the gutta-percha in the middle and coronal but not the apical portions is removed when the plugger is withdrawn; the apex is now 'corked'. The rest of the canal can be back-filled using the same heating device, gutta-percha plugs with pluggers, or more effectively with thermoplasticized injected gutta-

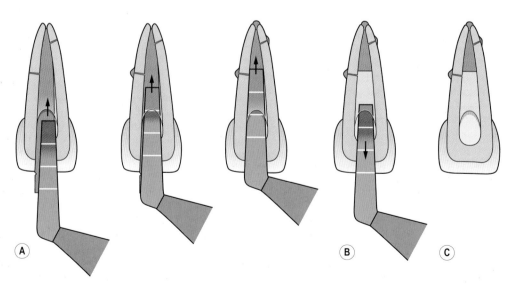

Figure 9.10 Continuous wave condensation. (A) Downpack. (B) Separation and withdrawal. (C) Apical 4–5 mm 'corked' with gutta-percha. (based on an original drawing by M Monteith).

percha devices such as the Elements Obturation Extruder (SybronEndo) or Obtura III Max (Obtura Spartan, East Earth City, MI, USA).

The continuous wave technique seems simple but the skills required take considerable time to master, particularly in teeth with confluent canal systems, so practice on extracted teeth is essential. No evidence is available to confirm whether the technique has an improved clinical outcome, but radiographs often show material forced into irregularities and lateral canals implying more complete filling. Unfortunately, the technique is also associated with material, most likely sealer, extruded beyond the foramen. As achieving apical patency is an essential step when preparing canals with a continuous taper and due to the high hydraulic pressure involved with this technique, extrusion of root filling material is a not uncommon result. The passage of sealer into the periapical region is a concern as, although evidence exists that it will be absorbed,[73] there is also evidence that it may cause inflammation in the tissues.

Rotating condenser

The use of an engine-driven rotating compactor to soften and condense gutta-percha vertically and laterally was described by McSpadden.[74] A rotating stainless steel instrument is used to generate frictional heat within the canal to plasticize a cold master gutta-percha cone and drive the thermomechanically plasticized gutta-percha apically. The method is termed thermatic condensation, with the original instruments discontinued. However, Gutta-Condensor (Dentsply Maillefer), which operates at 8000 rpm in a high torque handpiece and Thermal Lateral Condensor (Brasseler) are available.

The original technique involved the condenser being activated in the canal, alongside the master gutta-percha cone, at approximately 12 000 rpm without apical pressure. The gutta-percha is softened very rapidly and driven apically by advancing the condenser to about 2 mm from the termination of the preparation. As the apical region filled, the condenser backs-out of the canal and is slowly withdrawn while still rotating at the optimum speed. In large canals, the procedure is repeated with additional gutta-percha cones to fill any coronal deficiencies.

Following concerns about the unpredictable nature of the technique, particulary apical extrusion of root filling material and instrument fracture, the method was modified.[75] A hybrid technique combined the predictability of lateral condensation near the apex with the speed and efficacy of the condenser in the remainder of the canal. A master cone is cemented and lateral condensation of accessory points carried out in the apical 3–4 mm before using the compactor in the rest of the canal.

Modern condensers are manufactured from nickel-titanium, not just stainless steel, and used with gutta-percha

that has been pre-softened outside the mouth; these techniques are described later.

Extracanal heating techniques

These rely on gutta-percha being warmed and softened out of the mouth prior to its insertion into the root canal. All of these techniques are used with sealer.

Precoated carriers

An approach to filling canals using a carrier to introduce thermally softened gutta-percha into the root canal was described three decades ago.[76] The efficacy of this technique was based on the flow characteristics of a special α-phase gutta-percha and the ability of the carrier to transport and condense the gutta-percha.

The technique was commercially modified in 1989 and initially featured a series of metal carriers but plastic carriers are now used (Thermafil Endodontic Obturators, Dentsply Tulsa Dental). The carrier is precoated with gutta-percha (obturator) and when warmed, in a controlled manner in a dedicated oven, the material is sticky and adhesive with good flow characteristics. A series of instruments, plastic verifiers, are provided to check the diameter of the termination of the preparation and to simplify the selection of the correct size of obturator. There are also similar carrier-based systems made by other companies on the market.

The technique for using precoated carriers is simple,[77] but it is important to appreciate that the taper of the carriers is at least 0.04 and so root canal shaping procedures must take this into account. Following preparation and drying of the canal, an uncoated carrier or a verifier of the estimated size is inserted to the full working distance; a radiograph can confirm the position. If it passes down to the termination of the preparation without using force, the equivalent size of obturator is selected and the working distance marked with a silicone stop (Fig. 9.11). The canal is then coated with a small amount of sealer. The obturator is then placed in the conditioning oven for the appropriate time, removed and immediately seated into the canal. It should not be inserted so that the tip of the carrier reaches the apical extent of preparation; the aim is to ensure the tip of the carrier is 0.5 mm from this point leaving the apical region filled only with gutta-percha and sealer. The canal length must be measured accurately and the silicone stop on the obturator carefully positioned.

After the gutta-percha has cooled, the obturator is severed at the canal entrance with a bur and the handle discarded. The excess gutta-percha in the chamber is removed and the remainder condensed vertically to enhance the coronal seal; additional gutta-percha can be introduced if the canal morphology dictates. A disadvantage of these devices, particularly when a post-retained

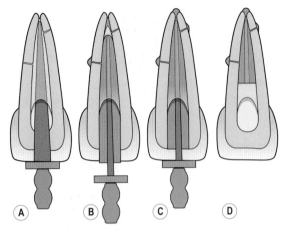

Figure 9.11 Precoated carrier obturation. (A) Verification of size with a blank carrier. (B) Selected carrier conditioned in oven, placed into canal and (C) inserted to length. (D) Excess removed (based on an original drawing by M Monteith).

restoration is planned, is the fact that the shaft of the carrier remains within the gutta-percha in the root canal. Although some studies have shown that this does not affect the apical seal,[78,79] one has reported substantially more leakage after immediate post preparation.[80] Another disadvantage is that the heat-softened gutta-percha may be stripped from the carrier and the apical portion of the canal is then occupied by the carrier instead of gutta-percha.

Most laboratory studies on precoated carriers suggest the technique is significantly faster than lateral condensation,[22,81,82] produces fillings of similar radiographic appearance[22,81] and an equivalent or better apical seal with both the original metal[81,83,84,85] and plastic carriers.[22,86,87,88,89] A minority of studies have reported that lateral condensation produced a better apical seal[90,91,92,93] In laboratory studies, the use of precoated carriers has been associated with an increased incidence of sealer and gutta-percha extrusion.[81,84,86] Although no reports have been published to confirm whether this phenomenon occurs in vivo, it seems this is not an uncommon clinical occurrence. A technique for back-filling with Thermafil Obturators following the initial placement of a cold master gutta-percha cone has been described, with extrusion of sealer and gutta-percha potentially eliminated using this method.[94]

Recent research showed that with more modern techniques of root canal preparation, the resultant sealer thickness can be significantly less than with lateral condensation.[95] The carriers may be in direct contact with the canal wall and not embedded entirely within gutta-percha.[86,92,96] Experiments with carriers made using Delrin® acetal resin (Polyoxymethylene) showed centreing of these prototype carriers in the canal and less canal wall contact.[97]

Concerns have also been expressed about the problems of removing carriers should retreatment be necessary.[98,99] The latest Thermafil Obturators feature a v-shaped groove in the shaft of the carrier which is aimed at facilitating removal. Newer research shows they may be removed from moderately curved canals using rotary nickel-titanium files.[100] Although precoated carriers are convenient they are relatively expensive and cannot be customized easily for specific canals.

A number of other techniques were developed where the operator could coat the carrier with gutta-percha at the chairside prior to insertion. With some systems, syringes of gutta-percha are provided, which are heated and then applied to a carrier. There is little data on the efficacy of these systems and many were subject to modifications or have been discontinued.

Thermoplastic delivery systems

The technique involves heating gutta-percha to a molten state and then injecting it into the root canal.[101] The delivery device deposits the softened gutta-percha into the canal; vertical condensation is required to ensure adaptation of the gutta-percha to the canal wall.

The ability of gutta-percha to adapt to the canal walls has been confirmed[102] and the method produces a seal comparable to lateral condensation,[101] although extrusion of root filling material may occur. In a commercially available delivery system (Obtura), the gutta-percha is heated to 160°C and delivered through the needle tip at approximately 60°C.[103] The original device has been superseded by the Obtura III Max system (Obtura Spartan), which has improved temperature control.

The high-temperature Obtura devices have been shown to produce clinically acceptable results (Fig. 9.12),[104,105] while a number of laboratory studies have demonstrated an apical seal as good as lateral condensation.[15,46] Warm injected gutta-percha can also penetrate dentinal tubules to an extent.[42] On the other hand, some studies have reported the apical seal to be less effective[106,107] and the incidence of gutta-percha under or over-extension to be high.[108]

Clinical experience and the results of various laboratory studies have emphasized the need to limit the enlargement of the foramen[109] and for the prepared canal to include a definite stop at the termination of the preparation.[110,111,112] The use of a sectional injection technique in which the gutta-percha is deposited and condensed in several increments rather than in one application has also been found to improve the apical seal as it allows better condensation of the material deposited apically.[113] Improvement of the apical seal has also been reported when a conventional master gutta-percha cone is cemented before injection of the heated gutta-percha.[114] Injection

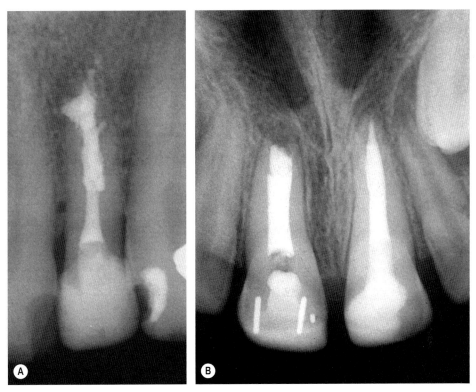

Figure 9.12 (A) Maxillary lateral incisor with communicating resorptive defects filled apically with vertically condensed warm gutta-percha and backfilled using an injection delivery system (reproduced courtesy of L Friedlander). (B) One-step apexification of maxillary right central incisor using an absorbable collagen matrix and injected thermoplasticized gutta-percha. The left central incisor was filled using lateral condensation.

delivery systems are very popular for back-filling the middle and coronal portions following vertical condensation or lateral condensation.

Operator-coated carrier-condenser

The original technique of thermatic condensation of gutta-percha used conventional gutta-percha cones and a rotating condenser to generate heat.[74] Concerns about instrument fracture, its inability to be used effectively in curved canals, excessive heat generation and lack of predictability led to the development of nickel-titanium condensers and a technique in which the condenser is coated with heat-softened gutta-percha prior to insertion into the canal (AlphaSeal, NT Company). The special gutta-percha was available in two formulations, one relatively viscous and the other more fluid. A number of methods could be used to obturate canals; one involved sealing a conventional master gutta-percha cone into the canal followed by the immediate use of a condenser coated with heat-softened gutta-percha.[115] Alternatively, the compactor can first be coated with the more viscous material and then with an additional layer of the more

fluid material. AlphaSeal has been superseded by the MicroSeal system (SybronEndo) (Fig. 9.13). The concept remains as before, but it has been enhanced by provision of master cones having a different gutta-percha formulation to the one that is warmed and injected onto the condenser. The manufacturer recommends the fitting of a cold master gutta-percha cone prior to the introduction of the warmed gutta-percha on the condenser.

Solvent-softened gutta-percha

Chloroform-softened gutta-percha has a long tradition in endodontics. Following extensive drying with alcohol, the root canal was filled with a solution of rosin (colophony) in chloroform into which was seated a master gutta-percha cone. The chloroform softened the surface of the gutta-percha and made it swell, and the rosin acted as a glue to make the mass stick to the canal walls. This method is taught with only minor modifications in Sweden.

The high degree of evaporation and the fluid nature of the rosin solution led to the development of chloropercha. Primarily a thick suspension of fine shavings of

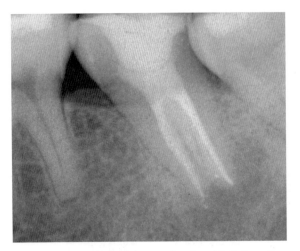

Figure 9.13 Mandibular left second molar with C-shaped canal; two main canals filled with MicroFlow master cone and warm gutta-percha. Reproduced courtesy of D Parmar.

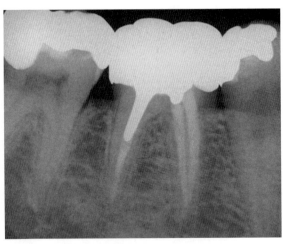

Figure 9.14 Mandibular right first molar with three canals filled with MTA. Material condensed by hand; 7 year review. Reproduced courtesy of G Bogen.

gutta-percha in chloroform, chloro-percha was modified by the addition of zinc oxide and metal salts to act as much as a conventional sealer as merely softening the points. Kloroperka is the best known formulation, with studies of its performance being reported to be favourable.[116]

Chloroform may also be used to customize master gutta-percha cones. This has been popularized as the chloroform dip technique.[117,118] The apical 2–5 mm of the master gutta-percha cone is dipped in chloroform for a few seconds and inserted into the canal to the termination of the preparation and then withdrawn and allowed to dry. The chloroform softens the outer layer of the gutta-percha so that when it is seated fully it takes up the shape of the apical portion of the canal. Since the volume of solvent is small and the thickness of gutta-percha affected is minimal there is, potentially, little shrinkage following solvent evaporation.[119] The customized cone is then cemented in place with a conventional sealer and the remainder of the canal filled with laterally condensed gutta-percha. The apical seal obtained with this technique is reported to be comparable with traditional cold lateral condensation.[120]

OTHER METHODS OF ROOT CANAL FILLING

Mineral Trioxide Aggregate

Mineral Trioxide Aggregate (MTA) is a powder that consists of hydrophilic particles that sets in the presence of moisture.[121] Hydration of the powder results in a colloidal gel with a pH of 12.5 that solidifies to a hard structure. Several in vitro and in vivo studies have shown that MTA has good sealing ability, is biocompatible, and promotes tissue regeneration when placed in contact with the dental pulp or periapical tissues.[122]

Clinical applications for MTA include capping of pulps with reversible pulpitis, apexification, surgical and non-surgical repair of root perforations and fractures, and as a root-end filling material. MTA has application as a root canal filling material without a core material, such as gutta-percha, if the difficulties of placement in the canal can be mastered (Fig. 9.14). MTA should be placed incrementally rather than introduced with a spiral filler, and condensed using condensers or modified finger pluggers to a depth of at least 4 mm. Ultrasound has been suggested as an aid to condensation, with a laboratory study indicating this can achieve a denser fill in curved, as well as straight canals.[123] Root fillings of MTA must be considered permanent, since a disadvantage is the set material is very hard and virtually impossible to remove.

The use of MTA as an apical plug for teeth with immature, open apices has been described.[122,124] The MTA creates a hard barrier and the remainder of the canal is then filled with MTA or the root reinforced by appropriate materials (Figs. 9.15 & 9.16). Treatment in one or two appointments in this manner avoids the long-term use of calcium hydroxide dressings which may dessicate and weaken the already thin dentine[125] while waiting for the formation of a hard tissue barrier. MTA may also be used to root fill the non-vital coronal aspect of a tooth with a horizontal root fracture, which presents a similar clinical challenge to a tooth with an open apex (Fig. 9.17).

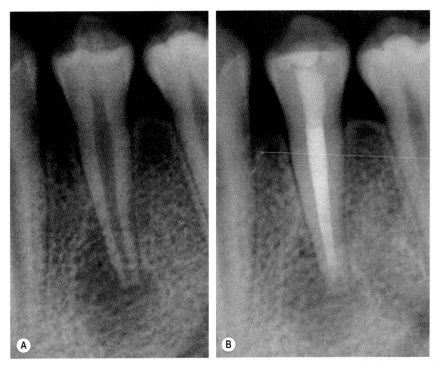

Figure 9.15 Mandibular left first premolar with immature apex and periapical lesion a result of pulp exposure of a dens evaginatus tubercle: (A) initial presentation. (B) canal filled with MTA and access cavity sealed with composite resin. Reproduced courtesy of M Gordon.

Hydrophilic polymers

The SmartSeal system (DRFP Ltd, Stamford, Peterborough, UK), introduced in 2007, uses a single master cone (SmartPoint) made of a polymer similar to that used in intraocular and contact lenses. The cones have a high filler content and are covered by a hydrophilic polymer sheath. They are designed to work in a 'wet' canal so that the polymer swells, to create a seal. An epoxy-amine-type sealer (SmartPaste) is used in conjunction with the SmartPoint. No special equipment is required and the cones are provided in a variety of tapers and sizes to match variable taper preparation instruments. Two points may be used to fill an oval canal. The radiographic appearance differs from gutta-percha, as the polymer sheath is not radiopaque. The system claims to be easier to handle and less technique sensitive than other obturation methods, with cost and time savings in both preparation and obturation. The material swells into the space available in the canal, the manufacturer claiming no damage (cracking) to the tooth. Unfortunately, there is insufficient independent data on this product to make specific recommendations.

Monoblocks

A key disadvantage of gutta-percha is that it does not adhere to dentine. Bonding of restorative materials to the enamel and dentine during the coronal restoration of teeth is now routine. A search for simpler methods of filling canals and alternatives to gutta-percha led to the investigation of low viscosity composite resins to seal all the entrances and walls of root canals in the late 1970s.[126] The introduction of fibre posts for restoring root filled teeth introduced the potential to, simultaneously, fill the root and also reinforce the tooth. The development of a polycaprolactone thermoplastic material (Resilon, Pentron Corp, Wallingford, CT, USA) with bioactive glass, bismuth and barium salts as fillers provided an alternative core material to gutta-percha. With handling characteristics very similar to gutta-percha, it has the potential to bond to suitable sealers.

Together with a UDMA-based sealer (e.g. Epiphany, Pentron Corp; RealSeal or RealSeal SE, SybronEndo) there is the potential to create a form of 'monoblock'[127] which has a single interface between the dentine of the root canal wall and the filling core. With the smear layer removed, a

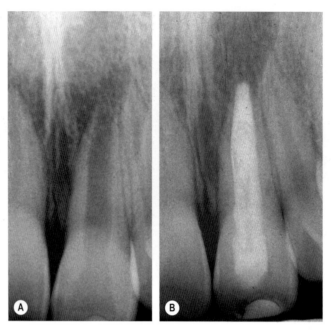

Figure 9.16 Maxillary left central incisor: (A) preoperative view showing open apex. (B) apex filled with MTA and the remaining canal space filled with composite.

primer is applied and the dual-cured sealer coated onto the dentine wall. Cones or thermoplasticized portions of core material are then inserted. The preliminary tests of these materials indicated less apical leakage[128] and an improvement in the strength of the tooth.[129] The work of other researchers has challenged the increase in fracture resistance offered by these systems,[130] the improved bond strength to dentine,[131-135] and also their sealing ability.[136,137,138] Many factors are involved in the success or failure of these systems, including the nature of the smear layer (if present), dentine tubule permeability, thickness of the sealer and polymerization contraction, with all self- and dual-cure adhesives having lower bond strengths than the light-activated varieties. In addition to the problem of contraction on setting, no polymer is considered entirely stable over time.

Carrier-type obturators, similar to Thermafil but pre-coated with Resilon instead of gutta-percha have recently come onto the market (RealSeal 1, SybronEndo). The other components of the system include blank carriers (verifiers) for determining the size of the obturator required, a conditioning oven and the self-etch resin sealer (RealSeal SE, SybronEndo). Together, the claim is that the obturator is 'warm-bonded' to the canal.

Another family of products designed with the 'mono-block' concept in mind is the Next system (Heraeus-Kulzer, Armonk, USA) consisting of Next Post/Obturators, fibreglass carriers tipped with Resilon, for straight canals. Where the subsequent restoration requires an intraradicular post and for curved canals, Next Tapered Obturators in which the carriers are resin rather than glass fibre can be used. Both types of obturators are bonded to the root dentine using a resin-based (Next) sealer and bonding agents.

Non-instrumentation technology

A non-instrumentation hydrodynamic method for root canal treatment has been described that allows the cleaning, disinfection and filling of the root canal system without the use of traditional instruments.[139,140,141] The canals are cleansed by irrigation with sodium hypochlorite under alternating pressure generated by a vacuum pump; the canals are not enlarged, and no smear layer is created. Filling of the canal system is performed using a vacuum pump that produces a negative pressure. When this is achieved, a valve is opened to a reservoir containing freshly mixed sealer and the material is sucked into the root canal system. Although laboratory and clinical studies of the technique were promising and the seal reported to be comparable to lateral condensation,[142,143,144] it has not materialized into a clinically viable technique.

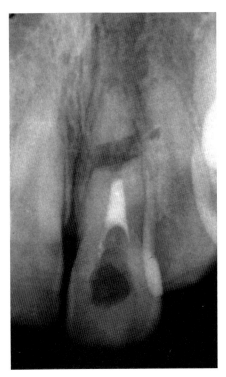

Figure 9.17 Maxillary left central incisor with horizontal root fracture. The non-vital coronal part of the canal has been filled with MTA; radiograph to check placement of MTA prior to restoration.

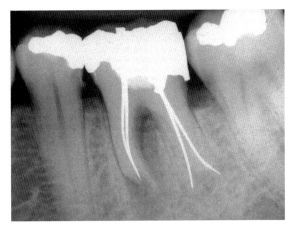

Figure 9.18 Mandibular left first molar filled with silver points. The tooth has two distal roots and inflammatory resorption is evident at the apex of the mesial root.

Silver points

Silver points were introduced in the 1930s to fill curved canals. At the time, because of the limitations of early canal preparation instruments, these canals were difficult to enlarge adequately to accept gutta-percha cones. Lacking rigidity in narrow, curved canals, gutta-percha cones will bend or deform. The more rigid silver points could be forced down narrow canals and provided the radiographic appearance of a dense radiopaque filling occupying the full length of the canal (Fig. 9.18). Unfortunately, this filling technique encouraged clinicians to pay less attention to thorough cleaning and shaping of the root canal system, often leaving debris and microorganisms present, leading to failure. Silver points have other disadvantages. They are round in cross-section, and few canals are round or can be made round, particularly coronally.[50] The seal will rely heavily on large volumes of sealer. Silver points are also prone to corrosion when exposed to tissue fluids or saliva. The corrosion products are toxic and may reach the periapical tissues and compound the problems caused by sealer dissolution. In addition, full length silver points could not be used in teeth where post-retained restora-

tions were planned; a sectional technique was devised to overcome this difficulty (Fig. 9.19). Finally, removal of silver points, particularly sectional silver points, for retreatment is also not easy. The use of silver points is not recommended.

Paste fillers

Paste fillers were introduced to speed up root canal treatment,[145] just as silver points were introduced to facilitate filling of narrow, curved canals. They also hark back to the dated concept of mummifying pulps. The paste fillers should not be confused with sealers or cements designed as luting agents for solid or semi-solid root canal filling materials.

Paste fillers contain strong disinfectants (e.g. paraformaldehyde) and anti-inflammatory agents (e.g. corticosteroids) and were introduced in the belief that their use could bypass the accepted principles of canal preparation, disinfection and filling. The proponents of paste fillers argued that the medicaments would eliminate microorganisms so that thorough cleaning and shaping were not necessary, and the anti-inflammatory agents would reduce the host response. The use of paste fillers is to be condemned as some patients (Fig. 9.20) suffered permanent injury as a result of toxic materials being passed into the periapical tissues and beyond.[146,147] Most of the paste fillers (Endomethasone, Septodont; N2, Indrag-Agsa, Bologna, Italy; SPAD, Quetigny, France) contain paraformaldehyde. If deposited in the periapical tissues this may give rise to severe inflammatory reactions and long-lasting or permanent injury, particularly to nerve bundles.[147,148]

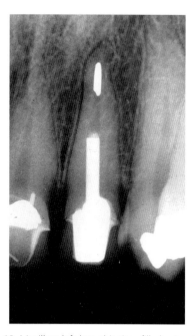

Figure 9.19 Maxillary left lateral incisor filled using the sectional silver point technique and restored with a cast post/core and a porcelain jacket crown.

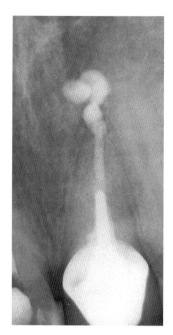

Figure 9.20 Maxillary left central incisor filled with paste material; a substantial quantity has been extruded into the periapical region.

Corticosteroid in paste fillers severely affects the defence responses of the periapical tissues by suppressing phagocytosis, providing the opportunity for microorganisms to multiply. Their use may, possibly, cause unwanted systemic side-effects.[149]

The application of paraformaldehyde to vital tissue will also result in traces of the material or its components being spread throughout the body.[24,150] Individuals may show a hypersensitivity response and the material may have both mutagenic and carcinogenic potentials.[151] A recent development is Endomethasone N (Septodont) which does not contain paraformaldehyde and claims greatly improved biocompatibility, but studies are lacking.

CORONAL RESTORATION

A variety of materials are used as provisional restorations between treatment visits.[152] There is much evidence to support the concept of coronal leakage[1] and the necessity to restore the tooth with a good quality, permanent coronal restoration[2,153,154] after root canal filling. Root filled teeth are vulnerable and do not survive unless they are properly restored.[155,156] Provided all the technical requirements of the root canal treatment have been achieved, a permanent coronal restoration should be placed without unnecessary delay.

FOLLOW-UP

It is essential to take a postoperative radiograph straight after completion of root canal filling. Immediately following root canal preparation and filling, teeth may be tender and it advisable to warn patients of this possibility.[157,158] Fortunately, the incidence of severe pain following root canal filling is low.[159,160] In most cases, any discomfort is mild and no active intervention is required. If severe pain occurs over an extended period then further investigation and diagnosis are necessary. In particular, the quality of treatment should be reviewed so that it can be established whether poor technique and/or procedural accidents may have contributed to the problem. Once the cause has been identified then the correct treatment can be instituted; this may be non-surgical or surgical retreatment.

Follow-up of root-filled teeth is important to ascertain treatment outcome. Firm guidelines for the timing of recalls are not possible as each case is different, but a clinical and radiographic check after 1 year is advisable.[161]

TREATMENT OUTCOME

The outcome of root canal treatment is assessed using a combination of clinical and radiological criteria:[161]

- the tooth should be functional with no signs of swelling or sinus tract
- the patient should be free from symptoms
- the radiographic appearance of the periapical tissues should either remain normal or return to normality.

While the patient's symptoms may improve, and signs such as a swelling or a draining sinus may disappear after root canal preparation and dressing, success or failure cannot be declared immediately. Large areas of periapical bone loss may take months or even years to heal completely, with extended review necessary especially for retreatment cases.[162] It may also take many months for bone loss to become obvious on radiographs in cases which are not successful.

LEARNING OUTCOMES

This chapter should allow the reader to:

- recognize the objectives of filling root canals
- understand the various materials and the different techniques for root canal filling, with the emphasis on the use of gutta-percha as the core material
- discuss the role and use of different types of root canal sealers
- appreciate newer materials for root canal filling including MTA and the 'monoblock' concept
- understand the shortcomings of older filling techniques, which although no longer recommended, are frequently encountered in clinical practice.

REFERENCES

1. Saunders WP, Saunders EM. Coronal leakage as a cause of failure in root canal therapy: a review. Endodontics and Dental Traumatology 1994;10:105–108.
2. Tronstad L, Asbjørnsen K, Døving L, et al. Influence of coronal restorations on the periapical health of endodontically treated teeth. Endodontics and Dental Traumatology 2000;16:218–221.
3. Whitworth J. Methods of filling root canals: principles and practices. Endodontic Topics 2005;12:2–24.
4. Wu M-K, Wesselink PR, Walton RE. Apical terminus location of root canal treatment procedures. Oral Surgery, Oral Medicine, Oral Pathology, Oral Radiology, Endodontics 2000;89: 99–103.
5. Buchanan LS. The standardized-taper root canal preparation – Part 1. Concepts for variably tapered shaping instruments. International Endodontic Journal 2000;33:516–529.
6. Byström A, Sundqvist G. Bacteriologic evaluation of the efficacy of mechanical root canal instrumentation in endodontic therapy. Scandinavian Journal of Dental Research 1981;89: 321–328.
7. Byström A, Claesson R, Sundqvist G. The antibacterial effect of camphorated paramonochlorophenol, camphorated phenol and calcium hydroxide in the treatment of infected root canals. Endodontics and Dental Traumatology 1985;1:170–175.
8. Peters LB, Wesselink PR, Moorer WR. The fate and the role of bacteria left in root canal tubules. International Endodontic Journal 1995;28:95–99.
9. Byström A, Happonen RP, Sjögren U, Sundqvist G. Healing of periapical lesions of pulpless teeth after endodontic treatment with controlled asepsis. Endodontics and Dental Traumatology 1987;3: 58–63.
10. Sjögren U, Figdor D, Persson S, Sundqvist G. Influence of infection at the time of root filling on the outcome of endodontic treatment of teeth with apical periodontitis. International Endodontic Journal 1997;30:297–306.
11. Trope M, Delano EO, Ørstavik D. Endodontic treatment of teeth with apical periodontitis: single visit vs. multivisit treatment. Journal of Endodontics 1999;25:345–350.
12. Weiger R, Rosendahl R, Löst C. Influence of calcium hydroxide intracanal dressings on the prognosis of teeth with endodontically induced periapical lesions. International Endodontic Journal 2000;33:219–226.
13. Weiger R, Axmann-Krcmar D, Löst C. Prognosis of conventional root canal treatment reconsidered. Endodontics and Dental Traumatology 1998;14:1–9.
14. Brownlee WA. Filling of root canals in recently devitalized teeth. Dominion Dental Journal 1900;12:254–256.
15. Hata G, Kawazoe S, Toda T, Weine FS. Sealing ability of thermoplasticized gutta-percha fill techniques as assessed by a new method of determining

apical leakage. Journal of Endodontics 1995;21:167–172.

16. Grossman LI, Oliet S, del Rio CE. Endodontic Practice. 11th edn. Philadelphia, PA, USA: Lea and Febiger; 1988:242–270.

17. Spångberg L, Langeland K. Biologic effects of dental materials. 1. Toxicity of root canal filling materials on HeLa cells in vitro. Oral Surgery, Oral Medicine, Oral Pathology 1973;35:402–414.

18. Ørstavik D, Mjör IA. Histopathology and X-ray microanalysis of the subcutaneous tissue response to endodontic sealers. Journal of Endodontics 1988;14:13–23.

19. Seltzer S, Soltanoff W, Smith J. Biologic aspects of endodontics. V. Periapical tissue reactions to root canal instrumentation beyond the apex and root canal fillings short of and beyond the apex. Oral Surgery, Oral Medicine, Oral Pathology 1973;36:725–737.

20. Ørstavik D. Weight loss of endodontic sealers, cements and pastes in water. Scandinavian Journal of Dental Research 1983;91:316–319.

21. Al-Dewani N, Hayes SJ, Dummer PMH. Comparison of laterally condensed and low temperature thermoplasticized gutta-percha root fillings. Journal of Endodontics 2000;26:733–738.

22. Dummer PMH, Lyle L, Rawle J, Kennedy JK. A laboratory study of root fillings in teeth obturated by lateral condensation of gutta-percha or Thermafil obturators. International Endodontic Journal 1994;27:32–38.

23. Grossman LI. An improved root canal cement. Journal of the American Dental Association 1958;56:381–385.

24. Tronstad L, Barnett F, Flax M. Solubility and biocompatibility of calcium hydroxide-containing root canal sealers. Endodontics and Dental Traumatology 1988;4:152–159.

25. Jacobsen EL, BeGole EA, Vitkus DD, Daniel JC. An evaluation of

two newly formulated calcium hydroxide cements: a leakage study. Journal of Endodontics 1987;13:164–169.

26. Limkangwalmongkol S, Abbott PV, Sandler AB. Apical dye penetration with four root canal sealers and gutta-percha using longitudinal sectioning. Journal of Endodontics 1992;18:535–539.

27. Schweikl H, Schmalz G, Stimmelmayr H, Bey B. Mutagenicity of AH26 in an in vitro mammalian cell mutation assay. Journal of Endodontics 1995;21:407–410.

28. Barkhordar RA, Nguyen NT. Paresthesia of the mental nerve after overextension with AH26 and gutta-percha: report of a case. Journal of the American Dental Association 1985;110:202–203.

29. Spångberg LSW, Barbosa SV, Lavigne GD. AH26 releases formaldehyde. Journal of Endodontics 1993;19:596–598.

30. Heling I, Chandler NP. The antimicrobial effect within dentinal tubules of four root canal sealers. Journal of Endodontics 1996;22:257–259.

31. Pitt Ford TR. The leakage of root fillings using glass ionomer cement and other materials. British Dental Journal 1979;146:273–278.

32. Friedman S, Löst C, Zarrabian M, Trope M. Evaluation of success and failure after endodontic therapy using a glass ionomer cement sealer. Journal of Endodontics 1995;21:384–390.

33. Wu M-K, Tigos E, Wesselink PR. An 18-month longitudinal study on a new silicon-based sealer, RSA RoekoSeal: a leakage study in vitro. Oral Surgery, Oral Medicine, Oral Pathology, Oral Radiology, Endodontics 2002;94:499–502.

34. Miletic I, Devcic N, Anic I, et al. The cytotoxicity of RoekoSeal and AH Plus compared during different setting periods. Journal of Endodontics 2005;31:307–309.

35. Leonardo MR, Flores DSH, de Paula e Silva FWG. A comparison study of periapical repair in dog's teeth using RoekoSeal and AH Plus root canal sealers: a histopathological examination. Journal of Endodontics 2008;34:822–825.

36. Zielinski TM, Baumgartner JC, Marshall JG. An evaluation of GuttaFlow and gutta-percha in the filling of lateral grooves and depressions. Journal of Endodontics 2008;34:295–298.

37. Kontakiotis EG, Tzanetakis GN, Loizides AL. A 12-month longitudinal in vitro leakage study on a new silicon-based root canal filling material (Gutta-Flow). Oral Surgery, Oral Medicine, Oral Pathology, Oral Radiology and Endodontology 2007;103:854–859.

38. Mader CL, Baumgartner JC, Peters DD. Scanning electron microscopic investigation of the smeared layer on root canal walls. Journal of Endodontics 1984;10:477–483.

39. McComb D, Smith D. A preliminary scanning electron microscopic study of root canals after endodontic procedures. Journal of Endodontics 1975;1:238–242.

40. Sen BH, Wesselink PR, Türkün M. The smear layer: a phenomenon in root canal therapy. International Endodontic Journal 1995;28:141–148.

41. Czonstkowsky M, Wilson EG, Holstein FA. The smear layer in endodontics. Dental Clinics of North America 1990;34:13–25.

42. Gutmann JL. Adaptation of injected thermoplasticized gutta-percha in the absence of the dentinal smear layer. International Endodontic Journal 1993;26:87–92.

43. Hovland EJ, Dumsha TC. Leakage evaluation in vitro of the root canal sealer cement Sealapex. International Endodontic Journal 1985;18:179–182.

44. Galvan DA, Ciarlone AE, Pashley DH, et al. Effect of smear layer removal on the diffusion permeability of human roots.

Journal of Endodontics 1994;20:83–86.

45. Drake DR, Wiemann AH, Rivera EM, Walton RE. Bacterial retention in canal walls in vitro: effect of smear layer. Journal of Endodontics 1994;20: 78–82.

46. Evans JT, Simon JH. Evaluation of the apical seal produced by injected thermoplasticized gutta-percha in the absence of smear layer and root canal sealer. Journal of Endodontics 1986;12:100–107.

47. Combe EC, Cohen BD, Cummings K. Alpha- and beta-forms of gutta-percha in products for root canal filling. International Endodontic Journal 2001;34:447–451.

48. Ingle JI. A standardized endodontic technique utilizing newly designed instruments and filling materials. Oral Surgery, Oral Medicine, Oral Pathology 1961;14:83–91.

49. Jungmann CL, Uchin RA, Bucher JF. Effect of instrumentation on the shape of the root canal. Journal of Endodontics 1975;1:66–68.

50. Schneider SW. A comparison of canal preparations in straight and curved root canals. Oral Surgery, Oral Medicine, Oral Pathology 1971;32:271–275.

51. Beatty RG. The effect of standard or serial preparation on single cone obturation. International Endodontic Journal 1987;20: 276–281.

52. Kerekes K. Evaluation of standardized root canal instruments and obturating points. Journal of Endodontics 1979;5:145–150.

53. Gordon MPJ, Love RM, Chandler NP. An evaluation of .06 tapered gutta-percha cones for filling of .06 taper prepared curved root canals. International Endodontic Journal 2005;38:87–96.

54. Yared GM, Bou Dagher FE. Elongation and movement of the gutta-percha master cone during initial lateral condensation. Journal of Endodontics 1993;19:395–397.

55. Allison DA, Weber CR, Walton RE. The influence of the method of canal preparation on the quality of apical and coronal obturation. Journal of Endodontics 1979;5: 298–304.

56. Van der Sluis LWM, Versluis M, Wu MK, Wesselink PR. Passive ultrasonic irrigation of the root canal: a review of the literature. International Endodontic Journal 2007;40:415–426.

57. Blum J-Y, Machtou P, Micallef J-P. Analysis of forces developed during obturations. Wedging effect: Part II. Journal of Endodontics 1998;24: 223–228.

58. Van der Burgt TP, Eronat C, Plasschaert AJM. Staining patterns in teeth discolored by endodontic sealers. Journal of Endodontics 1986;12:187–191.

59. Madison S, Zakariasen KL. Linear and volumetric analysis of apical leakage in teeth prepared for posts. Journal of Endodontics 1984;10:422–427.

60. Zmener O. Effect of dowel preparation on the apical seal of endodontically treated teeth. Journal of Endodontics 1980;6:687–690.

61. Wu M-K, Wesselink PR. A primary observation on the preparation and obturation of oval canals. International Endodontic Journal 2001;34:137–141.

62. Wu M-K, Kastáková A, Wesselink PR. Quality of cold and warm gutta-percha fillings in oval canals in mandibular premolars. International Endodontic Journal 2001;34:485–491.

63. De-Deus G, Reis C, Beznos D, et al. Limited ability of three commonly used thermoplasticized gutta-percha techniques in filling oval-shaped canals. Journal of Endodontics 2008;34:1401–1405.

64. Schilder H. Filling root canals in three dimensions. Dental Clinics of North America 1967;11: 723–744.

65. Yared GM, Bou Dagher FE. Apical enlargement: influence on the sealing ability of the vertical compaction technique. Journal of Endodontics 1994;20: 313–314.

66. Yared GM, Bou Dagher FE. Apical enlargement: influence on overextensions during in vitro vertical compaction. Journal of Endodontics 1994;20: 269–271.

67. Wong M, Peters DD, Lorton L. Comparison of gutta-percha filling techniques, compaction (mechanical), vertical (warm), and lateral condensation techniques, part 1. Journal of Endodontics 1981;7:551–558.

68. Khayat A, Lee SJ, Torabinejad M. Human saliva penetration of coronally unsealed obturated root canals. Journal of Endodontics 1993;19:458–461.

69. Hand RE, Huget EF, Tsaknis PJ. Effects of a warm gutta-percha technique on the lateral periodontium. Oral Surgery, Oral Medicine, Oral Pathology 1976;42:395–401.

70. Bailey GC, Cunnington SA, Ng L-Y, et al. Ultrasonic condensation of gutta-percha: the effect of power setting and activation time on temperature rise at the root surface – an in vitro study. International Endodontic Journal 2004;37:447–454.

71. Zmener O, Banegas G. Clinical experience of root canal filling by ultrasonic condensation of gutta-percha. Endodontics and Dental Traumatology 1999;15:57–59.

72. Buchanan LS. The Buchanan continuous wave of condensation technique. A convergence of conceptual and procedural advances in obturation. Dentistry Today October 1994;80–85.

73. Olsson B, Sliwkowski A, Langeland K. Subcutaneous implantation for the biological evaluation of endodontic materials. Journal of Endodontics 1981;7:355–367.

74. McSpadden J. Self-study course for the thematic condensation of gutta-percha. York, PA, USA: Dentsply; 1980.

75. Tagger M, Tamse A, Katz A, Korzen BH. Evaluation of apical seal produced by a hybrid root canal filling method combining lateral condensation and thermatic compaction. Journal of Endodontics 1984;10: 299–303.

76. Johnson WB. A new gutta-percha filling technique. Journal of Endodontics 1978;4:184–188.

77. von Schroeter C. Thermafil obturation technique: an overview from the practitioner's point of view. ENDO (London, England) 2008;2:43–54.

78. Rybicki R, Zillich R. Apical sealing ability of Thermafil following immediate and delayed post space preparations. Journal of Endodontics 1994;20:64–66.

79. Saunders WP, Saunders EM, Gutmann JL, Gutmann ML. An assessment of the plastic Thermafil obturation technique. Part 3. The effect of post space preparation on the apical seal. International Endodontic Journal 1993;26:184–189.

80. Ricci ER, Kessler JR. Apical seal of teeth obturated by the laterally condensed gutta-percha, the Thermafil plastic and Thermafil metal obturator techniques after post space preparation. Journal of Endodontics 1994;20: 123–126.

81. Dummer PMH, Kelly T, Meghji A, et al. An in vitro study of the quality of root fillings in teeth obturated by lateral condensation of gutta-percha or Thermafil obturators. International Endodontic Journal 1993;26:99–105.

82. Gutmann JL, Saunders WP, Saunders EM, Nguyen L. An assessment of the plastic Thermafil obturation technique. Part 1. Radiographic evaluation of adaptation and placement. International Endodontic Journal 1993;26:173–178.

83. Beatty RG, Baker PS, Haddix J, Hart F. The efficacy of four root canal obturation techniques in preventing apical dye penetration. Journal of the American Dental Association 1989;119:633–637.

84. Leung SF, Gulabivala K. An in vitro evaluation of the influence of canal curvature on the sealing ability of Thermafil. International Endodontic Journal 1994;27: 190–196.

85. McMurtrey LG, Krell KV, Wilcox LR. A comparison between Thermafil and lateral condensation in highly curved canals. Journal of Endodontics 1992;18:68–71.

86. Clark DS, ElDeeb ME. Apical sealing ability of metal versus plastic carrier Thermafil obturators. Journal of Endodontics 1993;19:4–9.

87. Dalat DM, Spångberg LSW. Comparison of apical leakage in root canals obturated with various gutta-percha techniques using a dye vacuum tracing method. Journal of Endodontics 1994;20:315–319.

88. Gutmann JL, Saunders WP, Saunders EM, Nguyen L. An assessment of the plastic Thermafil obturation technique. Part 2. Material adaptation and sealability. International Endodontic Journal 1993;26:179–183.

89. Xu Q, Ling J, Cheung GSP, Hu Y. A quantitative evaluation of sealing ability of 4 obturation techniques by using a glucose leakage test. Oral Surgery, Oral Medicine, Oral Pathology, Oral Radiology and Endodontology 2007;104: e109–e113.

90. Chohayeb AA. Comparison of conventional root canal obturation techniques with Thermafil obturators. Journal of Endodontics 1992;18: 10–12.

91. Haddix JE, Jarrell M, Mattison GD, Pink FE. An in vitro investigation of the apical seal produced by a new thermoplasticized gutta-percha obturation technique. Quintessence International 1991;22:159–163.

92. Lares C, ElDeeb ME. The sealing ability of the Thermafil obturation technique. Journal of Endodontics 1990;16: 474–479.

93. Ravanshad S, Torabinejad M. Coronal dye penetration of the apical filling materials after post space preparation. Oral Surgery, Oral Medicine, Oral Pathology 1992;74:644–647.

94. Da Silva D, Endal U, Reynaud A, et al. An in vitro study of a Thermafil backfilling technique. International Endodontic Journal 2002;35:88 Abstract R24.

95. Gulsahi K, Cehreli ZC, Kuraner T, Dagli FT. Sealer area associated with cold lateral condensation of gutta-percha and warm coated carrier filling systems in canals prepared with various rotary NiTi systems. International Endodontic Journal 2007;40:275–281.

96. Juhlin JJ, Walton RE, Dovgan JS. Adaptation of Thermafil components to canal walls. Journal of Endodontics 1993;19:130–135.

97. Pagliarini A, Riccardo R, Massimo C. An in vitro evaluation of a prototype Delrin carrier for the Thermafil obturation system. Quintessence International 2007;38(4): e195–e200.

98. Wilcox LR. Thermafil retreatment with and without chloroform solvent. Journal of Endodontics 1993;19:563–566.

99. Wilcox LR, Juhlin JJ. Endodontic retreatment of Thermafil versus laterally condensed gutta-percha. Journal of Endodontics 1994;20:115–117.

100. Royzenblat A, Goodell GG. Comparison of removal times of Thermafil plastic obturators using ProFile rotary instruments at different rotational speeds in moderately curved canals. Journal of Endodontics 2007;33: 256–258.

101. Yee FS, Marlin J, Krakow AA, Gron P. Three-dimensional obturation of the root canal using injection-molded, thermoplasticized dental gutta-percha. Journal of Endodontics 1977;3:168–174.

102. Torabinejad M, Skobe Z, Trombly PL, et al. Scanning electron microscopic study of root canal obturation using

thermoplasticized gutta-percha. Journal of Endodontics 1978;4:245–250.

103. Glickman GN, Gutmann JL. Contemporary perspectives on canal obturation. Dental Clinics of North America 1992;36: 327–341.

104. Marlin J. Injectable standard gutta-percha as a method of filling the root canal system. Journal of Endodontics 1986;12:354–358.

105. Sobarzo-Navarro V. Clinical experience in root canal obturation by an injection thermoplasticized gutta-percha technique. Journal of Endodontics 1991;17:389–391.

106. Bradshaw GB, Hall A, Edmunds DH. The sealing ability of injection-moulded thermoplasticized gutta-percha. International Endodontic Journal 1989;22:17–20.

107. LaCombe JS, Campbell AD, Hicks ML, Pelleu GB. A comparison of the apical seal produced by two thermoplasticized injectable gutta-percha techniques. Journal of Endodontics 1988;14: 445–450.

108. Mann SR, McWalter GM. Evaluation of apical seal and placement control in straight and curved canals obturated by laterally condensed and thermoplasticized gutta-percha. Journal of Endodontics 1987;13:10–17.

109. Richie GM, Anderson DM, Sakumura JS. Apical extrusion of thermoplasticized gutta-percha used as a root canal filling. Journal of Endodontics 1988;14:128–132.

110. Gatot A, Peist M, Mozes M. Endodontic overextension produced by injected thermoplasticized gutta-percha. Journal of Endodontics 1989;15:273–274.

111. George JW, Michanowicz AE, Michanowicz JP. A method of canal preparation to control apical extrusion of low-temperature thermoplasticized gutta-percha. Journal of Endodontics 1987;13:18–23.

112. Gutmann JL, Rakusin H. Perspectives on root canal obturation with thermoplasticized injectable gutta-percha. International Endodontic Journal 1987;20:261–270.

113. Veis A, Lambrianidis T, Molyvdas I, Zervas P. Sealing ability of sectional injection thermoplasticized gutta-percha technique with varying distances between needle tip and apical foramen. Endodontics and Dental Traumatology 1992;8: 63–66.

114. Olson AK, Hartwell GR, Weller RN. Evaluation of the controlled placement of injected thermoplasticized gutta-percha. Journal of Endodontics 1989;15:306–309.

115. Gilhooly RMP, Hayes SJ, Bryant ST, et al. Comparison of lateral condensation and thermomechanically compacted warm α-phase gutta-percha with a single cone for obturating curved root canals. Oral Surgery, Oral Medicine, Oral Pathology, Oral Radiology, Endodontics 2001;91:89–94.

116. Strindberg LZ. The dependence of the results of pulp therapy on certain factors. An analytic study based on radiographic and clinical follow-up examinations. Acta Odontologica Scandinavica 1956;21(Suppl. 4):1–175.

117. Beatty RG, Zakariasen KL. Apical leakage associated with three obturation techniques in large and small root canals. International Endodontic Journal 1984;17:67–72.

118. Keane KM, Harrington GW. The use of chloroform-softened gutta-percha master cone and its effect on the apical seal. Journal of Endodontics 1984;10:57–63.

119. Wong M, Peters DD, Lorton L, Bernier WE. Comparison of gutta-percha filling techniques: three chloroform-gutta-percha filling techniques, part 2. Journal of Endodontics 1982;8:4–9.

120. Smith JJ, Montgomery S. A comparison of apical seal: chloroform versus halothane-dipped gutta-percha cones.

Journal of Endodontics 1992;18:156–160.

121. Torabinejad M, Hong CU, McDonald F, Pitt Ford TR. Physical and chemical properties of a new root-end filling material. Journal of Endodontics 1995;21:349–353.

122. Torabinejad M, Chivian N. Clinical applications of mineral trioxide aggregate. Journal of Endodontics 1999;25:197–205.

123. Yeung P, Liewehr FR, Moon PC. A quantitative comparison of the fill density of MTA produced by two placement techniques. Journal of Endodontics 2006;32:456–459.

124. Witherspoon DE, Small JC, Regan JD, Nunn M. Retrospective analysis of open apex teeth obturated with mineral trioxide aggregate. Journal of Endodontics 2008;34:1171–1176.

125. Andreasen JO, Farik B, Munksgaard EC. Long-term calcium hydroxide as a root canal dressing may increase risk of root fracture. Dental Traumatology 2002;18:134–137.

126. Tidmarsh BG. Acid-cleansed and resin-sealed root canals. Journal of Endodontics 1978;4: 117–121.

127. Tay FR, Pashley DH. Monoblocks in root canals: a hypothetical or a tangible goal. Journal of Endodontics 2007;33:391–398.

128. Shipper G, Ørstavik D, Teixeira FB, Trope M. An evaluation of microbial leakage in roots filled with a thermoplastic synthetic polymer-based root canal filling material (Resilon). Journal of Endodontics 2004;30:342–347.

129. Teixeira FB, Teixeira ECN, Thompson JY, Trope M. Fracture resistance of roots endodontically treated with a new resin filling material. Journal of the American Dental Association 2004;135: 646–652.

130. Stuart CH, Schwartz SA, Beeson TJ. Reinforcement of immature roots with a new resin filling material. Journal of Endodontics 2006;32:350–353.

131. Gesi A, Raffaelli O, Goracci C, et al. Interfacial strength of Resilon and gutta-percha to

intraradicular dentin. Journal of Endodontics 2005;31: 809–813.

132. Hiraishi N, Papacchini F, Loushine RJ, et al. Shear bond strength of Resilon to a methacrylate-based root canal sealer. International Endodontic Journal 2005;38: 753–763.

133. Jainaen A, Palamara JEA, Messer HH. Push-out bond strengths of the dentine-sealer interface with and without a main cone. International Endodontic Journal 2007;40:882–890.

134. Sly MM, Moore BK, Platt JA, Brown CE. Push-out bond strength of a new endodontic obturation system (Resilon/Epiphany). Journal of Endodontics 2007;33: 160–162.

135. Üreyen Kaya B, Keçeci AD, Orhan H, Belli S. Micropush-out bond strengths of gutta-percha versus thermoplastic synthetic polymer-based systems- an *ex vivo* study. International Endodontic Journal 2008;41:211–218.

136. Paqué F, Sirtes G. Apical sealing ability of Resilon/Epiphany versus gutta-percha/AH Plus: immediate and 16-months leakage. International Endodontic Journal 2007;40:722–729.

137. Saleh IM, Ruyter IE, Haapasolo M, Ørstavik D. Bacterial penetration along different root canal filling materials in the presence or absence of smear layer. International Endodontic Journal 2008;41:32–40.

138. Shemesh H, van den Bos M, Wu M-K, Wesselink PR. Glucose penetration and fluid transport through coronal root structure and filled root canals. International Endodontic Journal 2007;40:866–872.

139. Lussi A, Nussbächer U, Grosrey J. A novel noninstrumented technique for cleansing the root canal system. Journal of Endodontics 1993;19: 549–553.

140. Lussi A, Messerli L, Hotz P, Grosrey J. A new non-instrumental technique for cleaning and filling root canals. International Endodontic Journal 1995;28:1–6.

141. Lussi A, Portmann P, Nussbächer U, et al. Comparison of two devices for root canal cleansing by the noninstrumentation technology. Journal of Endodontics 1999;25: 9–13.

142. Lussi A, Imwinkelried S, Hotz P, Grosrey J. Long-term obturation quality using noninstrumentation technology. Journal of Endodontics 2000;26: 491–493.

143. Lussi A, Suter B, Fritzsche A, et al. In vivo performance of the new non-instrumentation technology (NIT) for root canal obturation. International Endodontic Journal 2002;35:352–358.

144. Portmann P, Lussi A. A comparison between a new vacuum obturation technique and lateral condensation: an in vitro study. Journal of Endodontics 1994;20: 292–295.

145. Sargenti A, Richter SL. Rationalized Root Canal Treatment. New York, NY: AGSA, USA; 1965.

146. Alantar A, Tarragano H, Lefevre B. Extrusion of endodontic filling material into the insertions of the mylohyoid muscle. A case report. Oral Surgery, Oral Medicine, Oral Pathology 1994;78:646–649.

147. Allard KUB. Paraesthesia – a consequence of a controversial root-filling material? A case report. International Endodontic Journal 1986;19:205–208.

148. Ørstavik D, Brodin P, Aas E. Paraesthesia following endodontic treatment: survey of the literature and report of a case. International Endodontic Journal 1983;16:167–172.

149. Spector RG. Pharmacological properties of the glucocorticoids. International Dental Journal 1981;31:152–155.

150. Block RM, Lewis RD, Hirsch J, et al. Systemic distribution of [^{14}C]-labelled paraformaldehyde incorporated within formocresol following pulpotomies in dogs. Journal of Endodontics 1983;9:176–189.

151. Ørstavik D, Hongslo JK. Mutagenicity of endodontic sealers. Biomaterials 1985;6:129–132.

152. Naoum HA, Chandler NP. Temporization for endodontics. International Endodontic Journal 2002;35:964–978.

153. Kirkevang L-L, Ørstavik D, Hörsted-Bindslev P, Wenzel A. Periapical status and quality of root fillings and coronal restorations in a Danish population. International Endodontic Journal 2000;33:509–515.

154. Ray HA, Trope M. Periapical status of endodontically treated teeth in relation to the technical quality of the root filling and the coronal restoration. International Endodontic Journal 1995;28:12–18.

155. Heling I, Gorfil C, Slutzky H, et al. Endodontic failure caused by inadequate restorative procedures: Review and treatment recommendations. Journal of Prosthetic Dentistry 2002;87: 674–678.

156. Lynch CD, Burke FM, Riordain RN, Hannigan A. The influence of coronal restoration type on the survival of endodontically treated teeth. European Journal of Prosthodontics and Restorative Dentistry 2004;12: 171–176.

157. Chapman CR. New directions in the understanding and management of pain. Social Science and Medicine 1984;19:1261–1277.

158. George JM, Scott DS. The effects of psychological factors on recovery from surgery. Journal of the American Dental Association 1982;105:251–258.

159. Harrison JW, Baumgartner JC, Svec TA. Incidence of pain associated with clinical factors during and after root canal therapy. Part 2. Postobturation pain. Journal of Endodontics 1983;9:434–438.

160. Yesiloy C, Koren LZ, Morse DR, et al. Post-endodontic obturation pain: a comparative evaluation. Quintessence International 1988;19:431–438.

161. European Society of Endodontology. Quality guidelines for endodontic treatment: concensus report of the European Society of Endodontology. International Endodontic Journal 2006;39:921–930.

162. Fristad I, Molven O, Halse A. Nonsurgically retreated root-filled teeth- radiographic findings after 20–27 years. International Endodontic Journal 2004;37:12–18.

Chapter | 10 |

Surgical endodontics

J.L. Gutmann, J.D. Regan

SUMMARY

For more than a century surgical endodontics has been a mainstay for the retention of teeth that cannot be treated with nonsurgical endodontic procedures alone. However, recent advances in surgical techniques, based on better scientific understanding of the periradicular disease process, have enabled more predictable outcomes in treatment. Empirical decision-making of the past has been replaced by evidence-based principles. Coupled with the introduction of new instruments and magnification, refined principles of soft and hard tissue management, use of tissue regenerative techniques and materials, surgical endodontics has become a highly predictable procedure when practised by well-trained clinicians. Whilst there are a variety of endodontic surgical procedures, the primary

© 2009 Elsevier Ltd, Inc, BV
DOI: 10.1016/B978-0-7020-3156-4.00013-9

procedure is periradicular surgery, which includes curettage, root-end resection, root-end cavity preparation and root-end filling. This chapter will focus on the scientific basis for surgical endodontics, to provide a better understanding of the rationale for their application and to achieve predictable results in clinical practice.

INTRODUCTION

Research studies indicate that the outcome of non-surgical endodontic therapy is highly favourable with success rates of ninety percent or more being reported in recent decades.[1,2] However, despite these impressive statistics, occasionally, surgery may be indicated in order to achieve what was not possible with root canal treatment alone or to secure a biopsy for histological examination.

In recent years, advances in surgical techniques based on better scientific understanding of the periradicular disease process have facilitated greater success rates in endodontic surgical procedures.[3] Empirical decision-making in the past has been replaced by evidence-based principles. Coupled with the introduction of new instruments and magnification,[4] refined principles of soft and hard tissue management,[5] use of tissue regenerative techniques and materials[6] and enhanced principles of wound closure,[7] surgical endodontics has become a highly predictable procedure when practised by well-trained clinicians. The application of these principles and techniques by the endodontic specialist will ensure the retention of many teeth that may otherwise be considered non-salvageable.

The most common endodontic surgical procedure is periradicular surgery consisting of periradicular curettage, root-end resection, root-end preparation and root-end filling. Other procedures include perforation repair, root and tooth resection, crown-lengthening, intentional replantation, regenerative techniques, incision and drainage, and cortical trephination. This chapter will focus primarily on the essentials of periradicular surgery.

TREATMENT CHOICES

It is incumbent on the clinician to empower the patient to make the best decision based on sound scientific evidence. In order to provide for optimal treatment planning, an accurate assessment of the likely outcome of any potential treatment modality (non-surgical endodontic treatment, surgical endodontic treatment or extraction of the tooth followed by implant placement) is required.[8] Failure to fully understand the aetiology of the disease process will result in impaired clinical decision-making detrimental to the overall well being of the patient.

The best decision can be made when all available evidence is considered. A hierarchy of evidence exists with randomized-controlled trials at the peak of the evidence pyramid and case reports and personal opinions at the base. The adoption of evidence-based decision-making has greatly advanced clinical treatment planning in dentistry.

INDICATIONS FOR PERIRADICULAR SURGERY

Historically, most texts on endodontic surgery list multiple, 'cook-book' type indications for surgical intervention.[9,10] These often include instrument separation, apical fracture, inadequate root canal filling, and presence of a cyst. Advances in the understanding of the disease process involved in the development of apical periodontitis and in clinical techniques have eliminated most of these indications for surgery. Outcome studies of non-surgical root canal treatment versus surgical treatment have clearly shown a higher success rate with high quality non-surgical root canal treatment procedures using contemporary techniques. Unfortunately, most of the teeth referred to the specialist for surgical endodontic treatment would more appropriately have been treated non-surgically.[11] Periradicular tissues usually heal following removal of infection originating from the root canal system combined with the prevention of further contamination.[12,13] The main cause of failure following both non-surgical and surgical treatment is inadequate cleaning, shaping and filling of the root canal system.[14] Therefore, the routine selection of surgery without full case assessment, in particular the status of the root canal system, is unwarranted as is selection of surgery for the convenience of the clinician. Consequently, many of these types of cases would benefit tremendously from specialist assessment and management.

The indications for surgery must always be in the best interest of the patient and within the realm of the clinician's understanding and expertise.[15] These include the following; first, if failure has resulted from root canal treatment, and retreatment is impossible or would not achieve a better result, surgery may be indicated, e.g. non-negotiable canal, perforation or ledge with signs and/or symptoms. Secondly, if there is a strong possibility of failure with root canal treatment, surgery may be indicated, e.g. calcified canal with concomitant patient signs and/or symptoms. Thirdly, if a biopsy is necessary then again surgery is indicated. Contraindications to surgery are few and far between and are usually limited to patient (psychological and systemic), clinician (experience and expertise), and anatomical factors or complete lack of surgical access.

Table 10.1 General medical conditions

Hypertension	Coronary atherosclerotic disease
Stable angina	Myocardial infarction
	Chronic obstructive pulmonary disease
Anti-coagulant therapy	Cerebrovascular accident
Epilepsy	Diabetes
Adrenal insufficiency	Steroid therapy
Organ transplant	Impaired hepatic or renal function

PREOPERATIVE ASSESSMENT

The prognosis following surgery is dependent on careful patient assessment, evidence-based diagnosis and appropriate treatment planning.[16] Contraindications involving the patient's psychological or systemic conditions must be identified. Patient acceptance of, and cooperation with, the anticipated surgical procedure must be forthcoming. Procedures to minimize stress for patients who are particularly susceptible to pain and anxiety may be required.[5] General systemic factors, which usually require medical consultation, are listed in Table 10.1. As a general rule, no special precautions need to be taken when surgery is planned other than those that normally apply to routine dental procedures.[5]

Local factors are related to the management of both soft and hard tissues. These factors include the possible need to remove previous dental restorations that are failing and the need to revise the root filling beforehand as part of overall management of the case. If the quality of the existing root filling is doubtful, more favourable results have been obtained when the root canal system is retreated prior to surgical management.[17] The tooth must also be assessed for restorability, and its place in the overall treatment plan determined.

Radiological examination is essential, including assessment of previous radiographs, if available.[16] Radiographs from different angles should be taken, identifying the number, curvature and angle of the roots requiring surgery and the position of the apices relative to adjacent structures. Anatomical structures that may impair surgical or visual access to the surgical site must be identified. These include the mental foramen, zygomatic process, anterior nasal spine and external oblique ridge. The following factors are particularly important in a radiological assessment:

- relation of the apices to the inferior dental canal, mental foramen, the maxillary sinus or adjacent roots
- number of, and access to, the roots

- approximate length of the roots; this may sometimes be ascertained from the patient's records if non-surgical endodontic treatment had been performed
- approximate extent of any visible lesion.

Whilst traditional radiographic techniques provide the clinician with the necessary information needed to assess the surgical site adequately, occasionally, newer techniques such as computed tomography (CT) may be necessary. Computed tomography can be divided into two main categories based on acquisition X-ray beam geometry, fan beam CT and cone beam CT. With the newer cone beam CT, the entire volume of data is collected in a single rotation of a cone shaped X-ray source and sophisticated software is used to generate three-dimensional images at substantially lower radiation doses than traditional CT scanners. The three-dimensional images are invaluable in allowing the clinician to define the precise extent and location of a lesion that otherwise might be impossible to determine.

Communication with the patient concerning the need for surgery, outline of the procedure, anticipated difficulties and problems, the prognosis, preoperative medication or mouth rinses, postoperative care and long-term assessment is essential.[5] Provision of written information and instructions is beneficial and can help to allay some of the patient's fears.

The following pre-treatment regimens are recommended:

- A periodontal examination must be performed prior to surgery to assess for periodontal pockets and/or sinus tracts. Scaling and/or root planing may be required. The patient's oral hygiene practices should be assessed and good oral hygiene reinforced.
- Patients should be placed on chlorhexidine (0.12–0.2%) rinses in an attempt to reduce the oral microorganisms. These rinses should be performed one day prior to surgery, immediately before surgery and should continue for at least 2 to 3 days afterwards.[5]
- Patients can begin taking, if tolerated, non-steroidal anti-inflammatory medication one day prior to surgery, or at the latest one hour before treatment.
- Patients should be advised to refrain from smoking.
- If sedation (enteral or parenteral) is to be used, the patient must bring an accompanying person, who will be responsible for escorting the patient home and for compliance with postoperative instructions.

SURGICAL KIT

A plethora of instruments are available for endodontic surgical procedures. The dental industry has formed an effective partnership with clinicians allowing for the development of numerous new instruments. Many of these have been developed specifically for use by clinicians operating with a microscope; these include miniature surgical blades and mirrors, rear-venting surgical handpieces, ultrasonically energized root-end preparation tips and root-end pluggers (see later). Specific instruments should be chosen that facilitate the procedure according to the individual operator's requirements. Instruments must be sterile, sharp, undamaged and should enable the surgeon to maintain total control of the surgical site. A basic kit should contain the most commonly used instruments and should be readily supplemented with any other instrument considered necessary. Key instruments and their general uses are listed in Table 10.2 and illustrated in Figure 10.1.

Magnification and illumination in endodontic surgery

Visual aids such as loupes and the operating microscope provide the operator with excellent lighting and magnification.[18] The development of operating microscopes specifically for endodontics has been a recent advance that greatly enhances the operator's view of the surgical site. However, there is a steep learning curve associated with the use of the operating microscope and proficiency demands regular and continuous use. The enhanced vision facilitates the location of a multitude of anatomical features not easily visible to the naked eye. These include isthmuses, fins, and additional or accessory canals. In addition, fractures, perforations and resorptive defects are more easily identified and managed.

SURGICAL TECHNIQUE

Tissue anaesthesia and haemostasis

The ability to achieve profound anaesthesia and tissue haemostasis in the surgical site is essential. Profound anaesthesia will minimize or eliminate patient discomfort during the procedure and for a significant period thereafter, whilst good haemostasis will improve vision at the surgical site, improve root-end cavity preparation and filling, minimize surgical time, and reduce surgical blood loss, postsurgical haemorrhage and postsurgical swelling.[5] An anaesthetic solution containing a vasoconstrictor is indicated to achieve these objectives.[19]

The choice of the anaesthetic-vasoconstrictor combination is dependent on the health status of the patient and surgical needs. Lidocaine (lignocaine) with adrenaline

Table 10.2 Surgical kit
Presurgical assessment
Mirror & curved explorer
Straight & curved periodontal probes
Soft tissue incision, elevation & reflection
Sharp scalpels – Nos 15, 15c, 11, & 12
Micro scalpels
Broad-based periosteal elevator
Broad-based periosteal retractor
Tissue forceps
Surgical aspirator
Irrigating syringes & needles
Periradicular curettage
Straight & angled bone curettes
Small endodontic spoon curette
Periodontal curettes
Fine, curved mosquito forceps
Small, curved surgical scissors
Bone removal & root-end resection
Surgical length round and tapered fissure burs
Straight & angled bone curettes
Rear-venting high-speed handpiece
Contra-angle slow-speed handpiece
Root-end preparation/placement of root-end filling/finishing of resected root end
Ultrasonic or sonic unit with appropriate root-end preparation tips
Root-end filling material
Haemostatic agent (avoid bone wax)
Miniature material carriers & condensers
Small ball-ended burnisher
Paper points or fine aspirator tip
Small, fine explorer
Suturing and soft tissue closure
Surgical scissors
Haemostat or fine needle holders
Various suture types & sizes (USP 3-0 to 6-0)
Sterile gauze for soft tissue compression
Miscellaneous (or readily available)
Adequate aspiration equipment
Additional light source – Magnification
Root canal filling materials
Anaesthetic syringes, needles & local anaesthetic solution
Biopsy bottle containing transport medium

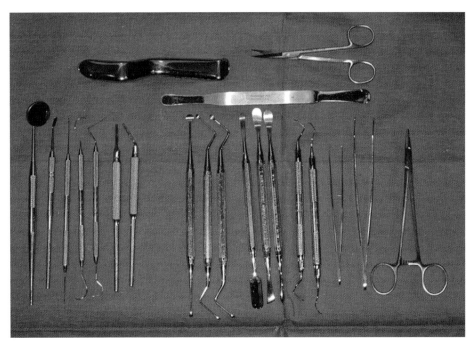

Figure 10.1 Basic instruments for periradicular surgery (see Table 10.2 for details).

(epinephrine) has long been recognized as an excellent anaesthetic agent for periradicular surgery because of its clinical success in producing profound and prolonged analgesia.[20] Although several studies support the efficacy of 2% lidocaine with 1:200000 to 1:100000 concentrations of adrenaline for profound anaesthesia,[21] clinical evidence suggests that a 1:50000 concentration provides better haemostasis.[22] The prolonged postoperative pain relief is due to the inhibition of peripheral neuronal discharges, which in turn, helps reduce the subsequent development of central sensitization.[23]

Assessment of the patient's systemic status is essential prior to the use of 2% lidocaine with adrenaline, especially 1:50000 adrenaline. This is important because lidocaine with adrenaline can elevate systemic plasma levels of the vasoconstrictor[24] although the haemodynamic response to this increase is still controversial.[25] The potential rise in adrenaline concentration suggests that high-risk patients should be carefully monitored. Great care should be taken during injection to prevent intravascular placement of the solution.[19] When an anaesthetic with 1:50000 adrenaline is unavailable, 1:80000 is clinically acceptable. While 2% lidocaine with 1:100000 adrenaline is recommended for regional nerve blocks prior to endodontic surgery, this level of vasoconstrictor does not suffice for local haemostasis at the surgical site. Haemostasis must also be established at the surgical site[26] by additional injections

supraperiosteally using 2% lidocaine with 1:50000 adrenaline.[27]

In healthy patients a dose of 2–4 ml is recommended. In the maxilla, achievement of both anaesthesia and haemostasis can be accomplished simultaneously. This requires multiple injections, depositing the solution throughout the entire submucosa superficial to the periosteum at the level of the root apices in the surgical site. The needle, with the bevel toward the bone, is advanced to the target site and, following aspiration, 0.5 ml of solution is deposited slowly (Fig. 10.2). The needle may be moved peripherally and similar, small amounts of solution deposited. Additional injections can be made to ensure that the entire surgical field has been covered. Slow, peripheral supraperiosteal infiltration into the submucosa promotes maximum diffusion (Fig. 10.3). In the mandible the anaesthetic–vasoconstrictor solution is injected slowly adjacent to the root apices, in addition to the block injection of the inferior alveolar nerve. Incisions that are made in alignment with the long axis of the supporting supraperiosteal vasculature coupled with careful elevation and reflection of the tissues, will minimize haemorrhage at the surgical site.[5]

The amount of anaesthetic solution containing 1:50000 adrenaline that is necessary to achieve anaesthesia and haemostasis is dependent on the surgical site, but 2.0 to 3.0 ml will usually suffice. The rate of injection can also

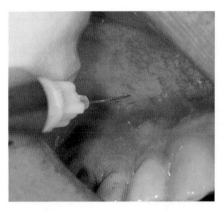

Figure 10.2 Placement of anaesthetic solution around the root apex of the tooth to be treated surgically.

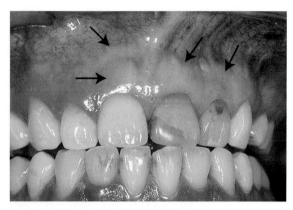

Figure 10.3 Slow and careful infiltration of the anaesthetic solution provides widespread and effective tissue haemostasis (delineated by arrows) for treatment of left maxillary central incisor.

influence the degree of haemostasis and anaesthesia obtained, with a rate of 1 to 2 ml/min recommended.[28] Injecting at higher rates will lead to localized pooling of solution, delaying and limiting diffusion into the adjacent tissues resulting in less than optimal anaesthesia and haemostasis. Predictable anaesthesia and haemostasis should be achieved prior to any incisions. Later attempts during surgery to improve anaesthesia and haemostasis are less successful. Following administration of the local anaesthetic, sufficient time must elapse prior to the initial incision (5–10 mins), to allow for proper vascular constriction throughout the surgical site. Other adjunctive agents are available to enhance the haemostasis during treatment. These will be discussed later in this chapter.

Soft tissue incision and reflection

Good surgical access requires predetermined, meticulous tissue flap design followed by the incision and elevation of the soft tissue from the underlying bone. The design of the tissue flap is crucial not only to surgical entry and management of the root structure, but also to healing of the surgical wound. The design of soft tissue flaps has received wide and varied attention. For years, the semilunar flap (Partsch incision) in the apical loose alveolar mucosa was recommended but this has now been largely superseded. Various flap designs have been advocated based on a biological approach to tissue management and wound healing. The range of contemporary surgical flap designs[5] is outlined in Table 10.3. There are strong biological reasons to consider the use of full muco-periosteal tissue flaps whenever possible (Table 10.3). Figures 10.4–10.9 detail diagrammatically each design,

whilst the subsequent text gives a brief description of their application.

Full mucoperiosteal tissue flap

The horizontal incision begins in the gingival sulcus, extending through the gingival fibres to the crestal bone. The scalpel blade is held in a near vertical position (Fig. 10.10). In the interdental region, the incision should pass through the mid-col area, separating the buccal and lingual papillae, and severing the gingival fibres to the depth of the interdental crestal bone (Fig. 10.11). This is critical to prevent sloughing of the papillae due to a compromised blood supply. Because of the shape of the embrasure space, it may be necessary to use a curved scalpel blade or a miniature surgical blade to follow the interproximal tooth contours (Fig. 10.11).

Vertical (releasing) incisions are used in the triangular and rectangular flap designs (Figs 10.4 & 10.5), and are vertically oriented passing between the roots of adjacent teeth and coursing parallel to the long axes of the roots. The incision should be over intact bone and to the depth of the bone. Vertical incisions should terminate at the mesial or distal line angles of teeth, and never in papillae or in the mid-root area. Incisions should be positioned to ensure that at closure, the re-apposed soft tissue will overlie solid bone.

The trapezoidal flap design (Fig. 10.6) incorporates angled releasing incisions and is not considered biologically acceptable for periradicular surgery because it cuts across the vertically positioned supraperiosteal vasculature and tissue-supportive collagen fibres. The horizontal or envelope flap design (Fig. 10.7) is often used for maxillary

Table 10.3 Periradicular surgical soft tissue flap designs

TYPE OF TISSUE FLAP	ADVANTAGES/DISADVANTAGES
Full mucoperiosteal	
Triangular	Maintains intact vertical blood supply.
Rectangular	Minimizes haemorrhage.
Trapezoidal	Primary wound closure & rapid healing.
Horizontal (envelope)	Allows survey of bone and root structure. Excellent surgical orientation. Minimal postoperative sequelae. May have loss of tissue attachment. May have loss of crestal bone height. Possibility of tissue flap dislodgement. Possible loss of interdental papilla integrity.
Limited mucoperiosteal	
Submarginal curved (semilunar)	Marginal & interdental papilla intact. Scarring.
Submarginal retangular (Luebke-Ochsenbein)	Unaltered soft tissue attachment. Adequate surgical access – may be compromised in posterior cases or cases with lateral root defects. Good healing potential. Disruption of blood supply. Possibility of tissue shrinkage. Delayed secondary healing/scarring. Limited orientation to apical region. Very limited in posterior surgery.
Papilla-base incision	Newer technique & relatively limited data. May interrupt blood supply leading to delayed healing. Difficult to perform. Good healing potential.

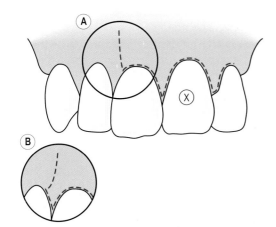

Figure 10.4 Triangular tissue flap design with single vertical releasing incision. The vertical releasing incision can be performed in different ways. Either (**A**) the incision leaves the interdental papilla intact or (**B**; insert) the incision includes the interdental papilla. In either case the incision line should meet the tooth at 90°.

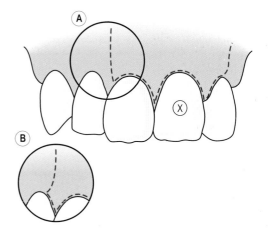

Figure 10.5 Rectangular tissue flap design with double vertical releasing incisions. As with the triangular flap design, variations can be used with the vertical incisions (A and B); a description has been included in Figure 10.4.

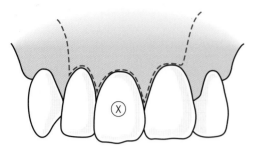

Figure 10.6 Trapezoidal tissue flap design. Note vertical releasing incisions are angled towards the base of the flap.

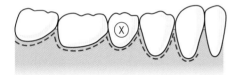

Figure 10.7 Horizontal tissue flap design. No vertical releasing incisions are used initially but they can be added later to enhance surgical access if necessary.

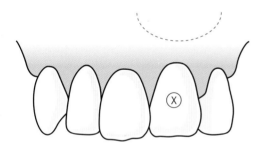

Figure 10.8 Semilunar tissue flap design. Note that the scope of this flap limits extension if necessary.

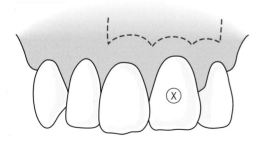

Figure 10.9 Luebke-Ochsenbein (submarginal) tissue flap design. This flap may have one or two vertical releasing incisions, or may be limited to a horizontal incision, only if sufficient surgical and visual access can be obtained.

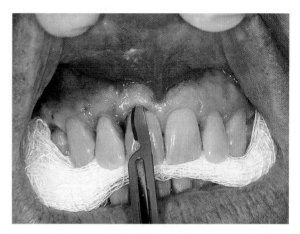

Figure 10.10 Intrasulcular incision with a no. 15 scalpel blade. Note the vertical position of the scalpel as it cuts through and releases the crestal fibres.

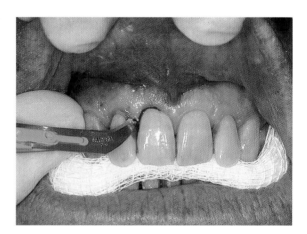

Figure 10.11 Use of a no. 12 scalpel blade to release the fibres of the interdental papilla. Note the depth and angulation of the blade.

or mandibular molars, or as palatal flaps. However, some type of releasing incision is generally incorporated, albeit not as long as that used with triangular or rectangular flaps.

Tissue reflection always begins in the attached gingiva of the vertical incision. The periosteal elevator is positioned to apply reflective forces in a lateral direction against the cortical bone while elevating the tougher fibrous-based tissue of the gingiva (Fig. 10.12). This also elevates the periosteum and its superficial tissues from the cortical plate. Subsequently, the elevator is directed coronally (Fig. 10.13) to elevate the marginal and interdental gingiva with minimal traumatic force (Fig. 10.14). All reflective forces should be applied to the bone and periosteum, with minimal forces on the gingival elements; this

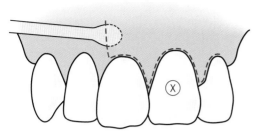

Figure 10.12 The periosteum is initially elevated by applying force against the cortical bone in the region of the attached tissues.

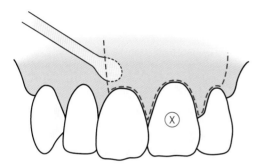

Figure 10.13 The periosteal elevator is subsequently moved coronally to elevate the marginal tissues.

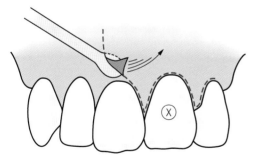

Figure 10.14 The entire tissue flap is elevated with minimal force being directed on the marginal and interdental gingival tissues.

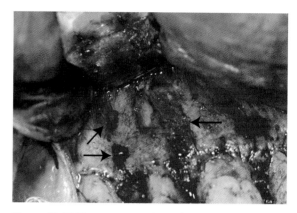

Figure 10.15 Tissue tags remain on the cortical bone after flap elevation (arrowed).

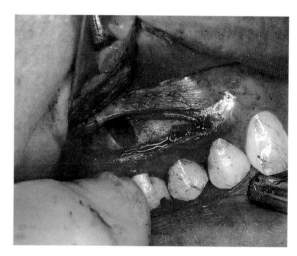

Figure 10.16 Pinching of the mucosal tissue with the periosteal retractor should be avoided during surgery.

is referred to as undermining elevation.[5] After tissue reflection, bleeding tissue tags are often seen on the cortical surface in the crestal region and between root eminences (Fig. 10.15). These tissue tags play an important role in healing so they should not be removed during surgery.

Adequate retraction of the tissue flap is necessary for surgical access to the periradicular tissues. The retractor must always rest on sound bone with light but firm pressure. Pinching of the soft tissue flap with the retractor must be avoided to minimize tissue damage and untoward postsurgical sequelae (Fig. 10.16). If this is not possible the reflected tissue must be elevated further or the tissue flap extended to release its attachment from the bone.

Limited mucoperiosteal tissue flap

These tissue flaps do not include the marginal and interdental gingiva. The horizontal incision of these flaps should be in the attached gingiva with the vertical incisions involving both the attached gingiva and alveolar mucosa. An absolute minimum of 2 mm of attached gingiva from the depth of the gingival sulcus must be present before this flap design is chosen. However, there is a very narrow limit for safe incision between the sulcular depth and the mucogingival junction in most patients, especially in the mandible.[29]

The rectangular submarginal flap design (Luebke-Ochsenbein flap) is formed by a scalloped horizontal incision in the attached gingiva and two vertical releasing incisions (Fig. 10.9). Scalloping reflects the contour of the marginal gingivae and provides an adequate distance from the depths of the gingival sulci. Here also, the vasculature and collagen fibres are severed. It may be used in maxillary anterior or posterior teeth in which reflection of marginal and interdental gingival is contraindicated because of tissue inflammation or aesthetic concerns with extensive fixed prostheses. Often, anatomical factors negate the use of a limited mucoperiosteal flap design.

Papilla-base flap

The papilla-base flap has been suggested[30] to prevent recession of the papilla. It consists of two releasing vertical incisions, connected by the papilla-base incision and intrasulcular incision in the cervical area of the tooth. A microsurgical blade that does not exceed 2.5 mm in width should be used, as intricate, minute movement of the surgical blade within the small dimensions of the interproximal space is crucial.

Two different incisions are made at the base of the papilla. An initial shallow incision severs the epithelium and connective tissue to the depth of 1.5 mm from the surface of the gingiva. The path is a curved line, connecting one side of the papilla to the other. The incision begins and ends perpendicular to the gingival margin. In the second step, the scalpel retraces the base of the previously created incision while inclined vertically, towards the crestal bone margin. The second incision, results in a split thickness flap in the apical third of the base of the papilla. From this point on moving apically, a full thickness mucoperiosteal flap is elevated. Whilst the papilla-base flap can result in predictable healing results, this technique is challenging to perform. Atraumatic handling of the soft tissues is of utmost importance in order to obtain rapid healing through primary intention. The epithelium of the partial thickness flap has to be supported by underlying connective tissue; otherwise, it will necrose and lead to scar formation. On the other hand, excessive thickness of the connective tissue layer of the split flap portion could compromise the survival of the buccal papilla left in place.[7]

Osseous entry and root identification

Prior to root-end resection and removal of any diseased soft tissue surrounding the root, bone may need to be removed to gain visual access to the surgical site. Removal of the bone is usually accomplished with a large round bur (ISO size 018 or 024), using a low- or high-speed

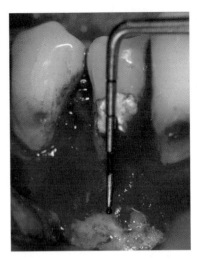

Figure 10.17 Placement of a calibrated periodontal probe to determine the approximate position of the root apex.

handpiece. The bone is removed in a brush-stroke fashion with copious irrigation, creating a window over the root apex. Adherence to this technique will reduce the heat produced during the osteotomy procedure, thereby minimizing the potential for damage to the living bone tissue. In many cases, the osteotomy may need to be started from a coronal position, moving apically once the root structure has been identified. Care should be taken to avoid removing cementum from the root surface in order to prevent resorption at a later date. Entry as close to the apex, however, is recommended, with the angle of entry facilitating visibility and surgical access. Measuring the approximate length of the root on the bone, as estimated from the preoperative radiological assessment, facilitates location of the root apex (Fig. 10.17).

The apex may also be identified during osseous palpation after soft tissue reflection. Where the bone is thin, or the root apex is prominent, a straight bone curette can be used in a rotating motion to penetrate the cortical plate and identify the root structure (Fig. 10.18). In cases with large periradicular lesions, the loss of the cortical plate of bone may directly expose the root apex. Once exposed, the bur can be used to create a larger window to outline the root apex. In those cases where the bone is thick and location of the apex is difficult, the same type of initial osseous penetration can be made and a sterile radiopaque object placed in the hole. A radiograph will then provide additional information on the location of the root apex.

Root structure can be differentiated from surrounding bone by texture (smooth and hard), lack of bleeding upon probing, outline (presence of periodontal ligament), and colour (yellowish). The perimeter of the root and its periodontal ligament may also be identified by painting 1% methylene blue dye on the surface.[31]

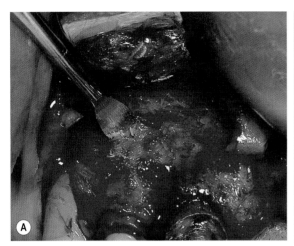
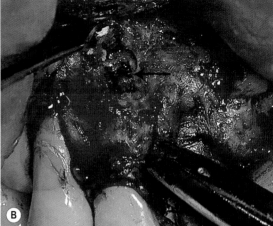

Figure 10.18 (**A**) Use of a straight curette to peel away the surface cortical bone. (**B**) Penetration through the bone with a curette alone to expose the root (arrowed). Note bone chips on curette.

Removal of diseased soft tissue (periradicular curettage)

This procedure can often be performed prior to, or in conjunction with, root-end resection. The purpose is to remove the reactive tissue.[32] Contrary to previous belief, every remnant of this soft reactive tissue need not be removed to avoid failure, as the tissue elements in the periphery of these lesions usually contain fibroblasts, vascular buds, new collagen and bone matrix. In cases where the soft tissue mass is exposed upon flap reflection or initial bone removal, curettage can proceed prior to root-end resection. In other cases, resection is necessary to gain access to most of the tissue.

Curettage is accomplished with straight or angled surgical bone curettes and periodontal curettes (Fig. 10.19). Initially the bone curettes are used to peel the soft tissue from the lateral borders of the bony crypt. This is performed with the concave surface of the curette facing the bony wall, applying pressure only against the bone (Fig. 10.20).[33] It is desirable to avoid penetration of the soft tissue as this may sever the vascular network, and increase local haemorrhage. Once the tissue is freed along the lateral margins, the bone curettes can be turned round and used in a scraping fashion along the deep walls of the crypt. This will detach the soft tissue from its lingual or palatal base. Once loosened, tissue forceps are used to grasp the tissue gently as it is teased from its position with a bone curette. The tissue sample is placed directly into a bottle of neutral buffered formalin or transport medium for biopsy. In cases requiring root-end resection prior to curettage, the root structure must be exposed sufficiently to minimize shredding of the soft tissues during resection. Despite profound anaesthesia at the surgical site as a

whole, it is often found that the centre of the periradicular lesion remains sensitive. This is explained by the proliferation of neural endings stimulated by inflammatory mediators.[34] Infiltration of local anaesthetic into the reactive tissue will invariably eliminate any residual sensation.

In the presence of large lesions, care must be exercised during curettage of the lateral surfaces of the bony crypt to avoid damage to adjacent roots and their pulpal vasculature. Presurgical radiographs should warn of this possibility, and tissue in these areas may need to be left in position. Caution is necessary to prevent damage to vital structures when operating close to the maxillary antrum, mental foramen, or mandibular canal. When soft tissue is adherent, either lingually to the root, or in the furcation region, periodontal curettes facilitate its removal. Periradicular curettage is normally performed in conjunction with resection of the root-end.[35]

Biopsy

It is evident from the literature that the vast majority of periradicular lesions are granulomas. However, a small percentage (0.7–5%) are reported to be different based on histological examination.[36] These 'other' lesions include odontogenic cysts (odontogenic keratocyst, dentigerous cysts,), non-odontogenic cysts (globulomaxillary cyst, nasopalatine cyst), ossifying fibroma, Pindborg tumour, Langerhans cell disease, or osteoblastoma to mention just a few. More seriously, however, are lesions that might be neoplastic. Many reports exist in the literature documenting cases of misdiagnosis.[37,38,39] Considering the potential gravity of this situation, it is widely agreed that tissue excised during surgical endodontic procedures should be sent for histological examination.[40]

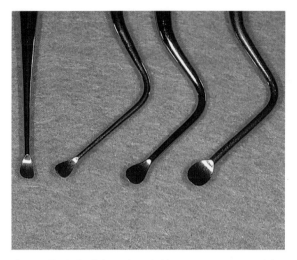

Figure 10.19 Straight and angled bone curettes are useful to manage the wide variety of challenges encountered in bone and soft tissue removal.

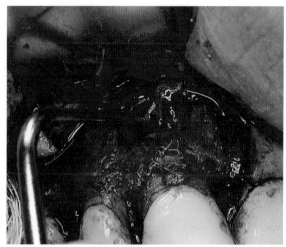

Figure 10.20 Use of the bone curette to peel the soft tissue lesion from the bone cavity.

Root-end resection

The term root-end resection refers specifically to the removal of the apical portion of the root. There are many indications for resection of the root-end during periradicular surgery, each designed to eliminate aetiological factors.

Historically, the technique of root-end resection involved the creation of a bevel on the root face, to improve surgical access and visibility.[35,41,42,43] The angle of resection was determined by the root inclination and curvature, number of roots, thickness of bone and position of the root in the bone. Current evidence indicates that reducing the angle of the bevel will reduce dentinal tubule exposure.[44] Based on the number of dentinal tubules communicating between the root canal and the resected root face, the angle of the bevel should be kept to a minimum.[44] A significant increase in leakage from the root canal system has been demonstrated as the bevel increased.[45] Ultrasonic instruments have been developed that greatly facilitate preparation along the long axis of the root and, therefore eliminate the need for extensive bevelling of the root face.

The root-end can be resected in one of two ways. First, after the root-end has been exposed, the bur (narrow straight fissure) is positioned at the desired angle and the root is shaved away, beginning from the apex, cutting coronally (Fig. 10.21). The bur is moved from mesial to distal, shaving the root to a smooth and flat finish until the entire canal system and root outline is exposed. As mentioned earlier, the root outline can be more easily visualized by staining the periodontal ligament with 1% methylene blue dye.[41] This approach allows for continual observation of the root-end during cutting. The second technique of resection is to predetermine the amount of

root-end to be resected. The bur and handpiece are positioned, and the apex is resected by cutting through the root from mesial to distal (Fig. 10.21). Once the apex is removed, the root face is gently shaved with the bur to smooth the surface and ensure complete resection and visibility of the root face. This technique works well when an apical biopsy is desired, or to gain access to significant amounts of soft tissue located lingual to the root. It is also the technique of choice in cases where the root-end is located in close proximity to structures such as the mental foramen or the inferior alveolar canal. The disadvantage however, is that this approach may remove more root structure than necessary.

The appearance of the root face following root-end resection will vary depending on the type of bur used, the external root anatomy, the anatomy of the canal system exposed at the particular angle of resection, and the nature and density of the root canal filling material. Various types of burs have been recommended for root-end resection;[5] each will leave a characteristic imprint on the root face, from rough-grooved and gouged to smooth.[46] To date, no study has determined the advantages of one type of bur over another, although for years clinical practice has favoured a smooth flat root surface.[47]

The level to which the root-end should be resected will be dictated by the following factors:[5]

- access and visibility to the surgical site
- position and anatomy of the root within the alveolar bone
- presence and position of additional roots, e.g. an additional palatal or lingual root
- anatomy of the cut root surface relative to the number of canals and their configuration

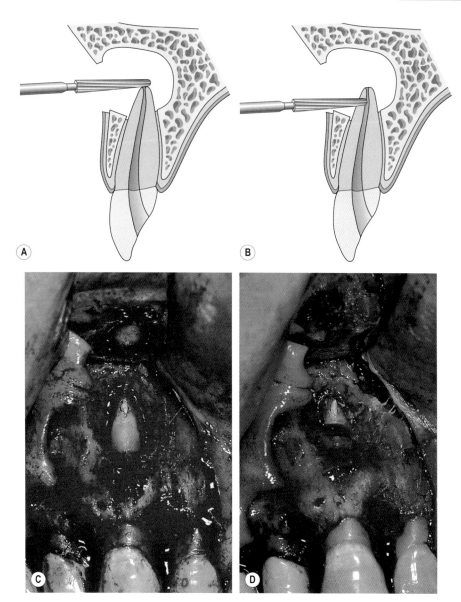

Figure 10.21 Diagrammatic representation of (A) root-end resection from the apex to coronal; (B) root-end resection when the amount of root to be resected has been determined. (C) Clinical case of root-end resection in which the amount of the root to be resected has been predetermined. (D) Resection of the root apex.

- need to place a root-end filling
- presence and location of a perforation
- presence of an intra-alveolar root fracture
- anatomical considerations, e.g. proximity of adjacent teeth, mental foramen or inferior dental canal, level of remaining crestal bone
- presence of significant accessory canals, which may dictate a more extensive resection.

Regardless of the rationale for the extent of root-end removal, there is no reason to resect the root to the base of a large periradicular lesion as was previously advised. Likewise, resection to the point where little (<1 mm) or no crestal bone remains covering the buccal aspect of the root may very well doom the tooth to failure (Fig. 10.22). On the other hand, omitting to remove sufficient root structure to be able to inspect the resected root face and

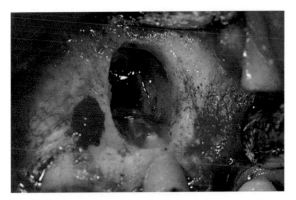

Figure 10.22 Severely angled resections, often coupled with large periradicular lesions, compromise the amount of remaining crestal bone.

place a root-end filling may also contribute to failure. Root canals or anastomoses may be missed, or may be improperly managed in confined spaces.

The complete root face must be identified and examined after resection. This is inspected, preferably under high magnification and good illumination, with a fine, sharp probe guided around the periphery of the root and the root canal. The external root anatomy will determine the ultimate shape of the cut root-end, such as oval, round, dumb-bell shaped, kidney-bean shaped, or tear-drop shaped (Fig. 10.23). The outline of the resected root-end will vary depending on the tooth, angle of any bevel and position of the cut on the root. However, the entire surface must be visible. If visibility is impaired, or the root has an unusual cross-section, 1% methylene blue dye can be placed on the root face for 5 to 10 seconds using a sterile sponge applicator and rinsed off with a stream of sterile water or saline. Cotton pellets should not be used as remnants of cotton fibres left in the surgical site have been shown to induce a foreign-body reaction in healing tissues.[5] The dye will stain the periodontal ligament dark blue, highlighting the root outline.[41] The shape of the exposed canal system will vary depending on the angle of the bevel and the canal anatomy at that level. Canal systems will generally assume a more elongated and accentuated shape with increasing angles of bevel (Fig. 10.24).

Also visible on most resected root-ends is the presence of root canal filling material and the interface between the filling material and the root dentine. Variations in quality of the filling will be seen in both the type of filling material and the nature of the filling technique (Fig. 10.25). Furthermore, the different burs used for resection will create discrepancies in the surface of the filling material and its adaptation to the canal walls. For example, coarse diamond burs will tend to rip and tear at the gutta-percha root canal filling, spreading the gutta-percha over the edge of the

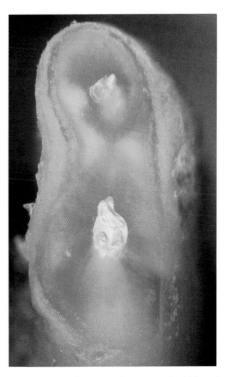

Figure 10.23 Resected root outline. Note the kidney bean shape along with position of the canals. No canal anastomosis is visible.

canal aperture and onto the resected root face (Fig. 10.26). Surface finishing with an ultra-fine diamond is recommended (Fig. 10.27) (Ultrafine no. 862-012 diamond bur, Brasseler, Savannah, GA, USA).

The presence of additional canals, anastomoses, fracture lines, and the quality of the apical adaptation of the root canal filling must be checked on the resected root surface (Fig. 10.28). If methylene blue dye has been used, it will also stain the periphery of the canal system and highlight fracture lines. A fibre-optic light can be aimed at, or behind, the root-end to enhance visibility.[9] Sometimes, it may be necessary to remove additional root structure to identify the canal system or, in the case of a fracture line, to observe its direction and extent.

A major area of concern following root-end resection and dentinal tubule exposure is the possibility that these tubules may serve as a direct source of contamination from the uncleaned root canal system into the periradicular tissues. Root-ends resected from 45° to 60° have as many as 28000 tubules/mm^2 immediately adjacent to the canal.[44] At the dentino-cemental junction, areas that may communicate with the root canal even in the presence of a root-end filling 13000 tubules/mm^2 are found. Likewise, due to angular changes in the tubules at the apex, there could be patent communication with the main canal if the

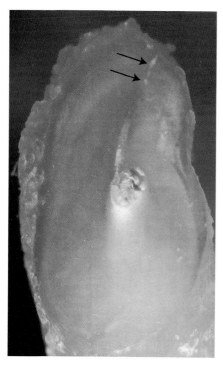

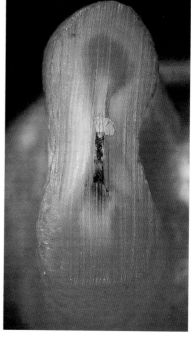

Figure 10.24 Angled resection reveals an extended canal space. Removal of additional root palatally will be necessary to manage the uppermost part of the canal system (arrowed).

Figure 10.25 Root-end resection reveals a poorly compacted gutta-percha filling. Voids filled with sealer are present between the gutta-percha cones and an anastomosis is present that is filled with tissue remnants (bluish colour).

depth of the root-end preparation in the buccal aspect of the cavity is insufficient.[48,49] Root-end resections in older teeth have shown less leakage than that seen in teeth from younger patients;[50] this corroborates with the findings of sclerosis and reduced patency in apical dentinal tubules.[51]

Another concern following root-end resection is the formation of a contaminated smear layer over the resected root-end (Fig. 10.29). This may serve as a source of irritation to the periradicular tissues, primarily preventing the intimate reformation of a layer of cementum against the resected tubules. A thicker smear layer is usually created when cutting without water spray,[52] or when using coarse diamond burs rather than tungsten carbide burs.[53] Therefore, it is recommended that root-end resection be performed under constant irrigation, which minimizes the dentinal smear layer. If diamond burs are used to resect the root, a medium grit is preferred, followed by a fine or ultrafine grit diamond.

Root-end cavity preparation

In order to seal the potential avenues of communication from the resected root-end to the canal system adequately, a root-end preparation should be made into the root

to the coronal extent of the resected apical tubules.[45] A depth of 2–4 mm is generally sufficient[43,54] depending on the angle of the resection. Increasing the depth of the root-end filling significantly decreases apical leakage.[45] The minimum depths for a root-end cavity, measured from the buccal aspect of the cavity, are 1.0, 2.1 and 2.5 mm for a 90°, 30° and 45° angle of resection, respectively.[45] Ideally, this preparation is made in the long axis of the root, parallel to the anatomical outline of the root, possesses adequate retention form, and encompasses all exposed orifices of the root canal system. If this is the case, then the depths indicated will be sufficient in all aspects of the preparation.

The final outline of the preparation will depend mainly on the anatomy of the exposed canal space, and in some cases, the nature of the root outline. For example, in maxillary central incisors, the shape of the root-end preparation will generally be round to oval in shape. In premolars or molars, it may be very elongated and narrow in conjunction with oval or round shapes.

Root-end preparations are best created with specially designed, ultrasonically energized instruments (Fig. 10.30). These ultrasonic tips eliminate many of the difficulties associated with root-end preparation with burs.

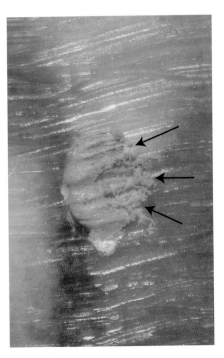

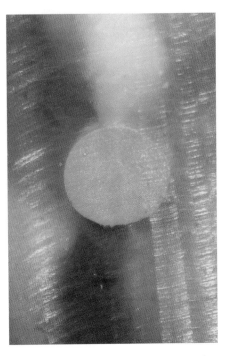

Figure 10.26 Rough surface of resected root after being cut with a coarse diamond. Note the gutta-percha has been dragged across the surface of the root (arrowed).

Figure 10.27 Smooth surface of resected root and root filling created with an ultrafine diamond and waterspray. Note the adaptation of the root filling material to the outline of the canal.

The small, angled tips allow for ultrasonic shaping of apical preparations parallel to the long axis of the root after minimal root-end resection and minimal bevelling of the root face (Fig. 10.31). They are effective in the debridement and enlargement of canal anastomoses and irregularities commonly found in molar roots (Fig. 10.32);[55] the ability of this technique to achieve better-shaped and cleaner root-end preparations as opposed to bur preparations has been highlighted.[56,57,58] The creation of clean, good quality root-end preparations can also been achieved with the use of sonic tips[59,60] and clinical experience would support the routine use of either of these newer techniques. However, a note of caution has been sounded by some authors,[61,62] who have demonstrated cracks in the root surface following use of ultrasonic root-end preparation instruments.

After root-end preparation the cavity should be irrigated with sterile saline or water. Small suction tips, made from 20- or 18-gauge needles that can be bent and adapted to a high-speed suction device, are used to remove fluid and debris from the cavity. Some clinicians prefer to use paper points to dry the preparation. The Stropko irrigator/drier device (Vista Dental, Racine, WI, USA) is a simple and effective means of drying the root-end preparation (Fig. 10.33A). Although rinsing the cavity with citric acid has

been recommended to remove the smear layer,[55] recent studies have indicated that this may actually enhance the amount of leakage after root-end filling.[62,63] Despite creating cleaner root-end cavity walls and assisting in debris removal, the routine use of citric acid is questionable. Following drying, the cavity must be inspected to ensure that it is clean and that it encompasses all of the canal extensions. Small mirrors have been designed specifically for this purpose (Fig 10.33B).

Root-end cavity filling

Irrespective of whether a root-end filling is placed or not, it is important that the canal system is cleaned and sealed as well as possible. In many cases this may necessitate that the old root canal filling should be revised prior to surgery. Under these circumstances, many cases may be successful without the need for a root-end filling.

In some cases, in which time is a factor, or cases in which there are persistent exacerbations between visits, root canal retreatment can be carried out at the time as surgery. The elevated tissue is reflected, the root apex exposed and resected. The canal preparation is performed with the file tips protruding through the resected root-end (Fig. 10.34A). Small aspirators can be placed next to the

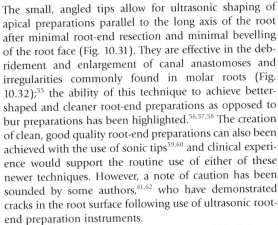

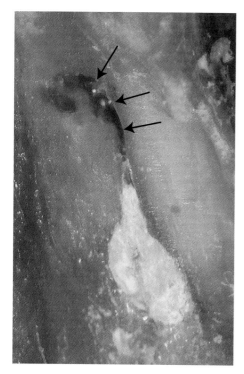

Figure 10.28 Resected root end. The main canal has been filled but the canal extension contains necrotic debris (arrowed). A root-end preparation and filling must be performed.

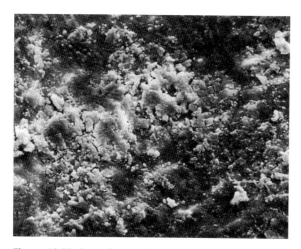

Figure 10.29 Smear layer on the resected root end.

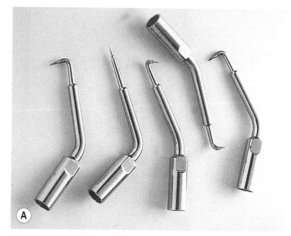

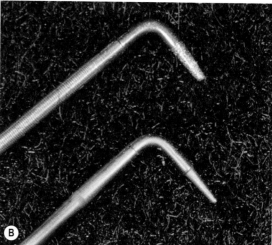

Figure 10.30 (A) Variously shaped and angled ultrasonic tips for preparing a root-end cavity. (B) Top, Berutti ultrasonic tip; bottom, EMS RE-2 tip.

apical opening to prevent root canal irrigant entering the bony cavity. After adequate preparation, the canal is dried with paper points. Filling should follow with a suitable material, and any excess removed (Fig. 10.34B). An ultrafine diamond bur or composite finishing bur can be run over the root surface with sterile water or saline spray (Fig. 10.34C). If the canal is filled properly, the result will be a very smooth, well-adapted root canal filling.

Prior to filling, the root-end cavity must be isolated to ensure moisture control. The appropriate use of vasoconstrictors will greatly reduce the blood flow in the surgical site but other supplementary agents are frequently used. Historically, bone wax was widely used; however, studies have shown that any wax particles retained in the surgical site will provoke a prolonged inflammatory reaction. In recent years, more biocompatible and biodegradable products have been developed; these include collagen-based products such as CollaPlug (Integra, Plainsboro, NJ, USA), CollaCote (Integra, Plainsboro, NJ, USA), Avitene (Davol Inc., Cranston, RI, USA) or Superstat (DPO

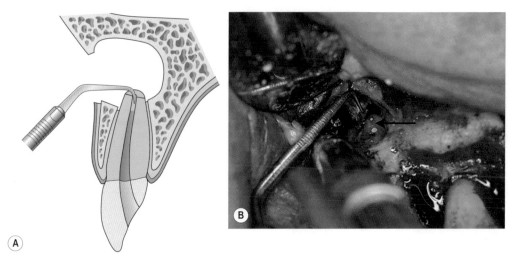

Figure 10.31 (A) Diagrammatic representation of root-end cavity preparation along the root axis using an ultrasonic tip. (B) An ultrasonic tip near the resected root end. Note good access and two canals (identified by gutta-percha) united by a thin white line – anastomosis (arrowed). Preparation of the anastomosis is essential.

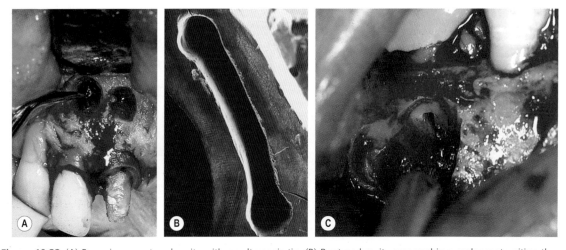

Figure 10.32 (A) Preparing a root-end cavity with an ultrasonic tip. (B) Root-end cavity prepared in a molar root uniting the two mesial canals through the anastomosis (SEM). (C) Ultrasonic root-end preparation in the mesial root of a mandibular molar.

Medical, Henderson, NV, USA) that can remain in the osseous cavity or be removed prior to closure (Fig. 10.35).[5] Non-collagen products include Surgicel (Johnson & Johnson, Piscataway, NJ, USA), Oxycel (Becton Dickinson, Sandy, UT, USA) and Gelfoam (Pfizer, New York, NY, USA). These products can exert their influence on haemostasis by stimulating the intrinsic clotting pathway and physically by creating a tamponading effect when packed into the crypt. Other less biocompatible products include Astringedent (Ultradent), Cut-Trol (Kisco, Wichita,

KS, USA), and ViscoStat (Ultradent); these are solutions of ferric sulphate, which must be removed from the bone cavity prior to tissue closure.[64,65] Haemostasis in periradicular surgery has been reviewed thoroughly.[66]

Root-end filling materials

The purpose of the root-end filling is to seal the canal system apically and prevent the egress of bacteria and

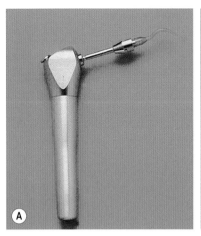
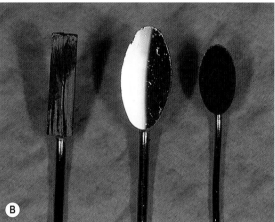

Figure 10.33 (A) Stropko irrigator. (B) Miniature mirrors.

bacterial products into the periradicular tissues. Presently, there are no commercially available materials that provide a perfect seal, therefore, the materials that are used must be prepared and placed carefully to ensure the best possible adaptation to the root-end cavity walls. When using modern materials as root-end fillings, adherence to manufacturers' recommendations in preparation, manipulation and placement is important. Table 10.4 lists current materials that are recommended for root-end filling. Amalgam has previously been the most widely used root-end filling material and has been associated with a reasonable level of success. However, problems have existed with corrosion and tissue argyria, persistence of apical inflammation, and long-term failure.[67] Coupled with concerns over the mercury component, it is recommended that more biocompatible materials be used and several clinical studies also support the use of alternative materials.[68–74]

Root-end filling materials commonly in use, or used in recent years include the following; amalgam, Intermediate Restorative Material (IRM), Super-Ethoxy Benzoic Acid (Super EBA), glass ionomer cement, dentine-bonded composite resin, Diaket, Mineral Trioxide Aggregate (MTA). Discussion will be restricted to those materials associated with the highest levels of success, both clinically and histologically. Evidence-based data from randomized clinical trials appears to indicate that two root-end filling materials, when used properly, will result in a high level of predictable clinical and radiographic healing.[75,76] These materials, IRM and MTA are discussed below.

Intermediate Restorative Material

Intermediate Restorative Material (IRM) is a resin reinforced zinc oxide–eugenol cement that has been shown to provide a better seal than amalgam, especially against the passage of microorganisms.[77] Healing of the periradicular tissues in the presence of IRM root-end fillings has been quite favourable.[77] Likewise, clinical studies have shown enhanced success with IRM root-end fillings (91%) compared with amalgam (75%) over long periods.[68] When using this material as a root-end filling, a higher powder-to-liquid ratio has been recommended to enhance placement, decrease setting time, reduce toxicity and reduce dissolution in tissue fluids.[78] Therefore, the use of IRM as a root-end filling material is recommended when mixed at a higher powder-to-liquid ratio.

Mineral Trioxide Aggregate

Mineral Trioxide Aggregate (MTA) is a relatively new material developed by Torabinejad and co-workers.[71,79,80,81] A series of studies have illustrated the useful properties of MTA as a root-end filling material including its biocompatibility, sealing properties and ability to promote tissue regeneration.[6,71,79,80] Additional studies have demonstrated the superior sealing properties of MTA over other root-end filling materials with either dye leakage, electrochemical testing[82] or endotoxin tracer tests.[83] The properties of this material have been shown to be relatively unaffected by blood contamination.[81] Complete regeneration of the periodontal apparatus has been demonstrated in some, but not in all cases.[70]

The cellular response to MTA has been shown to be more favourable than the response to IRM or amalgam. MTA promotes regeneration of the periradicular architecture.[84] However, the physical handling characteristics of MTA leave much to be desired. It is very difficult to deliver the material to the root-end cavity and to adequately compact it to the full length of the preparation. While moisture, such as bleeding, does not affect the setting ability of the material, it compounds the handling difficul-

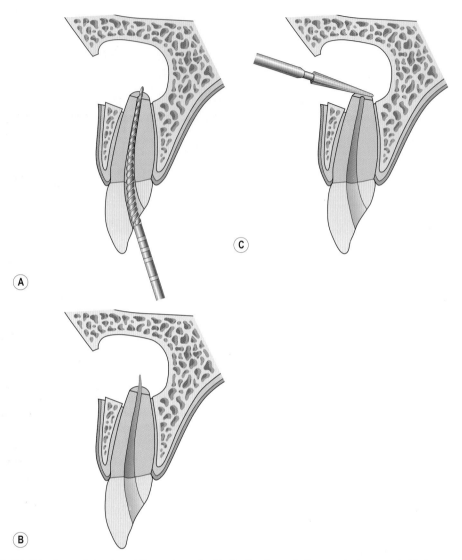

Figure 10.34 (A) Cleaning and shaping of the root canal with file tips through the resected root end. (B) Compaction of the gutta-percha filling with the tip through the root-end. (C) Removal of excess root filling material and finishing of the root surface with an ultrafine diamond bur.

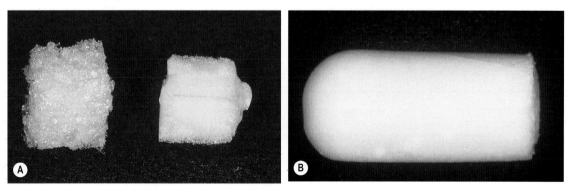

Figure 10.35 Collagen sponge materials for haemorrhage control in the apical bony cavity: (A) Hemofibrine – left; Hemocollagene – right. (B) Collaplug.

Table 10.4 Current root-end filling materials
Super EBA
Intermediate Restorative Material (IRM)
Glass ionomer
Diaket
Composite resin (dentine-bonded)
Mineral Trioxide Aggregate (MTA) – ProRoot® (regular and white)

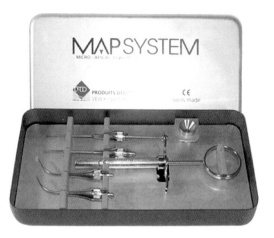

Figure 10.36 Miniature carriers, such as the MAP System, are used to carry small increments of root-end filling material.

ties. A number of instruments have been devised to facilitate the placement of the material such as the MAP system (Fig. 10.36), the Dovgan MTA carriers and the Lee MTA Pellet Forming Block. The usage of this material is greatly helped by ensuring that the powder/water ratio is correct. Following placement into the root-end cavity, the material can be effectively compacted using root-end pluggers and ultrasound transmitted by applying an ultrasonic instrument to the non-working part of the metal plugger. It is prudent to take a radiograph at this stage to confirm adequate placement of the material. MTA has a working time of approximately 3 to 4 hours and requires the presence of moisture for its final set.

Treatment of the root face

Removal of the smear layer and exposure of the apical collagen fibres is recommended after root-end resection, primarily to remove potentially contaminated debris and to enhance the healing environment for cemental deposition. Various agents have been recommended including phosphoric acid,[52,85] EDTA,[86] hydrochloric acid,[87,88] and citric acid.[89] The optimal exposure of collagen and demineralization occurs with a burnishing application of citric acid (pH 1.0) for 3 minutes.[90] Longer applications result in collagen denaturation. The peak activity pH of citric acid is 1.42.[91] Demineralization of resected root-ends with a two-minute burnishing of 50% citric acid at pH 1.0 resulted in a rapid and predictable layering of a cementoid type of material on the resected surface of dogs' teeth after 45 days.[92] No direct application to human teeth, under similar circumstances, has been studied, although the omission of an acid cleaner does not preclude the formation of a viable cementum layer.[93]

Recent studies have identified the use of the ferric ion, as an aqueous solution of 10% citric acid and 3% ferric chloride (10:3), to stabilize dentine collagen during the demineralization process;[94,95] however, applications were <30 seconds, as longer exposure increased demineralization and denaturation of the collagen. This approach has enhanced the bonding that occurs with restorative materials, and may also stimulate adhesion of the exposed, intact

collagen with fibrin and fibronectin[96] and the splicing of collagen with newly formed collagen fibrils[97] during the wound healing process. Further work on its use on the resected root-end is warranted.

The following treatment regimen is indicated for the resected root face after placement of a root-end filling, or root-end resection in which a well-condensed gutta-percha root filling is in place:

1. Finish the surface with an ultra-fine diamond or 30-flute tungsten-carbide composite-resin finishing-bur[55,98] (Fig. 10.37).
2. Burnish the surface gently with a weak acid cleaner (10%) for a short period (30 seconds).[98]

These procedures achieve the desired result of a smooth root face devoid of smear layer, regardless of the root or canal configuration type (Fig. 10.38). However, when using MTA as a root-end filling, such treatment of the root face is inappropriate. In these cases, the gross excess of MTA is removed with suction or spoon excavators and a saline-moistened sponge used to clean the root face.

Closure of the surgical site

Prior to repositioning the tissue flap, the underside of the reflected tissue, the surrounding bone, and the periradicular bone cavity should be inspected for debris. The surgical site is carefully flushed with saline, except where MTA has been used as the root-end filling. A radiograph is taken to ensure that all debris has been removed and that the goals of the surgical procedure have been accomplished. Final irrigation with saline is often warranted followed by tissue repositioning to the wound edges to ensure primary closure.

When surgery has been performed and there is a stable buccal cortical plate of bone to protect the root structure and no evidence of marginal periodontitis, tissue closure is straightforward. Intimate approximation of the healthy soft tissues and bone with sutures will suffice, and healing will occur uneventfully. Ideally, bony dehiscences or large fenestrations should be detected prior to surgery so that adjunct procedures such as guided-tissue regeneration can be planned (Fig. 10.39).[6,99,100,101] When there has been loss of the cortical bone, especially in the crestal region, or the presence of marginal periodontitis, the chances for long-term success are highly guarded.[102,103] Persistent periradicular inflammation following root-end surgery has been associated with marginal periodontitis at the time of surgery.[43]

Many clinicians will also apply gentle pressure to the repositioned tissue at this time to remove residual blood and to begin the intimate reattachment process. Gentle pressure can be applied using saline-soaked gauze squares. Suturing will be necessary in most cases. A variety of suturing techniques is frequently used and include interrupted, mattress, continuous or sling sutures. The suture is first placed in the flap and is then carried into the attached tissues. Whilst there is no one formula for the number of sutures and their position, the clinician must exercise judgement in their placement to ensure adequate and stable positioning, especially in the crestal region. Vertical incisions may require several sutures depending on the length and nature of the tissue (Fig. 10.40). Avoidance of postoperative gingival recession and delayed healing is dependent on correct suturing techniques and tissue handling.

A variety of suture materials are available each demonstrating advantages and disadvantages. Suture materials are either absorbable or non-absorbable. They can also be either monofilament or braided; the latter have a tendency to facilitate the movement of saliva and bacteria along the suture into the tissues. This property called 'wicking' contributes to irritation of the tissues and may delay healing. A list of suitable suture materials is shown in Table 10.5.

For years, silk sutures have been most widely used; their main disadvantage is bacterial colonization, which will delay healing. However, with proper suture placement, adequate cleaning of the surgical site by the patient, and timely suture removal in 48 to 72 hours, this problem can be minimized. Gut sutures can also be used, but their handling characteristics can be a challenge. A number of new synthetic suture materials are now available and may have relegated the silk suture to history. Materials such as polyglactin, polypropylene, polyethylene and Teflon (PTFE) cause minimal tissue reaction. With these newer monofilament synthetic materials, the preferred suture size for wound closure in periradicular surgery is either 5-0 or 6-0. Smaller 7-0 or even 8-0 sutures are advocated by some operators in particular situations such as the papilla-based incision.[30] Different needle sizes and shapes are

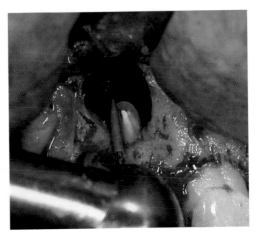

Figure 10.37 Smoothing of the resected root end with an ultrafine diamond.

often necessary due to osseous contours and tissue thickness. No single needle shape or radius is ideal for every situation. Thin tissue is often found along the vertical releasing incision and requires a small radius needle. Larger radius needles are generally used in the horizontal incision to facilitate passage interproximally.

Suture knots should always be placed away from the incision line to minimize microbial colonization in that area (Fig. 10.41). Sutured tissue should be cleaned routinely by the patient with chlorhexidine or warm saline rinses. Immediately following suturing, the tissue must be compressed with firm finger pressure for 3 to 5 minutes to ensure correct tissue position with a minimal blood clot between the bone and tissue flap (Fig. 10.42). During this time, the patient can be given postoperative instructions. All sutures should, ideally, be removed in 48 to 72 hours.

Postoperative radiological assessment

As previously indicated, a postoperative radiograph should be taken prior to closure of the surgical site; mistakes or deficiencies in techniques can be rectified easily at this point. In some cases, especially posterior teeth, angled radiographs should be considered. Radiographs taken with a film-holding device are preferred. When review examination radiographs are taken with the same device, healing can be assessed more accurately. Some points for the clinician to consider are:

- Is there any remaining unresected root structure, or have the wrong roots been inadvertently resected or damaged?
- Has any resected root tissue been left in the surgical site?
- Are the correct root ends surgically filled?

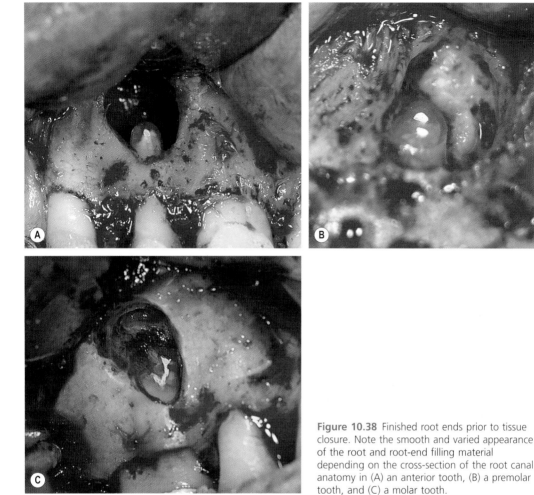

Figure 10.38 Finished root ends prior to tissue closure. Note the smooth and varied appearance of the root and root-end filling material depending on the cross-section of the root canal anatomy in (A) an anterior tooth, (B) a premolar tooth, and (C) a molar tooth.

- Do the root-end fillings appear adequate in depth and adaptation and appear well compacted?
- Is there scattered radiopaque material within the surgical site?
- Has root-end filling material been pushed into the maxillary sinus or mandibular canal?
- Is there evidence of a fracture that was not seen clinically?

Postoperative patient instructions

When the soft tissues are managed properly and surgical time is minimized, healing is generally uneventful. Careful attention to postoperative instructions is essential for patient comfort and tissue healing during the next few days. The following postoperative instructions should be given verbally and supported in writing for the patient's reference.

- Strenuous activity should be avoided, along with drinking alcohol and smoking.
- An adequate diet consisting of fruit juices, soups, soft foods and liquid food supplements should be consumed after the effects of the local anaesthesia have worn off. Avoid hard, sticky or chewy foods.
- Do not pull on, or unnecessarily lift the facial tissues.
- Oozing of blood from the surgical site is normal for the first 24 hours. Bleeding is managed by applying a gauze pack to the site. Slight and transient facial swelling and bruising may be experienced.
- Postsurgical discomfort is minimal but the surgical site will be tender and sore. The use of analgesics for

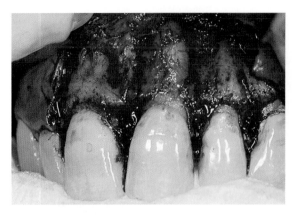

Figure 10.39 Loss of buccal cortical bone over the root of a left maxillary central incisor with a periradicular lesion. Correct treatment planning should be able to determine, or at least anticipate the presence of these defects prior to surgical entry.

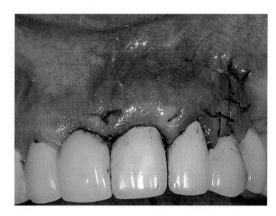

Figure 10.40 Close tissue flap approximation with minimal suturing and tissue damage.

Table 10.5 Suture materials

MATERIAL	ADVANTAGES/DISADVANTAGES
Black silk	Non-absorbable. Historically the most commonly used. Good handling characteristics. Braided; wicking effect delays healing.
Surgical gut (Collagen) Chromic acid treated surgical gut	Absorbable; manufacturing process determines longevity of catgut sutures. Treatment with chromic acid prolongs retention in tissues. Difficult to handle.
Nylon	Non-absorbable. Monofilament.
Polyglycolic Acid (PGA)	Absorbable. May be braided or monofilament.
Expanded polytetrafluoroethylene (PTFE) (GORE-TEX)	Single filament; smooth, strong. Non-porous surface; non-absorbable. Provokes little tissue reaction.
PTFE-coated polyester (Tevdek)	Non-absorbable. Usually braided.
Polyamide	Non-absorbable. Strong. Smooth, non-porous.

24 to 48 hours will help to alleviate this occurrence. Normally, continue with the analgesics given presurgically.

- For the first day, place ice packs with firm pressure directly on the face over the surgical site for 20 minutes and remove for 20 minutes. Repeat as necessary until retiring that evening.

- Chlorhexidine rinses should be used twice daily. On the day following surgery and for the next 3 to 4 days, warm hypertonic salt water rinses can be used every 1 to 2 hours if possible (half a teaspoon of salt in a glass of warm water).
- Sutures will be removed in 48 to 72 hours.
- Brushing of the surgical site is not recommended

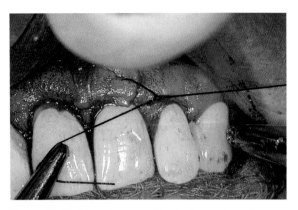

Figure 10.41 Suture knots must be kept away from the incision line to minimize infection of the wound.

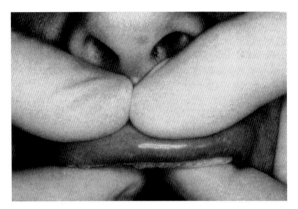

Figure 10.42 Compression of the tissue flap with gauge and light pressure is essential to minimize blood clot between tissue and cortical bone.

until the sutures are removed. Prior to that, the surgical area can be cleaned using a large cotton puff or ball saturated with warm salt solution.
* Telephone numbers are provided for your convenience should complications arise.

Postoperative examination and review

Review of the patient, both clinically and radiologically, is normally scheduled at 1 year. In most cases, osseous repair is virtually complete at this time; evidence of this as well as clinical healing has been considered as a valid criterion for success. Therefore, no additional follow-up may be necessary.[69,104,105] Failure to observe complete repair or delayed healing should warrant additional evaluation for as long as 4 years,[106] until repair is evident, or signs and symptoms indicate failure.

Radiological interpretation is highly variable and can easily be influenced by the quality and angulation of the film and processing irregularities. Therefore, the clinician should use a film-holding device for all follow-up radiographs. Likewise, familiarity with radiological classifications of healing (success/failure) is essential.[5,14,43] This will enable case outcome assessment to be based on a sound, logical and consistent decision-making process.[33]

PERIRADICULAR SURGERY OF PARTICULAR TEETH

Maxillary anterior teeth

Surgical access to maxillary anterior teeth is relatively straightforward due to root position in relation to the labial cortical bone. The lateral incisor may pose more of a challenge due to its common distopalatal root inclination and curvature. Deeper osseous penetration is often necessary and the root apex may impinge on the palatal cortical plate of bone. Common also in this region is the excessively long canine that requires extensive soft tissue elevation for access to the root end. Anatomical cross-sections after root-end resection usually reveal a round, oval or slightly oblong root outline with canals placed centrally on the root surface. As the apex of the lateral incisor is commonly positioned more towards the palatal, both the buccal and palatal cortical plates of bone may be destroyed from advancing periradicular disease or surgical intervention. This usually leads to a greater frequency of scar tissue (incomplete healing) as opposed to complete bony repair.

Maxillary premolars

Surgical access to single-rooted premolars is also straight-forward, with a minimal thickness of cortical plate covering the root apex. Complications generally occur when multiple roots are present, widely divergent in a bucco-palatal dimension, and/or the position of the maxillary sinus is such that penetration into the sinus cannot be avoided. Often, these teeth have buccal apices that have fenestrated the buccal cortex and access is relatively simple.

The resected root outlines of single-rooted premolars are oval, oblong, dumb-bell shaped or round. In multi-rooted premolars, canals are centrally placed and generally oval or circular on the resected root surface. In a two-canal, single-rooted premolar, two oval or round canals can be expected with an anastomosis. In this situation, the root-end cavity must encompass not only the canal openings but also the anastomosis, for which ultrasonic or sonic root-end preparation is particularly helpful.

183

Maxillary molars

When buccal fenestrations exist, surgical access to the buccal roots of maxillary molars is relatively easy. Depending on the position of the inferior border of the zygomatic process, extensive removal of bone may be necessary. Root outlines, after resection, are usually oval or circular for the distobuccal root and oblong, teardrop shaped, figure-of-eight shaped, or narrow and curved for the mesial buccal root. This root has a high incidence of two canals with an anastomosis, and therefore all orifices on the resected root face must be identified.

In palatal root surgery, soft tissue management is more difficult during reflection and retraction due to the thickness of the palatal flap and an irregular surface of the underlying cortical plate. Palatal roots have a tendency to curve towards the buccal and the root seldom fenestrate the bone at the apex. This often implies that large amounts of bone must be removed in a site that has restricted access and visibility. Penetration into the sinus is not uncommon. The greater palatine nerve and vessels will invariably be encountered with the palatal root of a second molar. Resected root outlines are generally oval, round or oblong, with the canal placed centrally on the root surface.

Mandibular anterior teeth

Surgical access to the root apices of mandibular anterior teeth is often difficult because of lingual tooth inclination, wide buccolingual roots, thick cortical bone apically with increased amounts of cancellous bone between the cortex and root, and root dehiscences in the coronal half of the root. It is common for the root apices of mandibular incisors to be in close proximity to each other, which may pose problems in root-end management. Resected root outlines are narrow, oblong, or figure-of-eight shaped, with canal space on the resected root usually narrow mesiodistally and wide buccolingually. The incidence of two canals or joining canals on the root surface is high after root-end resection.

Mandibular premolars

Surgical access to mandibular premolars is usually direct, except for the occasional presence of significant muscle attachments in the soft tissues and the mental foramen in the bone. Surgical entry is often from a superior direction to avoid the foramen, which is most commonly close to the second premolar. The thickness of the cortical bone overlying the root apices is variable depending on tooth inclination in the arch. Root outlines are generally oval to oblong in a buccolingual dimension, with a small incidence of multiple canals exiting on the resected root surface; preoperative radiographs should warn of this possibility.

Mandibular molars

Surgical entry through the cortical plate to mandibular molars can be straightforward, but is more often complicated by limited access, shallow vestibule, thick cortical plate, the external oblique ridge, root length, position and inclination. Although the apices of molar roots are inclined buccally,[9] the roots are often housed within a thick cortical plate of bone. Additionally, individual root variations and curvatures often place the apices in difficult to reach positions. Therefore, these anatomical problems must be considered during treatment planning. Radiological assessment is essential; the location of the mandibular canal must be identified through the use of angled films in a superior or inferior direction. Likewise, proximally angled films will provide information about the number and curvature of roots.

Root outlines after resection are oval, dumb-bell shaped, oblong, and wide in a buccolingual dimension. Canals often have anastomoses in both mesial and distal roots. The use of staining is strongly advised to improve visual definition. Root-end cavities, by necessity, are oblong encompassing the entire canal system as it exits on the resected root surface (Fig. 10.32).

General anatomical considerations

It is uncommon to penetrate the maxillary sinus during periradicular surgery. If this occurs, however, the opening must be protected to prevent debris entering the sinus during the management of the root end (Fig. 10.43). This can be done with collagen-based haemostatic agents as previously mentioned. Bone wax should not be used because it can be pushed into the sinus and evoke a significant foreign-body giant cell reaction along with delayed healing.[107] The postsurgical need for antibiotics or antihistamines has not been established.[33] Since primary closure can be achieved with soft tissue repositioning and suturing, an effective seal is obtained, avoiding the need for drug therapy.

The mental foramen also poses a challenge for many clinicians. Discussion with the patient at the treatment planning stage is essential to disclose the nature of the problem, the methods used to manage it, and the potential for untoward postoperative sequelae. The best way to manage this entity is to:

- identify its position
- plan surgical entry away from it
- use the periosteal retractor to protect the foramen and its contents during surgery
- avoid pinching the soft tissues with the retractor.

An additional concern with all periradicular surgery is the presence of fenestrations and dehiscences, along with large penetrating periradicular lesions, which have destroyed buccal and lingual cortical plates of

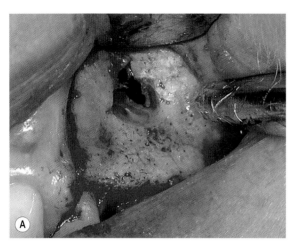
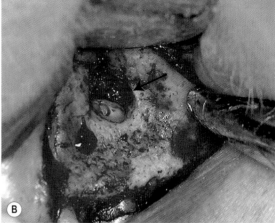

Figure 10.43 (A) Penetration into the maxillary sinus apical and distal to a premolar. (B) Blocking of the sinus perforation with a collagen sponge (arrowed). Note root-end preparation has been made with good haemorrhage control around the resected apex. Collagen was left in place to serve as a matrix for closure of the sinus perforation.

bone.[100,101,108] Previous studies have identified less than favourable results when the surrounding bone has been compromised.[102,103,105] Management of these osseous defects often requires a guided tissue/bone regenerative procedure, which is becoming more widespread. These situations should be diagnosed and treatment planned carefully; when appropriate, it is prudent to consider help from experienced specialists.

REPAIR OF PERFORATION

A root perforation is a mechanical or pathological communication formed between the supporting periodontal apparatus of the tooth and the root canal system. Non-surgical repair of root perforations is reasonably successful,[109,110,111,112] but when it fails or is impractical, surgery may be necessary. The surgical repair of root perforations is, generally more difficult than root-end procedures. Perforations pose greater radiological difficulties in identification, diagnosis and postsurgical assessment,[113] Surgical management of perforated roots depends on access to the defect and the relationship of the perforation to crestal bone and the epithelial attachment. Perforations have been classified according to their relationship to the epithelial attachment and the crestal bone – the 'critical crestal zone'.[114,115]

Perforations occurring in the apical third pose the least problem in surgical management and are generally amenable to root-end resection.[115,116,117,118] Mid-root per-

forations present a different set of challenges. Typically, they are not in line with the coronal aspect of the canal, and may only be identified by radiographs taken from different angles. Once identified, surgically, they can be managed like any root end (Figs 10.44 & 10.45). Access to the defect margins, however, is more difficult when the perforation is located on the proximal surface of the root, and it is necessary to ensure complete marginal adaptation of the sealant material while preventing its placement into the surrounding bone (Fig. 10.45). Access to lingual perforations is almost impossible on most teeth and other treatment options must be considered.

A common cause of perforation is due to post space preparation and placement.[115,119] Often the post must be removed prior to root repair and a shorter post placed. In some cases, the post may be ground down so that it lies inside the root and a filling material is placed to seal the perforation.

The prognosis for surgically repaired root perforations is based on a number of factors, similar to those for non-surgical repair of root perforations. Success is highly dependent on the following factors:

- Proximity of the perforation to the critical crestal zone. The prognosis for furcation perforations is very poor due to the potential for microbial contamination.
- Extent of microbial contamination of the perforation.
- Timely management of the perforation; the shorter the time interval between occurrence of the perforation and repair, the better the prognosis.

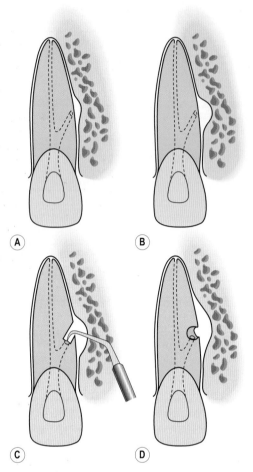

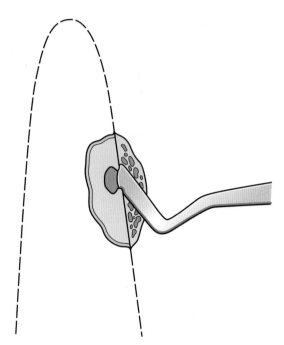

Figure 10.45 Repair of perforation. A flat plastic instrument or the convex side of a small curette is used to apply the filling material to the prepared cavity; it may also serve as a matrix, against which the filling material is compacted with pluggers.

Figure 10.44 Access to a mid-root proximal perforation. (A) Perforation; (B) access improved by careful removal of overlying bone; (C) creation of a cavity with an ultrasonic tip; (D) if necessary, additional bone can be removed to enhance access to the defect.

- Use of a biocompatible repair material. Any material that is cytotoxic will significantly reduce the prognosis. For example, the placement of phenolic compounds in the root canal after a perforation has occurred and before surgical repair, will cause irreparable damage to the periodontium at the perforation site. Likewise, the use of a cytotoxic material to seal the perforation will cause tissue damage.
- Sealing of the defect with minimal to no excess material in the surgical site that may cause persistent inflammation and possibly stimulate root resorption.
- Maintenance of optimal oral hygiene in the area of any perforation repair.

REPLANTATION/TRANSPLANTATION

Replantation is defined as replacing a tooth in its socket following deliberate or traumatic avulsion. In the case of surgical or deliberate removal of a tooth and its replacement, it is defined as intentional replantation.[120] Transplantation involves the transfer of a tooth from one alveolar socket to another either in the same or another person.[120]

Few true indications exist for choosing intentional replantation as a primary method of treatment.[5] The presence of calcified canals, separated instruments, non-negotiable root canals, perforations, or anatomical closeness of, e.g. the mandibular canal, are not valid indications for choosing intentional replantation. The patient's symptoms and signs, the strategic value of the tooth, and the overall dental condition, including arch continuity, occlusion, function, tooth restorability and periodontal status must be considered along with the patient's understanding and cooperation. Finally, awareness of the potential for adverse sequelae such as bone loss, tooth resorption and tooth fractures during extraction must be considered. When viewed from this perspective, the only true indication for intentional replantation is when there is absolutely no other treatment available to maintain a strategic tooth.[95,121,122] Even then it is essential that all phases of this planned procedure be communicated to the patient, in addition to providing a realistic appraisal of the treatment plan, sequelae, prognosis and alternatives.

Once a decision has been reached to perform intentional replantation, all efforts should be taken to ensure removal of all tissue debris within the tooth. Root canals must be as clean as possible, canals filled as far as possible, and the access opening closed with a permanent restoration. Occlusal adjustments and teeth cleaning should also be performed. Ideally, a two-person team should perform the procedure, one to remove the tooth and the other to assess and fulfil the endodontic needs of the tooth. The surrounding tissue is disinfected with an antiseptic solution. Elevators should be used to carefully loosen the tooth, minimizing injuries to the soft tissue, bone and root. If necessary, the extraction forceps can be wrapped with gauze to minimize damage to the root. Once removed the crown of the tooth is grasped with gauze sponges soaked in sterile saline. The socket is gently curetted to remove foreign debris. Care is exercised to avoid damage to the socket-retained periodontal fibres; gauze or cotton products should not be placed into the socket.

The extracted tooth is examined for fractures, extra roots or foramina, or any unusual anatomical configurations. Root ends are easily resected with a high-speed fine diamond bur under sterile saline spray. The nature of the canal system and its orifices are examined and if necessary, apically prepared with ultrasonics and filled. Time is of the essence with these procedures and all members of the team must be fully aware of their responsibilities and be skilled in their execution.

When the tooth is ready to be replaced in its socket, the walls should be gently rinsed with saline to remove the blood clot. Additionally the tooth is rinsed to remove any residual cotton fibres or debris from the root-end filling material. The tooth is teased carefully and slowly into its original position in the socket, allowing for the slow escape of the blood that has built up in the socket. Slight pressure is applied to the buccal and lingual cortical plates to ensure adaptation. The occlusion is rechecked, and a splint is placed if necessary. Often only a periodontal pack is necessary. If a splint is used the tooth must be in physiological function. Convenient splints can be made from soft, clear resin or nylon line that is acid-etched and cemented to the buccal surface. Splints are removed after 5 to 7 days.

The prognosis for intentionally replanted teeth is primarily dictated by the presence or absence of inflammatory and replacement resorption. Long-term studies provide mixed results with this technique, with 50–60% success over a 5 to 10 year period.[5,123]

REGENERATIVE PROCEDURES

A major factor influencing the prognosis of endodontic surgery is the complete loss of cortical bone overlying the root.[102,103] If the buccal or lingual cortical bone is lost or a naturally occurring dehiscence is revealed upon entry to the periradicular surgical site, the success rate is reduced.[17,102,103,105,124,125] When there is loss of the cortical plates both buccally and lingually, the success rate is reduced even further. In an attempt to improve the chance of success, regenerative procedures have been advocated as a means of encouraging formation of bone. Regenerative procedures have been used widely in periodontal surgery. Regeneration of the periradicular tissues subsequent to surgery or due to the ravages of disease processes implies replacement of the various components of the tissues in their appropriate locations, amounts and relationships to each other.[126] There are a number of clinical situations in endodontic surgery where regenerative procedures might be suitable.[6] These include:

- apical periodontitis without communication to the alveolar crest
- apical periodontitis with communication to the alveolar crest
- dehiscence
- proximal bone loss
- developmental grooves
- root or furcation bone loss caused by perforations
- cervical root resorption
- oblique root fracture
- ridge augmentation.

At present, the prognosis for regenerative procedures in endodontic surgery in patients is inconclusive. However, animal studies,[127,128,129,130] case reports[99,131,132,133,134] and empirical data would suggest that more favourable healing is likely when regenerative procedures are used. Unfortunately, successful regeneration can only be demonstrated histologically. Clinically, measurements such as gain in probing attachment level, decrease in probing depth and increased filling of the osseous defect have been used to measure and compare results.

Clinical techniques in regenerative procedures

In guided-tissue regeneration, the type of healing that occurs after surgery is considered to be determined by the cells that first repopulate the root surface;[135] this has been supported by experimental work.[136,137,138] Membrane therapy has resulted in predictable formation of new attachment by preventing gingival connective tissue and gingival epithelium from contacting the root surface.[139] Regenerative membrane procedures aim to delay the advance of rapidly growing epithelial cells in order to allow the more slowly growing progenitor cells from the bone and periodontal ligament to repopulate the root surface and produce a new connective tissue attachment. The objectives of membrane application in endodontic surgery are the following:[140]

- To facilitate tissue regeneration by creating an optimum environment (stable and protected wound).
- To exclude undesirable, fast-proliferating cells that interfere with desired tissue regeneration.

A classification for guided-tissue regeneration (GTR) application in endodontic surgery based on the location, extent and nature of the lesion has been proposed:

- Class I – bony defects located at the apex.
- Class II – apical lesions with concomitant marginal lesions.
- Class III – lateral or furcation lesions with or without a marginal lesion.

Two main types of membrane have been used, absorbable and non-absorbable. The first commercially available membrane was an expanded polytetrafluoroethylene (ePTFE) non-absorbable membrane (GORE-TEX, W.L. Gore & Associates, Flagstaff, AZ, USA). The use of GORE-TEX membrane necessitated a second surgical procedure to remove it. With the development of absorbable membranes, single visit surgical procedures became possible. Studies have subsequently shown that there is no significant difference in the healing with either type of membrane.[141]

The absorbable membranes can be either natural materials such as collagen (Biomend, Zimmer Dental, Carlsbad, CA, USA or Bio-Gide, Geistlich, Wolhusen, Germany) or synthetic polymers such as polyglactin. The natural materials are absorbed by enzymatic action while the synthetic materials are absorbed by hydrolysis. The use of an absorbable membrane (Bio-Gide) in combination with a bone substitute material (Bio-Oss, Geistlich) has been shown to stimulate substantial new bone and cementum formation with Sharpey's fibre attachment.[142] Histological evaluation suggests that the combined approach compares favourably with other regenerative treatment.

TREATMENT OUTCOME – AETIOLOGY AND EVALUATION

Although many studies have attempted to determine success–failure rates for periradicular surgery, none have been able to integrate fully all parameters of evaluation with techniques performed, materials used, patient compliance, clinician expertise, variability and interpretative skills. Attempts at multivariate analysis have provided some trends and correlations, but even these findings may only be applicable to specifically controlled cases.[105,143]

Success (complete healing) with periradicular surgery has been reported to range from very low levels to levels as high as 96.8%[143] using mixed populations, at frequently less than ideal percentages of review examinations and short follow-up periods. With longer follow-up periods of up to 8 years, a success rate of 91.5% has been achieved,[3] which correlates closely with other long-term prospective studies (91.2%).[144] Whilst significant variability in results makes comparisons of studies questionable, the identification of factors that have contributed to the success or failure of periradicular surgery is essential, and these should be integrated into all phases of case assessment and treatment.[145] Often the aetiology of failure may be difficult to identify, and may encompass a multitude of factors. For periradicular surgery, most failures can be attributed to specific causes. At the same time, when failure cannot be explained, uncertain aetiological factors and treatment may be speculated. Table 10.6 lists the aetiological factors often cited as valid, or uncertain in the failure of periradicular surgery.

Table 10.6 Factors influencing success or failure of periradicular surgery

Valid causes for surgical failure
Failure to debride the root canal space thoroughly.
Failure to seal the root canal space adequately.
Tissue irritation from toxic root canal or root-end fillings.
Failure to manage root canal or root-end materials properly.
Superimposition of periodontal disease.
Longitudinal root fracture.
Recurrent cystic lesion.
Improper management of the supporting periodontium.
Uncertain causes for surgical failure
Infected dentinal tubules.
Infected periradicular lesion.
Failure to use antibiotics when indicated.
Accessory or lateral canals.
Loss of alveolar bone.
Root resorption.
Timing of root canal filling (before or during surgery).
Type of root-end filling.

Table 10.7 Clinical evaluation of success and failure

Clinical success
No tenderness to percussion or palpation.
Normal mobility and function.
No sinusitis or paraesthesia.
No sinus tract or periodontal pocket.
No infection or swelling.
Adjacent teeth respond as expected to stimuli.
Minimal to no scarring or discolouration.
No subjective discomfort.
Clinical uncertainty
Sporadic vague symptoms.
Pressure sensation or feeling of fullness.
Low grade discomfort on percussion, palpation, or chewing.
Discomfort with tongue pressure.
Superimposed sinusitis focused on treated tooth.
Occasional need to use analgesics.
Clinical failure
Persistent subjective symptoms.
Discomfort to percussion and/or palpation.
Recurrent sinus tract or swelling.
Evidence or irreparable tooth fracture.
Excessive mobility or progressive periodontal breakdown.
Inability to chew on the tooth.

Table 10.8 Radiological evaluation of success and failure

Radiological success
Normal periodontal ligament width or slight increase.
Normal lamina dura or elimination of radiolucency.
Normal to fine-meshed osseous trabeculae.
No resorption evident.
Radiological uncertainty
Slight increase in periodontal ligament width.
Slight increase in width of lamina dura.
Size of radiolucency static or slight evidence of repair.
Radiolucency is circular or asymmetric.
Extension of the periodontal ligament into radiolucency.
Evidence of resorption.
Radiological failure
Increased width of the periodontal ligament and lamina dura.
Circular radiolucency with limited osseous trabeculae.
Symmetrical radiolucency with funnel-shaped borders.
Evidence of resorption.

Evaluation of success or failure following root-end surgery is limited to clinical and radiological examinations. Clinical criteria for success or failure are used most commonly and in conjunction with the radiological findings. The clinical outcome is classified into one of three categories at the time of review (Table 10.7). Patient assessment, however, must be made in conjunction with both clinical and radiological parameters of evaluation (Table 10.8). If the only goal of periradicular surgery is to retain the tooth in adequate clinical function, then many cases can be classified as successful. Many factors, however, such as case selection, evaluator bias, and patient factors can skew levels of success or failure. Likewise, many clinically symptom-free teeth may have histopathological changes at the root apices along with minimal or extensive radiological changes. Even in the presence of an apparently normal radiological appearance, a clinically symptom-free tooth may exhibit histopathological changes in the periradicular tissues. This is especially true adjacent on resected root surfaces which are difficult to assess radiologically.

RETREATMENT OF SURGICAL PROCEDURES

Not all surgery is successful, but when a case has been identified as failing, it is necessary to use all tests and information available to determine the cause prior to further surgery. Table 10.9 lists some of the more common unsuspected, anatomical and technical causes for failure. Not all of these causes are amenable to further surgery, and a tooth may require extraction and prosthetic replacement.

Very few studies have evaluated the results of periradicular surgery that was performed subsequent to previous surgical failure.[43,146] The success rates of repeat surgery were 50% or less with little subsequent alteration in healing after one year, but these figures

Table 10.9 Causes of surgical failure

Unsuspected
Root fracture not readily visible.
Post-hole perforation, especially on the buccal or lingual surface.
Instrument perforation coronal to the resected root end.
Persistent infection in the apically resected tubules.
Corrosion of previously placed amalgam root-end filling.

Anatomical
Fenestrations or dehiscences – loss of marginal bone.
Aberrant root anatomy or canal space.
Proximity of root of adjacent teeth.
Proximity of maxillary sinus.

Technical
Poor canal cleaning and filling.
Inadequate root-end resection.
Inadequate root-end preparation and filling.
Toxicity of root-end filling material.
Improper soft tissue management.

relate to discontinued techniques. In a recent, systematic review and meta-analysis of the outcomes of resurgery[14,63,105] there was a near equal distribution of the cases between the three outcome groups: 35.7 % healed successfully, 26.3% healed with uncertain results and 38% did not heal.

The primary reason for failure following periradicular surgery is the presence of infected debris in uncleaned and poorly filled canal spaces.[14,105] The primary cause of failure with root canal treatment has been identified as coronal leakage due to poor quality of the coronal restoration.[84,147] Therefore, it is essential to access, clean and fill as much of the canal space as possible and to seal thoroughly the coronal aspects of the root canal system before resorting to surgical intervention. Failing to adhere to this will inevitably result in failure.

LEARNING OUTCOMES

Upon completion of this chapter, the reader should be able to describe and discuss the:

- indications for periradicular surgery and the preoperative assessment process
- key instruments and their usage in surgical endodontics
- importance of tissue anaesthesia and haemostasis
- management of the soft tissue, including tissue flap design, tissue incision, elevation and reflection
- procedures for osseous entry and root identification in the various tooth groups
- rationale and techniques for the removal of soft tissue lesions and tissue biopsy
- rationale, techniques and instruments for root-end resection, root-end cavity preparation and root-end filling
- root-end filling materials available and the choice of material
- techniques for primary closure of the surgical site to minimize postoperative sequelae
- importance of the postoperative examination and case review, including radiographic assessment
- implications and anatomical concerns when considering periradicular surgery of particular teeth
- repair of tooth/root perforations and the rationale for tooth replantation or transplantation
- rationale for, and clinical techniques of, regenerative procedures that may be used in conjunction with periradicular surgery
- importance of assessing treatment outcome, including identification of adverse aetiological factors that may require the revision of previous surgical procedures.

REFERENCES

1. Naito T. Single or multiple visits for endodontic treatment? Evidence Based Dentistry 2008;9:24.

2. Suchina JA, Levine D, Flaitz CM, et al. Retrospective clinical and radiologic evaluation of nonsurgical endodontic treatment in human immunodeficiency virus (HIV) infection. Journal of Contemporary Dental Practice 2006;7:1–8.

3. Rubinstein RA, Kim S. Long-term follow-up of cases considered healed one year after apical microsurgery. Journal of Endodontics 2002;28:378–383.

4. Rubinstein R, Torabinejad M. Contemporary endodontic surgery. Journal of the

Californian Dental Association 2004;32:485–492.

5. Gutmann J, Harrison JW. Surgical Endodontics. St. Louis, MO, USA: Ishiyaku EuroAmerica; 1994.

6. Rankow HJ, Krasner PR. Endodontic applications of guided tissue regeneration in endodontic surgery. Oral Health 1996;86:3, 7–40, 33–35.

7. Velvart P, Peters CI. Soft tissue management in endodontic surgery. Journal of Endodontics 2005;31:4–16.

8. Doyle SL, Hodges JS, Pesun IJ, et al. Retrospective cross sectional comparison of initial nonsurgical endodontic treatment and single-tooth implants. Compendium of Continuing Education in Dentistry 2007;28:296–301.

9. Arens D, Adams WR, DeCastro RA. Endodontic Surgery Hagerstown. MD, USA: Harper & Row; 1981.

10. Ingle JI, Bakland LK. Endodontics. 4th ed. Malvern, PA, USA: Williams & Wilkins; 1994.

11. Doornbusch H, Broersma L, Boering G, Wesselink PR. Radiographic evaluation of cases referred for surgical endodontics. International Endodontic Journal 2002;35:472–477.

12. Maalouf EM, Gutmann JL. Biological perspectives on the non-surgical endodontic management of periradicular pathosis. International Endodontic Journal 1994;27:154–162.

13. Saunders WP, Saunders EM. Coronal leakage as a cause of failure in root-canal therapy: a review. Endodontics & Dental Traumatology 1994;10:105–108.

14. Rud J, Andreasen JO. A study of failures after endodontic surgery by radiographic, histologic and stereomicroscopic methods. International Journal of Oral Surgery 1972;1:311–328.

15. Gutmann JL. Clinical, radiographic, and histologic perspectives on success and failure in endodontics. Dental Clinics of North America 1992;36:379–392.

16. Bellizzi R, Loushine R. A Clinical Atlas of Endodontic Surgery. Chicago, IL, USA: Quintessence; 1991.

17. Forssell H, Tammisalo T, Forssell K. A follow-up study of apicectomized teeth. Proceedings of the Finnish Dental Society 1988;84:85–93.

18. Rubinstein R. Endodontic microsurgery and the surgical operating microscope. Compendium of Continuing Education in Dentistry 1997;18:659–668.

19. Jastak JT, Yagiela JA. Vasoconstrictors and local anesthesia: a review and rationale for use. Journal of the American Dental Association 1983;107:623–630.

20. Malamed SF. Handbook of Local Anesthesia. 3rd ed. St. Louis, MO, USA: Mosby-Year Book; 1990.

21. Gangarosa LP, Halik FJ. A clinical evaluation of local anesthetic solutions containing grades epinephrine concetrations. Archives of Oral Biology 1967;12:611–621.

22. Buckley JA, Ciancio SG, McMullen JA. Efficacy of epinephrine concentration in local anesthesia during periodontal surgery. Journal of Periodontology 1984;55:653–657.

23. Hargreaves KM, Keiser K. New advances in the management of endodontic pain emergencies. Journal of the Californian Dental Association 2004;32:469–473.

24. Troullos ES, Goldstein DS, Hargreaves KM, Dionne RA. Plasma epinepherine levels and cardiovascular response to high administered doses of epinepherine in local anesthesia. Anesthesia Progress 1987;34:10–13.

25. Hasse AL, Heng MK, Garret NR. Blood pressure and electrocardiographic response to dental treatment with local anesthesia. Journal of the American Dental Association 1986;113:639–642.

26. Bennett CR. Monheim's Local Anesthesia and Pain Control in Dental Practice. 7th ed. St. Louis, MO, USA: Mosby; 1984.

27. Gutmann JL. Parameters of achieving quality anesthesia and hemostasis in surgical endodontics. Anesthesia & Pain Control in Dentistry 1993;2:223–226.

28. Roberts DH, Sowray JH. Local analgesia in dentistry. 2nd ed. Bristol, UK: Wright; 1987.

29. Ainamo J, Loe H. Anatomical characteristics of gingiva. A clinical and microscopic study of the free and attached gingiva. Journal of Periodontology 1966;37:5–13.

30. Velvart P. Papilla base incision: a new approach to recession-free healing of the interdental papilla after endodontic surgery. International Endodontic Journal 2002;35:453–460.

31. Cambruzzi JV, Marshall FJ. Molar endodontic surgery. Journal of the Canadian Dental Association 1983;49:61–65.

32. Stashenko P. Role of immune cytokines in the pathogenesis of periapical lesions. Endodontics & Dental Traumatology 1990;6:89–96.

33. Gutmann JL. Principles of endodontic surgery for the general practitioner. Dental Clinics of North America 1984;28:895–908.

34. Byers MR, Wheeler EF, Bothwell M. Altered expression of NGF and P75 NGF-receptor by fibroblasts of injured teeth precedes sensory nerve sprouting. Growth Factors 1992;6:41–52.

35. Gutmann JL, Harrison JW. Posterior endodontic surgery: anatomical considerations and clinical techniques. International Endodontic Journal 1985;18:8–34.

36. Peters E, Lau M. Histopathologic examination to confirm diagnosis of periapical lesions: a review. Journal of the Canadian Dental Association 2003;69:598–600.

37. Burkes Jr EJ. Adenoid cystic carcinoma of the mandible masquerading as periapical inflammation. Journal of Endodontics 1975;1:76–78.

38. Copeland RR. Carcinoma of the antrum mimicking periapical pathology of pulpal origin: a case report. Journal of Endodontics 1980;6:655–656.

39. Hutchison IL, Hopper C, Coonar HS. Neoplasia masquerading as periapical infection. British Dental Journal 1990;168: 288–294.

40. Corcoran JF. The importance of periapical biopsy as a diagnostic tool in endodontics. Journal of Michigan Dental Association 1978;60:523–526.

41. Cambruzzi JV, Marshall FJ, Pappin JB. Methylene blue dye: an aid to endodontic surgery. Journal of Endodontics 1985;11: 311–314.

42. Luks S. Root end amalgam technic in the practice of endodontics. Journal of the American Dental Association 1956;53:424–428.

43. Rud J, Andreasen JO. Operative procedures in periapical surgery with contempraneous root filling. International Journal of Oral Surgery 1972;1:297–310.

44. Tidmarsh BG, Arrowsmith MG. Dentinal tubules at the root ends of apicected teeth: a scanning electron microscopic study. International Endodontic Journal 1989;22:184–189.

45. Gilheany PA, Figdor D, Tyas MJ. Apical dentin permeability and microleakage associated with root end resection and retrograde filling. Journal of Endodontics 1994;20:22–26.

46. Nedderman TA, Hartwell GR, Protell FR. A comparison of root surfaces following apical root resection with various burs: scanning electron microscopic evaluation. Journal of Endodontics 1988;14:423–437.

47. Molven O, Halse A, Grung B. Incomplete healing (scar tissue) after periapical surgery–radiographic findings 8 to 12 years after treatment. Journal of Endodontics 1996;22:264–268.

48. Beatty RG. The effect of reverse filling preparation design on apical leakage. Journal of Dental Research 1986;65:259, Abstract 805.

49. Vertucci FJ, Beatty RG. Apical leakage associated with retrofilling techniques: a dye study. Journal of Endodontics 1986;12:331–336.

50. Ichesco WR, Ellison RL, Corcoran JF, Krause DC. A spectrophotometric analysis of dentinal leakage in the resected root. Journal of Endodontics 1991;17:503–507.

51. Carrigan PJ, Morse DR, Furst ML, Sinai IH. A scanning electron microscopic evaluation of human dentinal tubules according to age and location. Journal of Endodontics 1984;10:359–363.

52. Pashley DH. Smear layer: physiological considerations. Operative Dentistry – Supplment 1984;3:13–29.

53. Brännström M. Smear layer: pathological and treatment considerations. Operative Dentistry – Supplment 1984;3: 35–42.

54. Barry GN, Heyman RA, Elias A. Comparison of apical sealing methods. A preliminary report Oral Surgery, Oral Medicine, Oral Pathology 1975;39:806–811.

55. Carr GB. Surgical Endodontics. In: Cohen S, Burns RC, editors. Pathways of the Pulp. 6th ed. St. Louis, MO, USA: Mosby-Year Book; 1994. p. 531–567.

56. Gutmann JL, Saunders WP, Nguyen L, et al. Ultrasonic root-end preparation. Part 1. SEM analysis. International Endodontic Journal 1994;27: 318–324.

57. Sultan M, Pitt Ford TR. Ultrasonic preparation and obturation of root-end cavities. International Endodontic Journal 1995;28: 231–238.

58. Sumi Y, Hattori H, Hayashi K, Ueda M. Ultrasonic root-end preparation: clinical and radiographic evaluation of results. Journal of Oral & Maxillofacial Surgery 1996;54:590–593.

59. Fong CD. A sonic instrument for retrograde preparation. Journal of Endodontics 1993;19:374–375.

60. Lloyd A, Jaunberzins A, Dummer PM, Bryant S. Root-end cavity preparation using the MicroMega Sonic Retro-prep Tip. SEM analysis. International Endodontic Journal 1996;29: 295–301.

61. Abedi HR, Van Mierlo BL, Wilder-Smith P, Torabinejad M. Effects of ultrasonic root-end cavity preparation on the root apex. Oral Surgery, Oral Medicine, Oral Pathology, Oral Radiology & Endodontics 1995;80:207–213.

62. Saunders WP, Saunders EM, Gutmann JL. Ultrasonic root-end preparation, Part 2. Microleakage of EBA root-end fillings. International Endodontic Journal 1994;27:325–329.

63. Peterson J, Gutmann JL. The outcome of endodontic resurgery: a systematic review. International Endodontic Journal 2001;34: 169–175.

64. Jeansonne BG, Boggs WS, Lemon RR. Ferric sulfate hemostasis: effect on osseous wound healing. II. With curettage and irrigation. Journal of Endodontics 1993;19: 174–176.

65. Lemon RR, Steele PJ, Jeansonne BG. Ferric sulfate hemostasis: effect on osseous wound healing. Left in situ for maximum exposure. Journal of Endodontics 1993;19:170–173.

66. Witherspoon DE, Gutmann JL. Haemostasis in periradicular surgery. International Endodontic Journal 1996;29:135–149.

67. Frank AL, Glick DH, Patterson SS, Weine FS. Long-term evaluation of surgically placed amalgam fillings. Journal of Endodontics 1992;18:391–398.

68. Dorn SO, Gartner AH. Retrograde filling materials: a retrospective success-failure study of amalgam, EBA, and IRM. Journal of Endodontics 1990;16:391– 393.

69. Jesslén P, Zetterqvist L, Heimdahl A. Long-term results of amalgam versus glass ionomer cement as apical sealant after apicectomy. Oral Surgery, Oral Medicine, Oral Pathology, Oral Radiology & Endodontics 1995;79:101–103.

70. Regan JD, Gutmann JL, Witherspoon DE. Comparison of Diaket and MTA when used as root-end filling materials to

support regeneration of the periradicular tissues. International Endodontic Journal 2002;35: 840–847.

71. Torabinejad M, Watson TF, Pitt Ford TR. Sealing ability of a mineral trioxide aggregate when used as a root end filling material. Journal of Endodontics 1993;19:591–595.

72. Torabinejad M, Smith PW, Kettering JD, Pitt Ford TR. Comparative investigation of marginal adaptation of mineral trioxide aggregate and other commonly used root-end filling materials. Journal of Endodontics 1995;21:295–299.

73. Torabinejad M, Hong CU, Lee SJ, et al. Investigation of mineral trioxide aggregate for root-end filling in dogs. Journal of Endodontics 1995;21:603–608.

74. Torabinejad M, Pitt Ford TR, McKendry DJ, et al. Histologic assessment of mineral trioxide aggregate as a root-end filling in monkeys. Journal of Endodontics 1997;23:225–228.

75. Chong BS, Pitt Ford TR, Hudson MB. A prospective clinical study of Mineral Trioxide Aggregate and IRM when used as root-end filling materials in endodontic surgery. International Endodontic Journal 2003;36:520–526.

76. Saunders WP. A prospective clinical study of periradicular surgery using mineral trioxide aggregate as a root-end filling. Journal of Endodontics 2008;34:660–665.

77. Pitt Ford TR, Andreasen JO, Dorn SO, Kariyawasam SP. Effect of IRM root end fillings on healing after replantation. Journal of Endodontics 1994;20:381–385.

78. Crooks WG, Anderson RW, Powell BJ, Kimbrough WF. Longitudinal evaluation of the seal of IRM root end fillings. Journal of Endodontics 1994;20:250–252.

79. Lee SJ, Monsef M, Torabinejad M. Sealing ability of a mineral trioxide aggregate for repair of lateral root perforations. Journal of Endodontics 1993;19:541–544.

80. Pitt Ford TR, Torabinejad M, McKendry D, Hong CU. Use of mineral trioxide aggregate for repair of furcal perforations. Oral Surgery, Oral Medicine, Oral Pathology, Oral Radiology, & Endodontics 1995;79:756–763.

81. Pitt Ford TR, Torabinejad M, Abedi HR, et al. Using mineral trioxide aggregate as a pulp-capping material. Journal of the American Dental Association 1996;127:1491–1494.

82. Torabinejad M, Higa RK, McKendry DJ, Pitt Ford TR. Dye leakage of four root end filling materials: effects of blood contamination. Journal of Endodontics 1994;20:159–163.

83. Tang HM, Torabinejad M, Kettering JD. Leakage evaluation of root end filling materials using endotoxin. Journal of Endodontics 2002;28:5–7.

84. Apaydin ES, Shabahang S, Torabinejad M. Hard-tissue healing after application of fresh or set MTA as root-end-filling material. Journal of Endodontics 2004;30:21–24.

85. Boyko GA, Melcher AH, Brunette DM. Formation of new periodontal ligament by periodontal ligament cells implanted in vivo after culture in vitro. A preliminary study of transplanted roots in the dog. Journal of Periodontal Research 1981;16:73–88.

86. Boyko GA, Brunette DM, Melcher AH. Cell attachment to demineralized root surfaces in vitro. Journal of Periodontal Research 1980;15:297–303.

87. Register AA. Bone and cementum induction by dentin, demineralized in situ. Journal of Periodontology 1973;44:49–54.

88. Ruse D, Smith DC. Adhesion to bovine dentin – surface characterization. Journal of Dental Research 1991;70:1002–1008.

89. Register AA, Burdick FA. Accelerated reattachment with cementogenesis to dentin, demineralized in situ. I. Optimum range. Journal of Periodontology 1975;46:646–655.

90. Codelli GR, Fry HR, Davis JW. Burnished versus nonburnished application of citric acid to human diseased root surfaces: the effect of time and method of application. Quintessence International 1991;22:277–283.

91. Sterrett JD. Optimal citric acid concentration for dentinal demineralization. Quintessence International 1991;22:371–375.

92. Craig KR, Harrison JW. Wound healing following demineralization of resected root ends in periradicular surgery. Journal of Endodontics 1993;19:339–347.

93. Meyers JP, Gutmann JL. Histological healing following surgical endodontics and its implications in case assessment: a case report. International Endodontic Journal 1994;27:339–342.

94. Molven O, Halse A, Grung B. Observer strategy and the radiographic classification of healing after endodontic surgery. International Journal of Oral & Maxillofacial Surgery 1987;16:432–439.

95. Weine FS. The case against intentional replantation. Journal of the American Dental Association 1980;100:664–668.

96. Polson A, Proye GT. Fibrin linkage: a precursor for new attachment. Journal of Periodontology 1983;54:141–147.

97. Ririe CM, Crigger M, Selvig KA. Healing of periodontal connective tissues following surgical wounding and application of citric acid in dogs. Journal of Periodontal Research 1980;15:314–327.

98. Gutmann JL, Pitt Ford TR. Management of the resected root end: a clinical review. International Endodontic Journal 1993;26:273–283.

99. John V, Warner NA, Blanchard SB. Periodontal-endodontic interdisciplinary treatment-a case report. Compendium of Continuing Education in Dentistry 2004;25:601–602, 4–6, 8; quiz 12–13.

100. Kellert M, Chalfin H, Solomon C. Guided tissue regeneration: an adjunct to endodontic surgery. Journal of the American Dental Association 1994;125: 1229–1233.

101. Pecora G, Kim S, Celletti R, Davarpanah M. The guided tissue regeneration principle in endodontic surgery: one-year postoperative results of large periapical lesions. International Endodontic Journal 1995;28: 41–46.

102. Hirsch JM, Ahlstrom U, Henrikson PA, et al. Periapical surgery. International Journal of Oral Surgery 1979;8:173–185.

103. Skoglund A, Persson G. A follow-up study of apicoectomized teeth with total loss of the buccal bone plate. Oral Surgery, Oral Medicine, Oral Pathology 1985;59:78–81.

104. Halse A, Molven O, Grung B. Follow-up after periapical surgery: the value of the one-year control. Endodontics & Dental Traumatology 1991;7:246–250.

105. Rud J, Andreasen JO, Jensen JF. A multivariate analysis of the influence of various factors upon healing after endodontic surgery. International Journal of Oral Surgery 1972;1:258–271.

106. Reit C. Decision strategies in endodontics: on the design of a recall program. Endodontics & Dental Traumatology 1987;3: 233–239.

107. Finn MD, Schow SR, Schneiderman ED. Osseous regeneration in the presence of four common hemostatic agents. Journal of Oral & Maxillofacial Surgery 1992;50:608–612.

108. Pinto VS, Zuolo ML, Mellonig JT. Guided bone regeneration in the treatment of a large periapical lesion: a case report. Practical Periodontics & Aesthetic Dentistry 1995;7:76–81; quiz 2.

109. Benenati FW, Roane JB, Biggs JT, Simon JH. Recall evaluation of iatrogenic root perforations repaired with amalgam and gutta-percha. Journal of Endodontics 1986;12:161–166.

110. Biggs JT, Benenati FW, Sabala CL. Treatment of iatrogenic root perforations with associated osseous lesions. Journal of Endodontics 1988;14:620–624.

111. Trope M, Tronstad L. Long-term calcium hydroxide treatment of a tooth with iatrogenic root perforation and lateral periodontitis. Endodontics & Dental Traumatology 1985;1: 35–38.

112. Walia H, Streiff J, Gerstein H. Use of a hemostatic agent in the repair of procedural errors. Journal of Endodontics 1988;14: 465–468.

113. Fuss Z, Assooline LS, Kaufman AY. Determination of location of root perforations by electronic apex locators. Oral Surgery Oral Medicine Oral Pathology Oral Radiology & Endodontics 1996;82:324–329.

114. Fuss Z, Trope M. Root perforations: classification and treatment choices based on prognostic factors. Endodontics & Dental Traumatology 1996;12: 255–264.

115. Regan JD, Witherspoon DE, Gutmann JL. Prevention, identification and management of tooth perforation. Endodontic Practice 1998;1:24–40.

116. Nicholls E. Treatment of traumatic perforations of the pulp cavity. Oral Surgery 1962;15:603–612.

117. Oswald RJ. Procedural accidents and their repair. Dental Clinics of North America 1979;23: 593–616.

118. Sinai IH. Endodontic perforations: their prognosis and treatment. Journal of the American Dental Association 1977;95:90–95.

119. Young GR. Contemporary management of lateral root perforation diagnosed with the aid of dental computed tomography. Australian Endodontic Journal 2007;33: 112–118.

120. American Association of Endodontists. Glossary of endodontic terms. 7th ed. Chicago, IL, USA: American Association of Endodontists; 2003.

121. Dumsha TC, Gutmann JL. Clinical guidelines for intentional replantation. Compendium of Continuing Education in Dentistry 1985;6:604–608.

122. Scott JN, Zelikow R. Replantation – a clinical philosophy. Journal of the American Dental Association 1980;101:17–19.

123. Andreasen JO, Rud J, Munksgaard EC. Atlas of Replantation and Transplantation of teeth. Fribourg, Switzerland: Mediglobe; 1989.

124. Mikkonen M, Kullaa-Mikkonen A, Kotilainen R. Clinical and radiologic re-examination of apicoectomized teeth. Oral Surgery, Oral Medicine, Oral Pathology 1983;55:302–306.

125. Persson G. Periapical surgery of molars. International Journal of Oral Surgery 1982;11:96–100.

126. Aukhil I. Biology of tooth-cell adhesion. Dental Clinics of North America 1991;35:459–467.

127. Bohning BP, Davenport WD, Jeansonne BG. The effect of guided tissue regeneration on the healing of osseous defects in rat calvaria. Journal of Endodontics 1999;25:81–84.

128. Dahlin C, Linde A, Gottlow J, Nyman S. Healing of bone defects by guided tissue regeneration. Plastic & Reconstructive Surgery 1988;81: 672–676.

129. Dahlin C, Gottlow J, Linde A, Nyman S. Healing of maxillary and mandibular bone defects using a membrane technique. An experimental study in monkeys. Scandinavian Journal of Plastic & Reconstructive Surgery & Hand Surgery 1990;24:13–19.

130. Douthitt JC, Gutmann JL, Witherspoon DE. Histologic assessment of healing after the use of a bioresorbable membrane in the management of buccal bone loss concomitant with periradicular surgery. Journal of Endodontics 2001;27:404–410.

131. Blomlöf L, Lindskog S. Cervical root resorption associated with guided tissue regeneration: a case report. Journal of Periodontology 1998;69:392–395.

132. Uchin RA. Use of a bioresorbable guided tissue membrane at an adjunct to bony regeneration in cases requiring endodontic surgical intervention. Journal of Endodontics 1996;22:94–96.

133. Zenobio EG, Shibli JA. Treatment of endodontic perforations using guided tissue regeneration and demineralized freeze-dried bone allograft: two case reports with 2–4 year post-surgical evaluations. Journal of Contemporary Dental Practice 2004;5:131–141.

134. Zorzano LA, Sanchez AL, Chacartegi JE, et al. Guided tissue regeneration procedure applied to the treatment of endodontic-periodontal disease: analysis of a case. Quintessence International 1997;28:87–91.

135. Melcher AH. On the repair potential of periodontal tissues. Journal of Periodontology 1976;47:256–260.

136. Karring T, Nyman S, Lindhe J. Healing following implantation of periodontitis affected roots into bone tissue. Journal of Clinical Periodontology 1980;7: 96–105.

137. Karring T, Nyman S, Gottlow J, Laurell L. Development of the biologic concept of guided tissue regeneration – animal and human studies. Periodontology 2000 1993;1:26–35.

138. Nyman S, Gottlow J, Karring T, Lindhe J. The regenerative potential of the periodontal ligament. An experimental study in the monkey. Journal of Clinical Periodontology 1982;9: 257–265.

139. Gottlow J, Nyman S, Karring T, Lindhe J. New attachment formation as the result of controlled tissue regeneration. Journal of Clinical Periodontology 1984;11: 494–503.

140. von Arx T, Cochran DL. Rationale for the application of the GTR principle using a barrier membrane in endodontic surgery: a proposal of classification and literature review. International Journal of Periodontics & Restorative Dentistry 2001;21: 127–139.

141. Caffesse RG, Mota LF, Quinones CR, Morrison EC. Clinical comparison of resorbable and non-resorbable barriers for guided periodontal tissue regeneration. Journal of Clinical Periodontology 1997;24: 747–752.

142. Camelo M, Nevins ML, Lynch SE, Shenk RK. Periodontal regeneration with an autogenous bone – Bio-Oss composite graft and a Bio-Gide membrane. International Journal of Periodontics & Restorative Dentistry 2001;21:109–119.

143. Rubinstein RA, Kim S. Short-term observation of the results of endodontic surgery with the use of a surgical microscope and Super-EBA as root-end filling material. Journal of Endodontics 1999;25:43–48.

144. Zuolo ML, Ferreira MO, Gutmann JL. Prognosis in periradicular surgery: a clinical prospective study. International Endodontic Journal 2000;33: 91–98.

145. Lim LM, Pascon EA, Skribner J, et al. Clinical, radiographic, and histological study of endodontic treatment failures. Oral Surgery, Oral Medicine, Oral Pathology 1991;71:603–611.

146. Nordenram A, Svardstrom G. Results of apicectomy. Swedish Dental Journal 1970;63:593–604.

147. Ray HA, Trope M. Periapical status of endodontically treated teeth in relation to the technical quality of the root filling and the coronal restoration. International Endodontic Journal 1995;28: 12–18.

Chapter | **11** |

Endodontics in primary teeth

A. O'Donnell

CHAPTER CONTENTS

SUMMARY

Endodontic treatment for deciduous teeth can be challenging due to the morphology of the root canal system, difficulties with correct diagnosis and behaviour management issues associated with a young patient. The vital, non-infected pulp should be preserved when appropriate. As with any endodontic treatment, the elimination of infection is critical to a successful outcome. There is a move away from formocresol and most paediatric dentists now prefer to use alternative medicaments. Root canal treatment of the infected primary tooth is, often, the best treatment option but it may be challenging and impractical to perform. A referral to a specialist may sometimes be necessary for endodontic management of primary teeth.

INTRODUCTION

The basic aims of endodontic treatment of primary teeth are similar to those for the permanent dentition: prevention or treatment of apical periodontitis, as well as the relief of associated symptoms including pain. It is generally accepted that primary molar teeth should be retained until they exfoliate naturally to avoid loss of space and crowding of the permanent dentition.

Although the response of primary teeth to infection is similar to that of adult teeth, morphological and physiological differences exist between primary and permanent teeth resulting in varying techniques for endodontic treatment. In addition, extra care must always be taken when carrying out endodontic treatment, especially on deciduous incisors. Parents must be warned of potential damage to the underlying permanent successor and the risks versus benefits discussed in full. A referral to a specialist paedodontic unit is sometimes necessary for endodontic management of primary teeth. When deciding on a suitable treatment plan for primary teeth, the clinician must consider whether the tooth should be saved with endodontic treatment or if extraction would be more advantageous. The following should be considered:

Factors related to the patient

- Patient cooperation – if a child is uncooperative or unable to cope with treatment in the dental chair, careful thought must be given to the potential benefits versus the risks of carrying out endodontic treatment under general anaesthesia. Although endodontic treatment enjoys a high success rate, the outcome cannot be guaranteed when there are compounding factors. If failure occurs, the child may

© 2009 Elsevier Ltd, Inc, BV
DOI: 10.1016/B978-0-7020-3156-4.00014-0

be subjected to a repeat general anaesthetic to remove the tooth.

- Medical history – certain medical conditions will determine whether endodontic treatment should be undertaken. Children who are immunosuppressed, e.g. receiving chemotherapy, are not suitable candidates for endodontic treatment as there is the concern regarding a potential source of infection in the deciduous tooth. In patients at risk of infective endocarditis, endodontic treatment in deciduous teeth is also not recommended. However, endodontic treatment may be the treatment of choice in patients with coagulation disorders to avoid the risk of bleeding associated with an extraction. Children whose medical history contraindicates general anaesthesia, and who are unable to tolerate an extraction under local anaesthesia, may sometimes be able to cope with root canal treatment under local anaesthesia. For any child with a relevant medical history, the medical team should be consulted before deciding on the best treatment option.
- Irregular attenders and poor parental attitude to dentistry – this may lead the clinician to decide against endodontic treatment due to the inability to carry out regular clinical and radiological follow-up.

Factors related to the dentition

- Extent of dental decay – if the decay is extensive and restoration following endodontic treatment will be difficult or impossible then extraction is the treatment of choice.
- Extent of periapical infection – if gross, pathological resorption has occurred or the infection is severe, extraction may be the best option.
- Condition of the rest of the dentition – if this is poor and patient's motivation to change diet and improve oral hygiene is not deemed to be high, extraction is usually recommended.
- Hypodontia – If there is no permanent successor, endodontic treatment may be the best option in order to keep the space for a future bridge or implant.[1] However, it is important to obtain orthodontic advice beforehand; the deciduous tooth may be best removed and, provided the timing is right, the space may be used orthodontically.
- Balancing in primary canines and first molars – if the contralateral tooth has been lost, it may be preferable to carry out a 'balancing' extraction rather than perform endodontic treatment, especially when the arch is crowded.
- Remaining natural lifespan of the tooth – it is generally accepted that primary molar teeth should be retained until they exfoliate naturally to avoid loss of space and crowding of the permanent dentition. However, if physiological root resorption has affected two-thirds or more of the roots, then endodontic treatment is not a sensible option as the tooth is close to being exfoliated.

TREATMENT OF PRIMARY TEETH

Primary teeth differ morphologically from their permanent successors both in shape and size; pulp space anatomy of primary teeth is covered in Chapter 4. In general, the enamel and dentine are thinner than in a permanent tooth. Pulpal changes in response to caries, therefore, occur more rapidly and even lesions that appear very minimal clinically can extend into the pulp (Fig. 11.1). Primary molars have fine tapered roots which are flattened mesiodistally to enclose a ribbon-like root canal system and their pulp chambers are relatively larger than permanent teeth. The single root canal may become partially calcified with age,[2] to produce several intercommunicating canals, thus making instrumentation of the radicular pulp space difficult. Many lateral canals have been reported to exist in the furcation of primary molar teeth,[3] and these may contribute to the early spread of infection from the pulp chamber to the interradicular area.[4]

The correct diagnosis of pulp disease is important as this will determine which endodontic treatment procedure will be required. The diagnosis is dependent on the combination of a good history, clinical and radiological examination. A clear history of clinical symptoms is especially difficult to obtain in young patients because they are usually unable to give an accurate pain history, and parental report is usually relied upon. Symptoms of irreversible damage will include a history of spontaneous pain, severe pain at night and pain on biting. The clinical examination should begin with assessing the extent of the caries. It has been reported that in the majority of primary molars with marginal ridge breakdown there is pulpal inflammation involving the pulp horn adjacent to the carious lesion.[5] The presence of abnormal tooth mobility, intraoral swelling, discharging sinus tracts and tenderness to pressure will also indicate periapical pathosis. In primary teeth, sensitivity testing has been shown to be an unreliable guide to the histological status of the pulp,[6,7,8] so a combination of the history, clinical and radiological examination provides an indication of the pulpal status.

If the child is cooperative, preoperative radiological examination is invaluable. This provides information regarding root morphology, periapical pathosis, resorption and calcifications, aiding diagnosis and assessment of any local contraindications to endodontic treatment. The treatment techniques that have been advocated for use on primary teeth may be grouped as follows:

- indirect pulp capping
- direct pulp capping

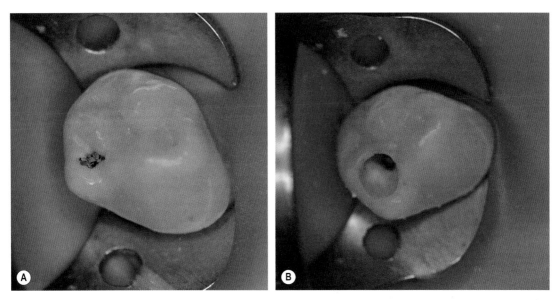

Figure 11.1 Carious deciduous molar. (A) The carious lesion appears minimal clinically. (B) Pulpal exposure following total caries removal. Reproduced courtesy of M.Vaidyanathan.

- pulpotomy
- pulpectomy.

In all cases, the administration of local anaesthesia and adequate tooth isolation, preferably with rubber dam, are advised. For vital maxillary teeth, infiltration anaesthesia is usually satisfactory, whereas a nerve block or intraligamentary injection may be more suitable for mandibular molar teeth. It cannot be overemphasized that a successful treatment outcome is dependent on correct diagnosis, appropriate technique and the provision of a definitive restoration, ideally a preformed metal crown, which will provide a good coronal seal.[9] All primary teeth that have had an endodontic procedure carried out should be followed up clinically and radiographically.

Indirect pulp capping

This is the term used to describe the placement of a dressing over residual carious dentine in an attempt to allow secondary dentine to be formed within the pulp chamber.[10] Exposure of the pulp is, therefore, avoided in teeth with deep carious lesions when there is no clinical or radiological evidence of pulpal or periapical disease. Removal of caries from the lateral wall ensures that there is an adequate seal between the tooth and the restoration so that microbes are deprived of the nutrients necessary for their survival.[11,12] Contraindications to this method of treatment include any evidence of an irreversibly inflamed or necrotic pulp such as a history of spontaneous pain, asso-

ciated swelling, tenderness to biting, or abnormal tooth mobility. Likewise, preoperative radiographs must be examined for pathological root resorption, pulp calcifications or periapical radiolucency, which if present, would necessitate less conservative treatment.

At the initial visit, all soft carious dentine is removed with a bur in a slow-speed handpiece or by hand with an excavator. The amelodentinal junction must be free from all softened carious dentine. The area of dentine over the site of a potential pulpal exposure is covered with a layer of hard setting cement containing calcium hydroxide (e.g. Dycal, Dentsply, Weybridge, Surrey, UK) and sealed with an overlying structural base of a quick-setting, reinforced zinc oxide–eugenol preparation (e.g. IRM, Dentsply) or glass ionomer cement. A success rate of 92% for indirect pulp capping with calcium hydroxide in primary incisors followed for 42 months has been reported,[13] and 96% in primary molars after 1 year.[14] Alternatively, an adhesive resin system may be used, directly over the dentine which has shown to have a success rate of 96% compared with 83% for calcium hydroxide.[15] Other studies have shown success when glass ionomer is placed over the dentine,[16] which offers the additional benefit of fluoride release. The final restoration can then be placed. The indirect pulp cap technique has been shown to be clinically more successful than formocresol pulpotomy,[17,18] and therefore, offers an alternative to the pulpotomy technique. Some authors have advocated a two-stage procedure where the tooth is re-opened 3 months later and further caries removal is performed.[18] Due to the

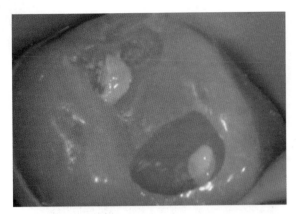

Figure 11.2 Pulp cap with calcium hydroxide. Reproduced courtesy of T.Kandiah.

high success of the one-stage indirect pulp cap, this is no longer necessary and regular review of tooth vitality is preferable to subjecting the patient to subsequent re-entry into the tooth.

Direct pulp capping

Direct pulp capping is generally not advocated for primary teeth due to limited evidence of success in the literature. Inflammation within the pulp can persist and is followed by necrosis or internal resorption. The only possible application of this technique is when pulp tissue has been mechanically exposed as a result of cavity preparation,[19] or when the tooth is close to exfoliation.[20] Calcium hydroxide is placed on the exposure and encourages formation of a dentine bridge below the exposure site in an attempt to maintain pulp vitality (Fig. 11.2). The technique should not be used for carious exposures.

The exposure site should be gently irrigated with a non-irritant solution, e.g. saline, to remove any debris that may impede healing and also to keep the pulp moist. The capping material should be flowed gently over the exposure and allowed to set. Various capping materials have been employed. Calcium hydroxide used alone or in conjunction with zinc oxide–eugenol, has been most widely investigated.[21,22] The use of dentine bonding systems has also been advocated and promising results have been reported.[19,23] The advantage is that a polymer film can be layered over an exposure site without displacing the pulp, and onto surrounding dentine where it permeates the tubules. Further work is required before these materials can be recommended as capping agents. A more promising material is Mineral Trioxide Aggregate (MTA), which is biocompatible and has good sealing properties.[24] Favourable results have been reported for MTA direct pulp capping on deciduous molars compared with calcium hydroxide;[25] and clinical case reports have also supported the use of MTA.[26] Following pulp capping and final resto-

ration, the tooth should be monitored clinically and radiologically for any signs of subsequent pulp necrosis or extensive resorption, indicative of treatment failure.

Pulpotomy

Vital (full coronal) pulpotomy involves the removal of the entire coronal pulp that has undergone irreversible inflammatory changes or necrosis, leaving remaining healthy vital tissue intact within the root canal system. The cut radicular pulp stumps are covered with a medicament which will result in either healing or 'fixation' of the tissue beyond the interface of dressing and radicular pulp. Vital pulpotomy provides the most suitable method for treating carious exposures in primary teeth without a history of spontaneous pain, swelling, sinus tract, any evidence of internal or external root resorption, or periapical pathosis. Its success is dependent on correct diagnosis, control of haemorrhage from the radicular pulp and achieving an excellent coronal seal. A preformed metal crown is the final restoration of choice as this minimizes the risks of tooth fracture and microleakage, and hence enhances the prognosis.

The basic technique consists of the following steps:

- Local anaesthesia and adequate isolation.
- Caries removal.
- Extend cavity so that entire roof of the coronal pulp chamber is removed.
- Rose head bur in a slow-speed handpiece or a hand excavator to remove coronal pulp tissue.
- Control haemorrhage with sterile cotton wool pledgets (if bleeding continues this may mean that initial diagnosis is incorrect and the pulp is irreversibly damaged, so pulpectomy is the treatment of choice).
- Placement of pulpotomy medicament (Fig. 11.3A).
- Coronal restoration of the tooth (Fig. 11.3B,C).
- Follow-up (Fig. 11.3D).

Electrosurgery may be used for pulpotomy procedures to either remove the pulp tissue or to control haemorrhage; the main advantage is that the need for any potentially toxic medicament can be avoided. However, it was reported that when electrosurgery was used to remove the entire coronal pulp and treat the remaining stumps, root resorption occurred.[27] An alternative method may be to remove the coronal pulp mechanically and treat the remaining pulp stumps electrosurgically[28] in order to avoid excessive heat dissipation. Although a clinical and radiological success rate of 99% has been demonstrated at 2 years,[29] the electrosurgical pulpotomy technique is still experimental and not widely adopted. Lasers have also been suggested as an alternative instrument but some studies have shown carbonization, necrosis and inflammation of the pulp with little evidence of repair.[19,30,31] A study on laser pulpotomy versus the formocresol

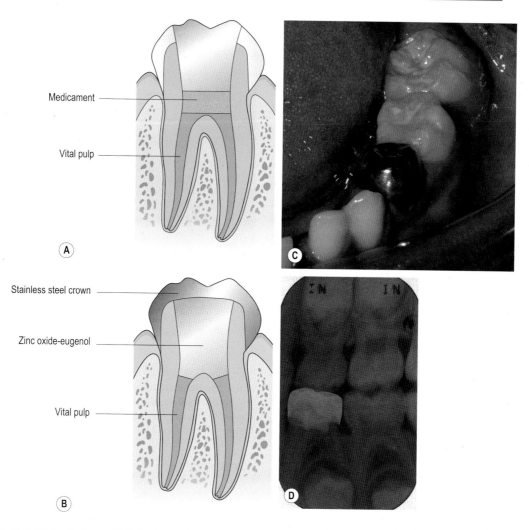

Medicament

Vital pulp

(A)

Stainless steel crown

Zinc oxide-eugenol

Vital pulp

(B)

(C)

(D)

Figure 11.3 Vital pulpotomy. (A) Following caries and coronal pulp removal, medicament is placed; (B) the pulp chamber is then filled with zinc oxide-eugenol cement and the tooth restored with a preformed metal crown (based on the original drawings by A Muir). (C) Clinical view of a preformed stainless steel crown. (D) Example of a follow-up radiograph. Reproduced courtesy of M.Vaidyanathan.

technique carried out on caries-free primary molar teeth, which were scheduled for extraction reported comparable results.[32] Due to limited evidence, the expense involved and the success of alternative techniques, lasers are rarely used for pulpotomies in children.

Medicaments

Medicaments are used in endodontic treatment of primary teeth as wound dressings, tissue fixatives, disinfectants and inflammatory suppressants. A systematic review of the literature on the relative effectiveness of various medicaments and techniques for treating primary molar teeth

with decay involving the pulp found that the evidence available did not support the superiority of one type of treatment over another.[33] Therefore, the choice of treatment is very much dependent on clinical presentation and the individual operator.

Formocresol

Buckley[34] formulated a solution containing equal parts of formalin and tricresol. A commercial solution containing 19% formaldehyde, 35% cresol in a glycerine/water vehicle (Buckley's formocresol, Cosby laboratories, Burbank, CA, USA), was later developed as a suitable medicament for the treatment of pulpally exposed primary teeth. The aim of this treatment technique is to fix the coronal portion of the radicular pulp and to maintain vitality of the remaining apical portion.[35,36] Formocresol acts through its aldehyde group and binds to the amino acids of protein and bacteria to prevent autolysis and hydrolysis so rendering tissue inert.[37]

Over the years, there has been increasing concern about the toxicity, both local and systemic, of formocresol. Experimental evidence has shown that sufficient formocresol was absorbed systemically from multiple pulpotomy sites in an experimental animal to induce early tissue injury in the kidneys and liver.[38,39,40] However, it was argued that due to the quantity normally used in man, the risk is much less and may therefore be negligible. A definite relationship between formocresol pulpotomies in primary teeth and enamel defects on their permanent successors has been demonstrated,[41] but not confirmed in other studies.[42,43] In addition, carcinogenic and mutagenic properties have been recognized, which together with local and systemic effects, have led to the use of a 20% (1 : 5) diluted solution.[44,45] The International Agency for Research on Cancer (IARC) classified formaldehyde as a carcinogen in 2004. Case control and cohort studies of workers exposed to formaldehyde daily have shown an association between formaldehyde exposure and nasopharyngeal cancer and leukaemia. This has raised questions as to the continuing use of formocresol in children. The use of alternative medicaments has been debated within the literature due to alternative methods being shown to be equally successful clinically.[46,47,48] Although a recent evaluation of the research regarding safety of formaldehyde concluded that there was inconsequential risk of carcinogenesis associated with formaldehyde use in paediatric pulp therapy,[49] there is continuing unease. There is a growing movement away from using formocresol and most paediatric dentists now prefer to use alternative medicaments. Nevertheless, the clinician should always consider each case individually and involve parents in the decision-making process when treatment planning.

Glutaraldehyde

Glutaraldehyde has been investigated as an alternative fixative to formocresol because of its lower toxicity.[50] Glutaraldehyde is a larger molecule than formaldehyde, and as a result diffusion through the tissues is reduced. When 2% unbuffered glutaraldehyde was used, over 96% clinical success was reported after 42 months.[51,52] A 90% clinical success rate was reported after 1 year, where 2% buffered glutaraldehyde was applied for 5 minutes in pulpotomies.[53] At follow-up after 2 years there was a failure rate of 18% as a result of internal resorption;[54] the authors concluded that the relatively high failure rate reported in this study does not justify recommending a 2% buffered glutaraldehyde solution as a substitute to formocresol.

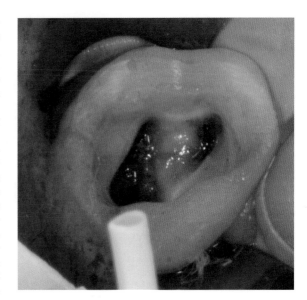

Figure 11.4 Ferric sulphate pulpotomy. The appearance of the pulp stumps following application of this medicament. Reproduced courtesy of T.Kandiah.

Although glutaraldehyde was proposed as a replacement for formocresol, questions remain about its safety.[36] On a weight-for-weight basis there is little difference in toxicity between formocresol and glutaraldehyde.[55]

Ferric sulphate

Ferric sulphate is commonly used in dentistry for control of bleeding during surgery or for gingival retraction. When applied directly to pulp tissue, a ferric ion-protein complex is formed which blocks the cut vessels mechanically. Although not a fixative, having only bacteriostatic properties, ferric sulphate is used to control haemorrhage by gentle intermittent application of a 15.5% solution for up to 15 seconds (Fig. 11.4). A zinc oxide–eugenol base is then placed to cover the pulp stumps, prior to the coronal restoration.

A better clinical success rate was reported, after 1 year, when 15.5% ferric sulphate was compared with 1:5 diluted formocresol.[56] However, the preliminary report from another study was that there was no difference between the two medicaments.[57] Following these results, the ferric sulphate technique was subjected to further clinical investigation with a longer follow-up period, and found to perform well.[58] Recent systematic reviews have concluded that the treatment outcome with either formocresol or ferric sulphate is similar.[59,60] The short application time is a clear advantage when treating children, and hence, ferric sulphate is considered an alternative to formocresol.

Calcium hydroxide

Although the application of pure calcium hydroxide to the cut pulp stumps after haemorrhage control was previously favoured for pulpotomy of primary teeth,[61] the work of Magnusson[62] cast doubt on the use of this material in primary teeth. However, later studies indicated that if a carefully controlled technique is used, then calcium hydroxide may produce long-term results which are comparable with those obtained with formocresol.[21,22,63] Calcium hydroxide in its pure, powder form is a clinically acceptable alternative when strict selection criteria are used.[64] The critical factor is the level of inflammation in the pulp and attempts have been made to assess this objectively by measuring prostaglandin levels;[65] however, this work is still experimental.

A well-conducted randomized controlled trial comparing the relative effectiveness of formocresol, ferric sulphate, laser and calcium hydroxide reported equally successful results with formocresol, ferric sulphate and laser. Only calcium hydroxide performed significantly worse and hence, considered less appropriate for pulpotomies.[66] Other studies have shown that calcium hydroxide does not perform well as a pulpotomy medicament when compared with available alternatives.[67] This could be due to the reported high incidence of internal resorption noted in calcium hydroxide pulpotomies. The rate of such 'pathological' resorption compared with 'physiological' resorption should be borne in mind when using this criterion to classify a pulpotomy as a 'failure'.

Mineral Trioxide Aggregate

Mineral Trioxide Aggregate (MTA) was originally formulated as a root-end filling material in apical surgery.[68] It is available in either grey or white forms and is, chemically, similar to Portland cement (mixture of dicalcium silicate, tricalcium silicate, tricalcium aluminate, gypsum and tetracalcium aluminoferrite), but made radiopaque due to the addition of bismuth oxide.[69] It is biocompatible, has a high compressive strength, good sealing ability and the potential to induce the formation of a hard tissue barrier. The setting time of MTA has been reported to vary from 45 to 175 minutes[70] Due to this long setting time, the initial compressive strength is low. Glass ionomer or composite resin can be placed directly over MTA with no adverse reactions.[71,72] It is, therefore, advisable to restore the tooth immediately with a preformed metal crown or a composite resin restoration. Following its successful application in endodontics for permanent teeth, MTA was suggested as also being suitable for endodontics in primary teeth. The MTA powder is mixed with sterile water to form a paste. This is then placed over the pulp stumps once haemostasis has been achieved. It has been recommended as an alternative to formocresol for pulpotomies in primary teeth[73,74,75] and the reported success rates are

greater than 90%. Studies have also compared MTA to formocresol and calcium hydroxide.[67] A small study compared the use of formocresol, ferric sulphate, calcium hydroxide and MTA in primary molar pulpotomies and showed no significant difference in the success of any of the medicaments.[63] However, internal root resorption, seen with both ferric sulphate and formocresol, was not observed in the MTA treated teeth.[20] MTA is relatively expensive when compared with other pulpotomy medicaments which may limit its more widespread use.

Corticosteroids

Corticosteroid may be used to suppress pulpal inflammation for the short-term purpose of desensitising the pulp. Ledermix (Haupt Pharma GmbH, Wolfratshausen, Germany), a corticosteroid-antibiotic dressing may be useful in treating the inflamed, but not infected pulp, when it is too painful to allow pulp tissue removal. Ledermix is placed directly over the exposed pulp followed by a temporary dressing. The tooth is then revisited a week or so later and pulp removal is then carried out. Corticosteroid compounds should only be used in carefully selected cases and never as a substitute for proper treatment.

Antibiotics

Recently, the concept of 'Lesion Sterilization and Tissue Repair' (LSTR) was developed in which a combination of antibiotics is employed to disinfect the infected root canal system. A study on primary teeth with infected root canals and periapical lesions in which a mixture of antibiotics (metronidazole, ciprofloxacin, and minocycline) was placed at the orifices of root canals or in the pulp chamber reported promising results.[76] However, research is limited and this technique is not recommended at present.

Bone morphogenic proteins

Bone morphogenic proteins (BMP) is a family of growth factors that was discovered following the observation that demineralized bone matrix can stimulate new bone when implanted in an ectopic site such as muscle.[77] With the development of molecular biology, these factors were isolated and their physiological roles investigated. A number of BMP are capable of inducing reparative dentine and recombinant human BMP have been used experimentally.[78] These materials would have clear advantages in pulpotomy techniques, producing a biological barrier without concern regarding toxicity.

Pulpectomy

Non-vital primary teeth may be retained successfully when this technique is employed but it may be technically dif-

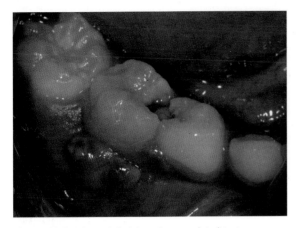

Figure 11.5 A buccal draining abscess related to two carious deciduous molars.

ficult to carry out due to the fine ribbon-like canals and the high incidence of accessory canals. Pulpal necrosis, alveolar swelling, interradicular or periapical radiolucency are not contraindications to this treatment modality. Root canal treatment provides the most satisfactory method of retaining the restorable primary tooth where infection extends to the radicular pulp and extraction remains the only other option. The whole procedure may be completed in one visit when there is no infection, or over two visits if infection is present (Fig. 11.5).

Once any initial pain or swelling has been relieved, an access cavity is prepared under rubber dam isolation. The use of local anaesthesia is recommended as some vital tissue could still be encountered in the root canal system. Any pulp tissue in the root canal system is removed, and the canals are cleaned with small files (sizes 15 and 20) to within 2 mm of the radiographic apex. Sodium hypochlorite solution (1%) should be used to irrigate the canals and achieve chemical dissolution of any remaining pulp tissue. An alternative is chlorhexidine (0.2%) but this has no tissue solvent properties. The canals are then dried with paper points and filled. If treatment is carried out over two visits and if required, the canals are dressed with non-setting calcium hydroxide and a temporary filling.

There is no agreed consensus as to the preferred root canal filling material, but it should have the following properties:

- non-irritant to the periapical tissues and the underlying, developing permanent tooth;
- resorption at a rate similar to that of the deciduous tooth;
- antiseptic properties.

Resorbable materials based on zinc oxide–eugenol, calcium hydroxide and iodoform paste have been used successfully.[79,80,81] Vitapex (Neo Dental, Federal Way, WA, USA), a premixed calcium hydroxide and iodoform paste, has also been recommended as a root canal filling material for primary teeth[82] and has been shown to be clinically superior to zinc oxide-eugenol,[79] as has another iodoform-based material (Kri paste).[83]

The chosen filling material should be mixed to a creamy consistency and carried into the canals using a pressure syringe, spiral root canal filler, or if mixed to a stiffer consistency, packed into the canal with pluggers. Various filling techniques including the Lentulo spiral filler and the Jiffy tube pressure syringe have been compared for filling root canals of primary teeth; the Lentulo spiral was found to perform best.[84] After root canal filling, the pulp chamber should be packed with a suitable cement, and the tooth restored with a preformed metal crown. Teeth that have had a pulpectomy should be followed up clinically and radiologically; if failure occurs, extraction should be considered. Pulpectomy can also be considered to be an alternative to current pulpotomy techniques when treating vital primary teeth with carious exposure.

LEARNING OUTCOMES

After completing this chapter the reader should be able to understand and discuss the:

- endodontic challenges of treating the primary dentition and the patient management issues associated with the young patient;
- importance and difficulties of correct diagnosis and its influence on treatment planning;
- factors to consider when deciding whether endodontic treatment is appropriate or not;
- various endodontic treatment procedures for primary teeth;
- medicaments used in endodontic treatment of primary teeth;
- importance of eliminating infection in order to secure a successful endodontic treatment outcome.

REFERENCES

1. Rodd H, Waterhouse PJ, Fuks AB, et al. Pulp therapy for primary molars. International Journal of Pediatric Dentistry 2006;16(Suppl 1):15–23.

2. Hibbard ED, Ireland RL. Morphology of the root canals of the primary molar teeth. Journal of Dentistry for Children 1957;24:250–257.

3. Winter GB. Abscess formation in connection with deciduous molar teeth. Archives of Oral Biology 1962;7:373–379.

4. Wrbas KT, Kielbassa AM, Hellwig E. Microscopic studies of accessory canals in primary molar furcations. ASDC Journal of Dentistry for Children 1997;64:118–122.

5. Duggal MS, Nooh A, High A. Responses of the primary pulp to inflammation: a review of the Leeds studies and challenges for the future. European Journal of Paediatric Dentistry 2002;3:111–114.

6. McDonald RE. Diagnostic aids and vital pulp therapy for deciduous teeth. Journal of the American Dental Association 1956;53:14–22.

7. Mumford JM. Pain perception threshold on stimulating teeth and the histological condition of the pulp. British Dental Journal 1967;123:427–433.

8. Asfour MA, Millar BJ, Smith PB. An assessment of the reliability of pulp testing deciduous teeth. International Journal of Paediatric Dentistry 1996;6:163–166.

9. Holan G, Fuks A, Keltz N. Success rate of formocresol pulpotomy in primary molars restored with stainless steel crown vs amalgam. Pediatric Dentistry 2002;24: 212–216.

10. Shovelton DS. The maintenance of pulp vitality. British Dental Journal 1972;133:95–101.

11. King JB, Crawford JJ, Lindahl RL. Indirect pulp capping: a bacteriologic study of deep carious dentine in human teeth. Oral Surgery, Oral Medicine, Oral Pathology 1965;20:663–671.

12. Handelman SL. Therapeutic use of sealants for incipient or early caries in children and young adults. Procedings of Finnish Dental Society 1991;87:463–475.

13. Coll JA, Josell S, Nassof S, et al. An evaluation of pulpal therapy in primary incisors. Pediatric Dentistry 1988;10:178–184.

14. Al Zayer MA, Straffon LH, Feigal RJ, Welch KB. Indirect pulp treatment of primary posterior teeth: a retrospective study. Pediatric Dentistry 2003;25:29–36.

15. Falster CA, Araujo FB, Straffon LH, Nor JE. Indirect pulp treatment: in vivo outcomes of an adhesive resin system vs calcium hydroxide for the protection of the dentin-pulp complex. Pediatric Dentistry 2002;24:241–248.

16. Massara MLA, Alves JB, Brandao PRG. Atraumatic restorative treatment: clinical, ultrastructural and chemical analysis. Caries Research 2002;36:430–436.

17. Farooq NS, Coll JA, Kuwabara A, Shelton P. Success rates of formocresol pulpotomy and indirect pulp therapy in the treatment of deep dentinal caries in primary teeth. Pediatric Dentistry 2000;22:278–286.

18. Vij R, Coll JA, Shelton P, Farooq NS. Caries control and other variables associated with the success of primary molar vital pulp therapy. Pediatric Dentistry 2004;26:214–220.

19. Ranly DM, Garcia-Godoy F. Current and potential pulp therapies for primary and young permanent teeth. Journal of Dentistry 2000;28:153–161.

20. Fuks AB. Current concepts in vital primary pulp therapy. European Journal of Paediatric Dentistry 2002;3:115–120.

21. Schröder U, Szpringer-Nodzak M, Janicha J, et al. A one-year follow-up of partial pulpotomy and calcium hydroxide capping in primary molars. Endodontics and Dental Traumatology 1987;3:304–306.

22. Turner C, Courts FJ, Stanley HR. A histological comparison of direct pulp capping agents in primary canines. ASDC Journal of Dentistry for Children 1987;54:423–428.

23. Kopel HM. The pulp capping procedure in primary molar teeth 'revisited'. ASDC Journal of Dentistry for Children 1997;65:327–333.

24. Torabinejad M, Chivian N. Clinical applications of mineral trioxide aggregate. Journal of Endodontics 1999;25:197–205.

25. Tuna D, Olmez A. Clinical long-term evaluation of MTA as a direct pulp capping material in primary teeth. International Endodontic Journal 2008;41:273–278.

26. Bodem O, Blumenshine S, Zeh D, Koch MJ. Direct pulp capping with mineral trioxide aggregate in a primary molar: a case report. International Journal of Paediatric Dentistry 2004;14:376–379.

27. Shulman ER, McIver FT, Burkes EJ. Comparison of electrosurgery and formocresol as pulpotomy techniques in monkey primary teeth. Pediatric Dentistry 1987;9:189–194.

28. Ruemping DR, Morton Jr TH, Anderson MW. Electrosurgical pulpotomy in primates – a comparison with formocresol pulpotomy. Pediatric Dentistry 1983;5:14–18.

29. Mack RB, Dean JA. Electrosurgical pulpotomy: a retrospective human study. ASDC Journal of Dentistry for Children 1993;60:107–114.

30. Jukic S, Anic I, Koba K, et al. The effect of pulpotomy using CO2 and Nd:YAG lasers on dental pulp tissue. International Endodontic Journal 1997;30:175–180.

31. Shoji S, Nakamura M, Horiuchi H. Histopathological changes in dental pulps irradiated by CO2 laser: a preliminary report on laser pulpotomy. Journal of Endodontics 1985;11:379–384.

32. Elliot RD, Roberts MW, Burkes J, Phillips C. Evaluation of the carbon dioxide laser on vital human primary pulp tissue. Pediatric Dentistry 1999;21: 327–331.

33. Nadin G, Goel BR, Yeung CA, Glenny AM. Pulp treatment for extensive decay in primary teeth. Cochrane Database Systematic Review 1, 2003;CD003220.

34. Buckley JP. A rational treatment for putrescent pulps. Dental Review 1904;18:1193–1197.

35. Sweet CA. Procedure for treatment of exposed and pulpless deciduous teeth. Journal of the American Dental Association 1930;17: 1150–1153.

36. Waterhouse PJ. Formocresol and alternative primary molar pulpotomy medicaments: a review. Endodontics and Dental Traumatology 1995;11:157–162.

37. Loos PJ, Han SS. An enzyme histochemical study of the effect of various concentrations of formocresol on connective tissues. Oral Surgery, Oral Medicine, Oral Pathology 1971;31:571–585.

38. Myers DR, Shoaf HK, Dirksen TR, et al. Distribution of 14C-formaldehyde after pulpotomy with formocresol. Journal of the American Dental Association 1978;96:805–813.

39. Myers DR, Pashley DH, Whitford GM, et al. The acute toxicity of high doses of systemically administered formocresol in dogs. Pediatric Dentistry 1981;3: 37–41.

40. Myers DR, Pashley DH, Whitford GM, McKinney RV. Tissue changes induced by the absorption of formocresol from pulpotomy sites in dogs. Pediatric Dentistry 1983;5:6–8.

41. Pruhs RJ, Olen GA, Sharma PS. Relationship between formocresol pulpotomies on primary teeth and enamel defects on their permanent successors. Journal of the American Dental Association 1977;94: 698–700.

42. Mulder GR, Van Amerongen WE, Vingerling PA. Consequences of endodontic treatment of primary teeth. Part II. A clinical investigation into the influence of formocresol pulpotomy on the permanent successor. Journal of Dentistry for Children 1987;54: 35–39.

43. Rolling I, Poulsen S. Formocresol pulpotomy of primary teeth and occurrence of enamel defects on the permanent successors. Acta Odontologica Scandinavica 1978;36:243–247.

44. Fuks AB, Bimstein E. Clinical evaluation of diluted formocresol pulpotomies in primary teeth of school children. Pediatric Dentistry 1981;3:321–324.

45. Morawa AP, Straffon LH, Han SS, Corpron RE. Clinical evaluation of pulpotomies using dilute formocresol. ASDC Journal of Dentistry for Children 1975;42: 360–363.

46. Duggal M. Formocresol alternatives. British Dental Journal 2009;206:3.

47. Milnes AR. Formocresol revisited. British Dental Journal 2008;205:62.

48. Srinivasan V, Patchett CL, Waterhouse PJ. Is there life after formocresol? Part I – a narrative review of alternative interventions and materials. International Journal of Paediatric Dentistry 2006;16:117–127.

49. Milnes AR. Persuasive evidence that formocresol use in pediatric dentistry is safe. Journal of Canadian Dental Association 2006;72:247–248.

50. S-Gravenmade EJ. Some biochemical considerations of fixation in endodontics. Journal of Endodontics 1975;1:233–237.

51. Garcia-Godoy F. Clinical evaluation of glutaraldehyde pulpotomies in primary teeth. Acta Odontologica Pediatrica 1983;4:41–44.

52. Garcia-Godoy F. A 42 month clinical evaluation of glutaraldehyde pulpotomies in primary teeth. Journal of Pedodontics 1986;10:148–155.

53. Fuks AB, Bimstein E, Klein H. Assessment of a 2% buffered glutaraldehyde solution in pulpotomized primary teeth of school children: a preliminary report. Journal of Pedodontics 1986;10:323–330.

54. Fuks AB, Bimstein E, Guelmann M, Klein H. Assessment of a 2 percent buffered glutaraldehyde solution in pulpotomized primary teeth of schoolchildren. Journal of Dentistry for Children 1990;57:371–375.

55. Feigal RJ, Messer HH. A critical look at glutaraldehyde. Pediatric Dentistry 1990;12:69–71.

56. Fei AL, Udin RD, Johnson R. A clinical study of ferric sulfate as a pulpotomy agent in primary teeth. Pediatric Dentistry 1991;13: 327–332.

57. Fuks AB, Holan G, Davis J, Eidelman E. Ferric sulfate versus diluted formocresol in pulpotomized primary molars: preliminary report. Pediatric Dentistry 1994;16:158–159 (Abstract).

58. Fuks AB, Holan G, Davis JM, Eidelman E. Ferric sulfate versus dilute formocresol in pulpotomized primary molars: long-term follow up. Pediatric Dentistry 1997;19:327–330.

59. Loh A, O'Hoy P, Tran X, et al. Evidence based assessment: evaluation of the formocresol vs ferric sulphate primary molar pulpotomy. Pediatric Dentistry 2004;26:401–409.

60. Peng L, Ye L, Guo X, et al. Evaluation of formocresol versus ferric sulphate primary molar pulpotomy: a systematic review and meta-analysis. International Endodontic Journal 2007;40:751–757.

61. Berk H. Effect of calcium-hydroxide methyl cellulose paste on the dental pulp. Journal of Dentistry for Children 1950;17:65–68.

62. Magnusson B. Therapeutic pulpotomy in primary molars – clinical and histological follow up. 1. Calcium hydroxide paste as wound dressing. Odontologisk Revy 1970;21:415–431.

63. Sonmez D, Sari S, Cetinbas T. A comparison of four pulpotomy techniques in primary molars: a long-term follow-up. Journal of Endodontics 2008;34:950–955.

64. Waterhouse PJ, Nunn JH, Whitworth JM. An investigation of the relative efficacy of Buckley's formocresol and calcium hydroxide in primary molar vital pulp therapy. British Dental Journal 2000;188:32–36.

65. Waterhouse PJ, Whitworth JM, Nunn JH. Development of a

method to detect and quantify Prostaglandin E2 in pulpal blood from cariously exposed, vital primary molar teeth. International Endodontic Journal 1999;32: 381–387.

66. Huth KC, Paschos E, Hajeck-Al-Khatar N, et al. Effectiveness of 4 pulpotomy techniques – randomised controlled trial. Journal of Dental Research 2005;84:1144–1148.

67. Moretti AB, Sakai VT, Oliveira TM, et al. The effectiveness of mineral trioxide aggregate, calcium hydroxide and formocresol for pulpotomies in primary teeth. International Endodontic Journal 2008;41:547–555.

68. Torabinejad M, Hong CU, McDonald F, Pitt Ford TR. Physical and chemical properties of a new root-end filling material. Journal of Endodontics 1995;21:349–353.

69. Camilleri J, Montesin FE, Brady K, et al. The constitution of mineral trioxide aggregate. Dental Materials 2005;21:297–303.

70. Srinivasan V, Waterhouse P, Whitworth J. Mineral trioxide aggregate in paediatric dentistry. International Journal of Paediatric Dentistry 2008;19:34–47.

71. Ballal S, Venkateshbabu N, Nandini S, Kandaswamy D. An in vitro study to assess the setting and surface crazing of conventional glass ionomer cement when layered over partially set mineral trioxide aggregate. Journal of Endodontics 2008;34:478–480.

72. Tunc ES, Sonmez IS, Bayrak S, Egilmez T. The evaluation of bond strength of a composite and a compomer to white mineral trioxide aggregate with two different bonding systems. Journal of Endodontics 2008;34:603–605..

73. Aeinehchi M, Dadvand S, Fayazi S, Bayat-Movahed S. Randomised controlled trial of mineral trioxide aggregate and formocresol for pulpotomy in primary molar teeth. International Endodontic Journal 2007;40:261–267.

74. Eidelman E, Holan G, Fuks AB. Mineral trioxide aggregate vs. formocresol in pulpotomized primary molars: a preliminary report. Pediatric Dentistry 2001;23:15–18.

75. Holan G, Eidelman E, Fuks AB. Long-term evaluation of pulpotomy in primary molars using mineral trioxide aggregate or formocresol. Pediatric Dentistry 2005;27:129–136.

76. Takushige T, Cruz EV, Asgor Moral A, Hoshino E. Endodontic treatment of primary teeth using a combination of antibacterial drugs. International Endodontic Journal 2004;37:132–138.

77. Urist M. Bone formation by autoinduction. Science 1965;150:893–899.

78. Nakashima M. Induction of dentin formation on canine amputated pulp by recombinant human bone morphogenic proteins (BMP)-2 and -4. Journal of Dental Research 1994;73:1515–1522.

79. Kopel HM. Pediatric endodontics. In: Ingle JI, Bakland LK, editors. Endodontics, 4th edn. USA: Williams and Wilkins Malvern, PA; 1994. p. 835–867.

80. Mortazavi M, Mesbahi M. Comparison of zinc oxide eugenol and vitapex for root canal treatment of necrotic primary teeth. International Journal of Paediatric Dentistry 2004;14:417–424.

81. Cerqueira DF, Mello-Moura AC, Santos EM, Guades-Pinto AC. Cytotoxicity, histopathological, microbiological and clinical aspects of an endodontic iodoform-based paste used in pediatric dentistry: a review. Journal of Clinical Pediatric Dentistry 2008;32:105–110.

82. Kubota K, Golden BE, Penugonda B. Root canal filling materials for primary teeth: a review of the literature. Journal of Dentistry for Children 1992;58:225–227.

83. Holan G, Fuks AB. A comparison of pulpectomies using ZOE and KRI paste in primary molars: a retrospective study. Pediatric Dentistry 1993;15:403–407.

84. Aylard SR, Johnson R. Assessment of filling techniques for primary teeth. Pediatric Dentistry 1987;9:195–198.

Chapter | 12 |

Endodontic aspects of traumatic injuries

H.E. Pitt Ford

SUMMARY

Correct diagnosis and treatment planning are fundamental to successful endodontic management of traumatized teeth. The preservation of pulpal vitality in a young tooth is very important for further development and maturation, allowing the tooth to attain structural strength, otherwise it is very liable to fracture. The elimination of infection during root canal treatment is critical to achieving a successful outcome. The introduction of Cone Beam Computed Tomography (CBCT) is a valuable new development in the diagnosis of complex traumatic injuries. The efficiency of root canal treatment of non-vital immature teeth has greatly improved with the more widespread use of Mineral Trioxide Aggregate. Better illumination and magnification through the use of an operating microscope facilitates the management of complex cases, which may be best referred to a specialist centre. Clinicians should always bear in mind the possibility of non-accidental injury in cases of trauma.

INTRODUCTION

This chapter is principally concerned with the endodontic aspects of traumatic injuries of the teeth, and does not

© 2009 Elsevier Ltd, Inc, BV
DOI: 10.1016/B978-0-7020-3156-4.00015-2

attempt to cover dental traumatology comprehensively. For this, reference should be made to a textbook on dental traumatology or to current guidelines.[1,2,3] Since most general practitioners see only a small number of patients with traumatic dental injuries, it may be appropriate to refer the more complex injuries to a colleague with specialist experience.

When a tooth has been damaged through trauma, a good history and thorough examination are essential to ensure a correct diagnosis and the best treatment outcome. The status of the pulp of all involved teeth must be assessed, and their vitality maintained wherever possible. Many injured teeth are immature, and their development and maturation depend on maintaining pulp vitality. It should be borne in mind that vital teeth may not respond to sensitivity testing immediately after an accident. Maintaining dental pulp vitality is covered in Chapter 5.

HISTORY, EXAMINATION AND IMMEDIATE MANAGEMENT

A dental injury should always be treated as an emergency. Management of any severe bleeding or respiratory problems takes priority. Any period of unconsciousness, amnesia, headache, nausea or vomiting may indicate cerebral involvement, and the patient should be referred immediately for medical examination and appropriate care.[1,4] It is important to give a full explanation of the extent of the injury and the prognosis to anxious parents. Inconsistencies between the history and the injuries sustained, particularly if accompanied by late presentation, should alert the clinician to the possibility of non-accidental injury.[1]

A full account of when, where, and how the injury occurred must be recorded. The circumstances of the accident may have legal implications and a photograph may be especially useful. The time interval between injury and presentation can influence the choice of treatment, and may be critical to the success of replantation of avulsed teeth. The place where the injury happened may suggest possible contamination of open wounds and the need for tetanus prophylaxis. The way the injury occurred may give some indication of the type and the extent. Any previous injury or treatment should be recorded. The medical history must be reviewed as this may influence treatment planning, for example, if the patient suffers from an immunological or blood disorder. The current National Institute for Health and Clinical Excellence (NICE) guidelines state that antibiotic prophylaxis against infective endocarditis is not recommended for patients undergoing dental procedures; however, it is essential to keep up to date with current guidelines and to liaise with the patient's medical practitioner where appropriate.[5] There is further coverage on this subject in Chapter 2.

The clinical examination should include assessment of the soft tissues and facial skeleton. Disturbances to the occlusion are investigated as these may indicate jaw fracture or condylar displacement. Any soft tissue injury is noted and the possible presence of a foreign body considered; radiographic examination may be necessary to locate this. Injuries to the oral mucosa are investigated, especially bleeding from the gingival sulcus; lacerations may occur with displaced teeth; bleeding from a non-lacerated gingival margin may indicate periodontal damage. The probing depths of the gingival sulci are recorded. It should always be remembered that the effect of an injury may not be confined to the visibly affected teeth, and adjacent, apparently unaffected teeth should always be included in the examination and investigations. Infractions, fractures, pulpal exposures, mobility or displacement are noted along with any colour changes. A dark discolouration immediately after the injury indicates haemorrhage within the pulp space. There may be potential for repair and, therefore, this is not an indication for root canal treatment. If, however, the tooth becomes dark some months after the injury this usually indicates pulp necrosis. Yellow discolouration some time after the injury is associated with pulp calcification and is not an indication for root canal treatment, even if there is no response to sensitivity testing.[6] Lost pieces of fractured teeth should be accounted for; in case they are embedded in soft tissue, or have been swallowed or inhaled. Thermal sensitivity of the teeth may be a consequence of exposed dentine or pulp. Mobility and percussion testing should be carried out as they may indicate damage to the supporting tissues.

Response to pulp sensitivity testing should be recorded. Some injured teeth may have the potential to recover but may not respond for up to 2 years after trauma;[7] the results of sensitivity tests will provide a baseline for later comparison. A negative response to sensitivity testing should not, therefore, be taken as an indication for root canal treatment. Blood flow in severely luxated teeth has been shown some time ahead of their pulps responding to electric pulp testing.[7,8,9] In assessing vitality of luxated teeth it is not unusual for the findings to be contradictory.[61] Radiographic examination of permanent teeth should include a paralleling technique periapical film of each affected tooth using a film holder to standardize projections for later comparison. For luxation injuries a further film, with the tube rotated horizontally, is often helpful.[11] If a root fracture is suspected in the maxillary incisor region an occlusal radiograph should be taken. If an immature tooth has been non-vital for some time, its development will have been arrested, leaving the pulp space larger than would be expected. For primary teeth an occlusal film alone is usually sufficient. Cone Beam Computed Tomography (CBCT) is a very valuable new devel-

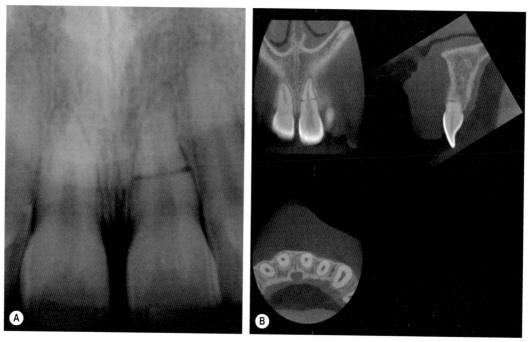

Figure 12.1 Maxillary left central incisor. (A) Radiograph showing the horizontal root fracture. (B) Cone beam CT scanning gives a more comprehensive three-dimensional view of the fracture (reproduced courtesy of S Patel).

opment in the diagnosis of traumatic injuries; the three-dimensional picture gives much more information than a standard radiograph[12–16] (Fig 12.1).

Following a thorough clinical and radiographic examination, a diagnosis is made for each injured tooth. The importance of this cannot be overstated. The outcome of treatment is dependent on a correct diagnosis as inappropriate treatment may readily be initiated at this stage.[1,17] The prognosis should be considered and the value, or otherwise, of endodontic treatment determined. Newer treatment methods, such as the introduction of Mineral Trioxide Aggregate (MTA) (ProRoot MTA, Dentsply, Weybridge, Surrey, UK) have resulted in a reduced number of treatment visits, less stressful and demanding of patients who have sustained dental injury. Also, methods of strengthening the cervical region of immature teeth reduce the risk of loss through fracture (see later). A tooth is the best space maintainer and, provided it is free of infection, its retention preserves alveolar bone for later restoration.

Soft tissue injuries should be cleaned and sutured if necessary, and any tooth fragments embedded in the lips removed. Exposed dentine is covered and pulp exposures treated; displaced teeth are repositioned and splinted when appropriate. If a permanent tooth has been avulsed, the socket is irrigated with saline to remove blood clot, and the tooth replanted and splinted. These injuries are

covered in more detail later. If the patient is very upset, it may be better to delay non-urgent treatment until a subsequent visit. In the case of a traumatically exposed pulp, inflammation has been shown not to extend beyond 3–4 mm after several days.[18] Unless unavoidable, it is most important not to remove the pulp of an immature tooth which has the potential for further maturation.

TYPES OF INJURY

Trauma may cause the following damage to the teeth:

- infraction of enamel
- fracture of enamel
- fracture of enamel and dentine
- fracture of enamel and dentine with pulp exposure
- crown-root fracture involving enamel, dentine, cementum and pulp
- intra-alveolar root fracture
- concussion
- subluxation
- extrusive luxation
- lateral luxation
- intrusive luxation
- avulsion.

Sudden contact of upper and lower teeth caused by, for example, a blow to the mandible can result in damage to posterior teeth. These injuries are rare but can result in a range of damage, from minimal loss of hard tissue to vertical crown-root fracture or avulsion.

EFFECTS OF TRAUMA ON THE DENTAL TISSUES

Many traumatized teeth are immature. These teeth have large pulp spaces and short, wide dentinal tubules. Infection may, therefore, readily spread to the pulp if the crown is fractured. This may lead to loss of vitality due to severance or crushing of the apical vessels during luxation injuries. The pulp of an avulsed tooth may also become infected via the apex, if contaminated. Teeth depend on a vital pulp in order to develop their potential maturity and strength. A tooth that loses its vitality while immature is always prone to fracture, especially in the cervical region of the root.[19]

The cementum on the root surface may be damaged by luxation injuries; the natural repair mechanism involves limited surface resorption. However, where there is extensive damage to the cementum, ankylosis associated with replacement resorption is a frequent complication. If infection from the pulp complicates damage to cementum, then external inflammatory root resorption may be very rapid, particularly in immature teeth.[1,2]

MANAGEMENT OF PRIMARY TEETH

When a primary tooth is injured, a major consideration is avoidance of damage to the successional tooth. This may occur either mechanically at the time of injury, during treatment, or as a result of infection.[1,20] Young children may not be very cooperative, particularly after a traumatic injury when the soft tissues are sore, swollen and bruised, therefore, immediate treatment may need to be limited.

Fractures

Crown fractures

Enamel fractures should be smoothed, while fractures into dentine should be covered. If the pulp has been exposed and if there is sufficient cooperation, a partial pulpotomy and restoration may be carried out with a view to preserving pulp vitality; this does not need to be at the emergency visit.[18,21] Otherwise, extraction of the tooth may be indicated. The technique of pulpotomy is covered in the section on permanent teeth. Root canal treatment of primary teeth has been covered in Chapter 11. An

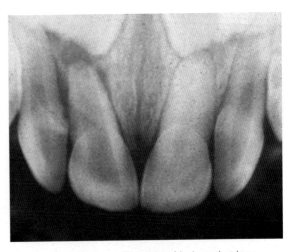

Figure 12.2 Primary maxillary central incisors that have suffered a traumatic injury. The maxillary left incisor has responded with calcification of the pulp space, while the right incisor has developed an abscess.

infected primary tooth should not be left untreated as the infection may cause damage to the permanent successor (Fig. 12.2).

Intra-alveolar root fracture

This is less common in primary teeth than in permanent teeth. Active intervention is rarely required. If the coronal fragment is very loose and at risk of being inhaled or grossly displaced, or if pulp necrosis and infection develop, extraction is usually indicated; however, the apical fragment is normally left *in situ* to resorb naturally and to avoid surgical damage to the developing permanent successor.

Luxation injuries

In general, a conservative approach to management is adopted with primary teeth. Laterally luxated primary teeth are frequently repositioned naturally in time by occlusal and muscular forces. If a laterally luxated tooth interferes with the occlusion, the injury is mild and there is no risk to the permanent successor, it may be carefully repositioned.[1,22] If the root apex is directed palatally towards the developing permanent tooth then it should be extracted atraumatically. If a tooth is very mobile and in danger of inhalation, or if occlusal interference is too great, it should be extracted. Intruded teeth will usually re-erupt albeit sometimes over several months. If the pulp becomes non-vital and infected, root canal treatment may be considered (see Ch. 11). Replantation of avulsed primary teeth is not normally carried out because of the potential risk of direct physical damage to the developing permanent tooth, or damage from later infection of the pulp of the primary tooth.

Tooth discolouration

Pulp damage is a frequent complication of injuries, and as a result primary teeth may discolour. Immediate discolouration indicates bleeding in the pulp and the possibility of repair. Later darkening of the tooth signifies pulp necrosis and if there is associated infection, root canal treatment or extraction is indicated. Later yellow discolouration indicates pulp canal obliteration and no intervention is required (Fig. 12.2).

MANAGEMENT OF PERMANENT TEETH

Fractures

Infractions and fracture of enamel

Infraction of enamel rarely requires operative treatment, but the pulpal status should be monitored. Infection may very rarely enter the pulp through enamel infractions. There is no effective treatment to avoid this. Fractures of enamel may be either smoothed or repaired with composite resin. The likelihood of pulp canal obliteration or pulp necrosis occurring is low for both enamel infractions and enamel fractures.[23] The chance of pulp damage is increased if there is associated luxation of the tooth.[24]

Fracture of enamel and dentine

In children, trauma to anterior teeth commonly affects sound teeth, which frequently have large pulps and wide dentinal tubules. Any injury that exposes dentine can,

therefore, result in damage to the pulp. Fractures involving dentine open up numerous dentinal tubules. If left untreated, microbial plaque will grow on the exposed surface and cause pulpal inflammation, which may lead to pulp necrosis. The early placement of a restoration prevents permanent pulp damage and relieves sensitivity. The use of etched and bonded composite resin restores the appearance and does not hinder subsequent monitoring of pulp vitality (Fig. 12.3). This has been shown to seal more effectively than conventional glass ionomer cement.[25] Restoration of the contour of the tooth may be left until a later visit. A fractured fragment may be successfully reattached with composite resin retained by etched enamel. The likelihood of pulp canal obliteration or pulp necrosis occurring is low following fractures involving dentine, provided the dentine tubules are effectively covered.[1,23] The chance of pulp damage is increased if there is associated luxation of the tooth.[24,26]

Fracture of enamel and dentine with pulp exposure

Immature teeth

If this type of injury occurs in a young patient whose permanent tooth is immature, then treatment is directed at maintaining pulp vitality to allow continued tooth maturation; this considerably improves the long-term prognosis of the tooth by reducing the risk of subsequent root fracture.[19] Permanent incisor teeth have been shown to reach maturity at the age of about 13 years. The pulp can usually be treated conservatively as it has a good blood supply and rarely becomes necrotic.[27,28] Partial pulpotomy is the treatment of choice.[18,27,29,30,31] The advantages of partial pulpotomy over pulp capping are that inflamed pulp tissue and adjacent infected dentine are removed, and that the pulp dressing is placed in a cavity where it can be covered by a protective base. If the

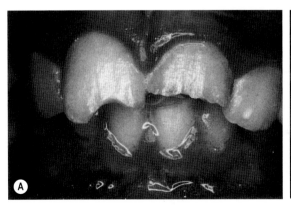
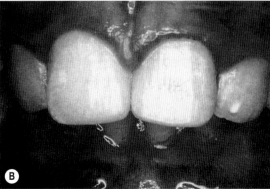

Figure 12.3 (A) Fractured incisal edges of maxillary central incisors exposing dentine. (B) Restoration of incisal edges using composite resin retained by etched enamel.

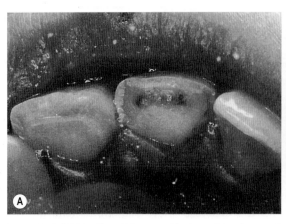
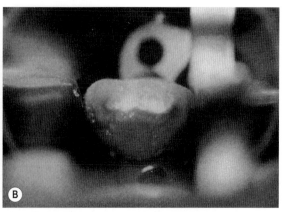

Figure 12.4 (A) Maxillary right central incisor with a fracture involving the pulp. (B) After placement of medicament in the partial pulpotomy preparation.

restoration is lost, the cavity dressing should not be displaced.

Local anaesthesia is necessary to carry out a pulpotomy. The tooth is isolated with rubber dam to exclude salivary contamination; retention of rubber dam on an immature tooth is facilitated by a suitable clamp (e.g. Ash EW, Dentsply). A small cavity approximately 2 × 2 mm is cut in the fractured dentine surface at the exposure site, with the periphery of the cavity floor in dentine (Fig. 12.4). Pulp removal is usually confined to the superficial 2 mm since infection does not normally extend beyond this level.[18] The pulp is best removed with a bur in the turbine handpiece using copious water spray; this causes less damage than a bur at slow-speed or an excavator.[29,30,32] Haemorrhage is arrested using a cotton pellet soaked in saline and the wound is covered with MTA.[31,33,34,35,36] Over this is placed a layer of resin-modified glass ionomer cement, before restoring the tooth with composite resin. Should the composite resin be lost the restoration within the cavity should remain intact. MTA has been shown to give better results than calcium hydroxide in this situation.[31,33] Alternatively, the cavity may be restored with a calcium hydroxide base (either a slurry which is subsequently compressed and dried with cotton wool or a hard setting base material) and a resin-modified zinc oxide-eugenol cement (IRM, Dentsply) followed by glass ionomer cement.

The coronal contour should then be restored with etched-retained composite resin. A hard tissue barrier should form beneath the dressing.[29,30,34,35] The tooth should be reviewed after six months, and then at least annually for several years, to ensure continued pulp vitality by regular pulp testing, and continued root development by examination of radiographs. Should the restoration fail, it must be replaced immediately in order to prevent infection of the pulp via the pulpotomy site, as

the hard tissue barrier is usually porous.[18] This treatment has a high success rate; the pulp may be expected to remain vital and healthy.[18,27,29] There is no need for root canal treatment subsequent to pulpotomy, unless necrosis and infection develop.[32]

Mature teeth

Where crown fracture of a mature tooth involves the pulp, conservative treatment by partial pulpotomy should still be considered as the first treatment option. However, where the entire clinical crown has been lost, pulpal extirpation, root canal filling and construction of a post-retained crown is usually indicated.

Crown-root fracture involving enamel, dentine, cementum and pulp

In this type of extensive tooth fracture, the coronal fragment is usually retained by a limited amount of periodontal ligament. These teeth may have a poor prognosis, especially if the fracture line is a long way subgingival on the palatal aspect. When the patient first presents, the coronal fragment is often loose and painful to bite on. It is usually necessary to give local anaesthesia to allow removal of the fragment and to assess the extent of the fracture. If time does not allow this, the fragment may be bonded temporarily to the tooth to minimize discomfort. Where the fracture does not extend far subgingivally, it is often possible to restore the tooth without crown lengthening. Otherwise periodontal surgery to expose the margin of the fracture, or orthodontic extrusion, will need to be considered. In an immature permanent tooth with an exposed pulp, where the fracture does not extend far subgingivally, pulpotomy should be carried out (as described above). Where loss of the root is more extensive, the tooth will be difficult to restore and is likely to have a poor long-term prognosis. While its loss will be planned for, in the longer term, it may be possible to carry out a pulpotomy, restoring the supragingival contour with composite resin and retain the tooth while the dentition continues to develop.

In a mature tooth where the fracture is superficial, pulpotomy may still be the first line of treatment, or it may be more appropriate to carry out root canal treatment and restore the tooth with a post-retained crown. If the fracture is deeper, it will be difficult to isolate the tooth for root canal treatment, and orthodontic extrusion of the root followed by crown lengthening will need to be considered before restoration by a post-retained crown.[1] When the fracture is very deep, there may be insufficient root remaining to support a restoration even after orthodontic extrusion; such teeth are also more likely to fail subsequently. Where the prognosis is very poor, extraction of the remaining root should be considered if it is infected;

otherwise, elective decoronation may be used to preserve the alveolar ridge.

Intra-alveolar root fracture

Intra-alveolar root fractures are relatively uncommon, and fortunately, often occur without the complication of microbial contamination from the mouth. The coronal fragment may be mobile with the fulcrum coronal to the apex, and may be extrusively or laterally luxated. The tooth should be examined carefully for any periodontal injury whereby the gingival sulcus communicates with the fracture; this substantially reduces the prognosis. Diagnosis of intra-alveolar root fracture is made by radiological examination with two films, taken at different vertical angles. Root fractures are more frequently observed on an occlusal film than a film taken with a paralleling technique (Fig. 12.5). CBCT has greatly contributed to diagnosis of complex fractures, as it gives a three-dimensional view.[14,15,16]

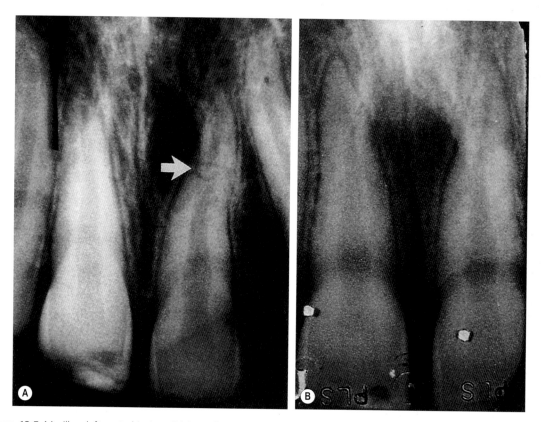

Figure 12.5 Maxillary left central incisor. (A) Part of an occlusal radiograph more easily demonstrates an intra-alveolar root fracture (arrowed) than (B) a paralleling-technique radiograph on which the fracture is more difficult to see.

The apical fragment almost without exception remains vital, and does not require treatment. This is, therefore, in effect a luxation injury of the coronal fragment. If there is no mobility or displacement, immediate treatment is not required and the fractured root should heal with hard tissue formation; the pulp is likely to remain vital. Teeth that have fractures remote from the gingival sulcus have the best long-term prognosis (Fig. 12.5). If the fracture is close to the neck of the tooth, the prognosis will be poorer, but extraction need not be indicated, unless there is a communication between the gingival sulcus and the fracture line. Teeth with a transverse fracture have a poorer long-term prognosis than those with an oblique fracture because of the risk of future displacement[37,38] (Fig. 12.6).

If the tooth is displaced or mobile, immediate treatment consists of repositioning the coronal fragment and splinting if it is very mobile, typically, for approximately 4 weeks. Recent work has failed to show a correlation between splinting method, duration and healing.[38] No displacement of the coronal fragment and preserved vitality of the pulp are highly indicative of fracture healing.[37,38,39] A splint should allow physiological movement to avoid ankylosis. The patient is advised to use a chlorhexidine mouthwash to maintain oral hygiene, and the tooth reviewed at the time of intended splint removal. Pulp sensitivity is checked. Where there is no response, the tooth should be reviewed clinically at 3-monthly intervals. Where no vital response is obtained, provided there is no tenderness to palpation, nor a sinus tract, pulp testing should be carried out at 3 and then 6-monthly intervals either until a response occurs, or evidence of pulp necrosis appears. Radiographic review should normally be restricted to once or twice yearly unless there is a risk of external inflammatory root resorption.

The most favourable response is uniting of the two fragments by hard tissue laid down both in the root canal and on the root surface. A less favourable but still satisfactory outcome is continued pulp vitality in the coronal fragment but no union of the fragments. The sharp edges at the fracture line become rounded by remodelling, and connective tissue and/or bone lie between the fragments; the space between the fragments may increase with continued alveolar growth in younger patients. Often the pulp in the coronal fragment calcifies and radiologically shows an obliterated pulp space; the pulp may not respond to sensitivity testing.[40,41] Pulp canal obliteration itself is not an indication for root canal treatment.[1,42]

Pulp necrosis occurs in approximately 20% of intra-alveolar root fractured teeth and is associated with initial coronal displacement, lack of pulp sensitivity after the accident, coronal position of the root fracture, a communication with the gingival sulcus, maturity of the root and coronal fracture.[37,38,39,41] Pulp necrosis is invariably confined to the coronal fragment.[1] As well as the loss of response to thermal and electrical stimuli, there is frequently radiolucency in the bone around the tooth at the fracture line (Fig. 12.7). Root canal treatment should be carried out in the coronal fragment alone unless there is definite evidence to implicate involvement of the apical fragment. Following cleaning of the canal in the coronal fragment, a well-packed dressing of calcium hydroxide may be placed, if required, to assist disinfection of the canal; MTA is subsequently placed in the first 3–4 mm at the fracture line, followed, if desired, by back filling with gutta-percha (see section on root filling of immature teeth for method)[35] (Fig. 12.7). This treatment has a high success rate.[43] If there is an inadequate stop at the apical end of the coronal fragment, the first 1–2 mm may be packed with calcium hydroxide, or a sterile resorbable material (e.g. Surgicel, Johnson and Johnson Medical Ltd., Gargrave, N. Yorks, UK) may be inserted to limit extrusion of MTA at the fracture site. It is not normally practical to attempt to root treat both fragments. If the apical fragment is non-vital surgical removal is indicated.

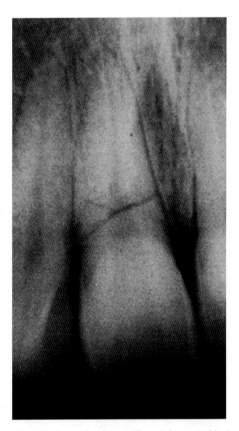

Figure 12.6 Radiograph of a maxillary right central incisor with a horizontal root fracture close to the gingival margin. The pulp responded to electric pulp testing one year after trauma; however, the long-term prognosis is poor.

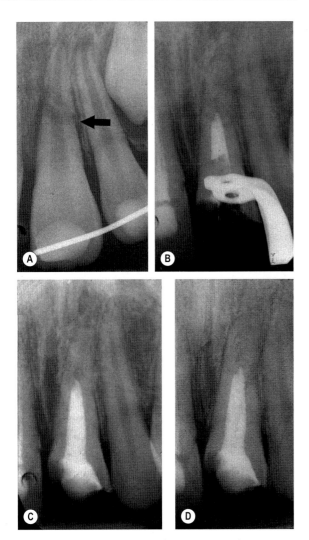

Figure 12.7 (A) The maxillary left central incisor has a root fracture in the mid-third and has been splinted; there is a radiolucency at the fracture line (arrowed). (B) The root canal of the coronal fragment has been disinfected and filled with MTA to the fracture line. (C) The neck of the tooth has been filled with etched and bonded composite resin. (D) One year later, healing has taken place and further calcification has occurred in the apical fragment indicating that it is still vital.

Luxation injuries

A luxation injury is characterized by damage to the supporting tissues of the tooth and the tooth may be displaced. There may be interruption of the vessels and nerves at the apex. The prognosis for pulp recovery is reduced if there is a concomitant crown fracture as this is a possible route for entry of microbes. Luxation injuries are the most common type of dental injury.[44]

Concussion

This is an injury to the supporting tissues without loosening or displacement of the tooth. Lasting pulp damage is rare, especially in an immature permanent tooth, although the tooth may not respond to sensitivity testing for some months.

Subluxation

The tooth is loosened in its socket but not displaced. With subluxation there is unlikely to be severance of the blood vessels supplying the pulp, giving a good possibility of pulp survival. Pulp survival rate is 90% for immature teeth and 75% for mature teeth.[11] It is essential to allow the pulp time for recovery before deciding to remove it.

Extrusive luxation

If this is severe the pulpal vessels and nerves are usually severed. In an immature tooth that is repositioned soon after injury, revascularization, followed by obliteration of the pulp space, is the likely outcome; in a mature tooth pulp necrosis is more common.[11] External inflammatory root resorption may occur following pulp necrosis.

Lateral luxation

The tooth is displaced laterally and the apex may be locked into bone. This can be diagnosed by percussion, when the tooth gives a high ringing tone. This crushing injury causes damage to the supporting structures. The labial plate of bone may also be fractured. Pulpal healing may be expected in 70% of immature teeth[11] (Fig. 12.8). Revascularization will take some weeks but return of functioning nerve fibres may take a year or more;[45] therefore, root canal treatment should not be undertaken unless there is positive evidence of pulpal infection. In mature teeth that have suffered a severe luxation injury pulpal healing is unlikely, and therefore, root canal treatment is indicated, except in cases where follow-up can be assured to observe for possible recovery. Damage to the supporting structures makes both inflammatory and replacement external root resorption frequent complications of lateral luxation.[11]

A laterally luxated tooth may need to be disimpacted from its new position, under local anaesthesia if necessary, to allow correct repositioning. If the apex is displaced labially, repositioning is most readily achieved from behind the patient, by pressing with the thumb on the impacted apex. The tooth may be splinted with a flexible splint for 2–3 weeks (Fig. 12.9). The patient is recommended to use a chlorhexidine mouthwash during the early stages of healing. Radiographs are taken at one month to check for signs of disease, especially external inflammatory root resorption. If there are signs of this, the pulp should be

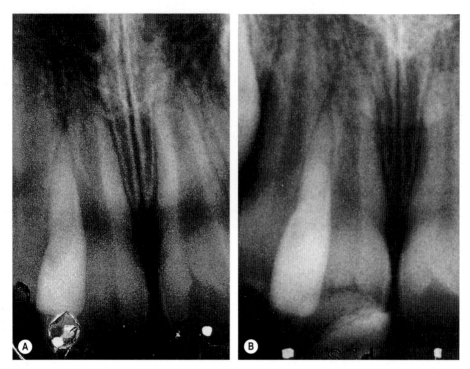

Figure 12.8 (A) The immature maxillary right central incisor was luxated. (B) One year later the root has continued to form.

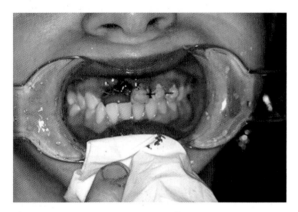

Figure 12.9 Emergency treatment after a traumatic injury. The maxillary right central incisor was avulsed and lost. The maxillary left central incisor was luxated and has been repositioned and splinted.

removed promptly and the pulp space disinfected. Root canal treatment should then be carried out (see later). If no signs of disease are observed, the patient is reviewed again after 2, 3, 6 months and 1 year. Pulp sensitivity is assessed at each period using thermal and electric tests; electric pulp testing often does not produce a

response in the early period after luxation injury. Concurrent with return of sensitivity, there may be evidence of pulp canal obliteration (Fig. 12.10), which is very common in laterally luxated teeth.[46] This causes a yellowish coronal discolouration and the tooth may cease to respond to sensitivity testing but it is not an indication for root canal treatment. In about 4% of luxated teeth periapical radiolucency, together with discolouration and absence of sensitivity, is a temporary phenomenon and disappears as healing progresses. This is known as transient apical breakdown.[47]

Intrusive luxation

This is a severe injury; the tooth is forced into its socket, so crushing the supporting structures and the blood vessels and nerve fibres that supply the pulp. The tooth is likely to be wedged in the supporting bone, therefore displaying a lack of mobility and a ringing note on percussion. Radiographs will show obliteration of the periodontal ligament space. Many immature teeth will re-erupt spontaneously, but if there is no evidence of this after 3 weeks, rapid orthodontic repositioning should be undertaken. Access to the clinical crown must be available for endodontic treatment should this become necessary. Severe intrusions may require surgical repositioning, taking great care

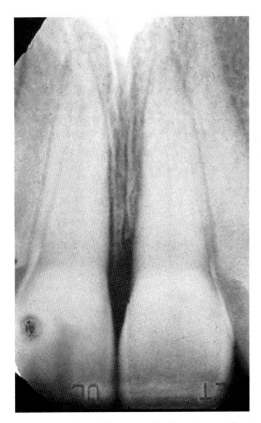

Figure 12.10 Both maxillary central incisors have suffered luxation injuries and have responded with calcification of the pulp spaces.

not to damage the cementum in the cervical area.[3] Pulp necrosis is a very frequent complication of intrusion; 60% of immature teeth become non-vital.[11] Immature teeth should, therefore, be observed for signs of pulp vitality returning or complications developing. The regime for reviewing intrusions is similar to that for other luxations. If evidence of pulp necrosis or infection appears, root canal treatment should be undertaken (see below). Mature teeth do not re-erupt and almost without exception become non-vital; endodontic treatment consists of pulp extirpation, disinfection of the pulp space, dressing with calcium hydroxide for a short period and subsequent root canal filling.

Radiographs should be taken frequently to check for the presence of external inflammatory root resorption. Another complication of intrusion is a high incidence of replacement resorption,[11] as a result of damage to the cementum. This can be diagnosed by percussion and radiologically. Intrusion is a severe injury, which may be best referred for specialist care.

Avulsion

The tooth is completely displaced from its socket, and should be replaced as soon as possible, preferably at the site of the accident. Immature avulsed teeth, which have been replanted immediately or correctly stored until emergency treatment can be obtained, have a reasonable prognosis for pulp revascularization and periodontal healing; mature teeth do not revascularize.[1] Both external inflammatory and replacement resorption are frequent complications.[48,49,50]

The avulsed tooth needs careful handling while it is out of the mouth to prevent damage to the periodontal ligament. It should not be allowed to dry out, and if necessary is best kept in cold milk. The patient should be taken immediately to an experienced practitioner, who should decide whether replantation of the tooth is appropriate.[2] The medical history must also be considered as to whether replantation is appropriate, and whether any special precautions may be required. The tetanus status should be checked if the accident took place outdoors. The tooth is examined, without touching the root to avoid damage to the periodontal ligament, and dirt rinsed off with saline; under no circumstances should it be scrubbed or severe periodontal ligament damage will occur. It is helpful to note the length of the tooth for future endodontic treatment. It may be necessary to take a radiograph of the socket to check that no tooth fragment remains. Local anaesthesia may not always be needed; the socket is syringed with saline to remove any clot, and the tooth gently repositioned into its socket; the position is then confirmed radiographically. The tooth is splinted for 7–10 days, using a flexible splint. For optimal healing it is essential to avoid infection, therefore, in the days following replantation the patient should use a chlorhexidine mouthwash to maintain oral hygiene. Current guidelines also recommend the administration of systemic antibiotics for the avulsed tooth.[2] Tetracycline is the first choice, doxycycline twice a day for 7 days at appropriate dose for the patient's age and weight.[2] However, the risk of discolouration of permanent teeth must be considered before systemic administration of tetracycline; it is not recommended for patients under 12 years of age. Phenoxymethyl penicillin (Pen V) may be used as an alternative to tetracycline provided the patient is not allergic to it.

With an immature tooth with an open apex, there is a good chance of pulp revascularization, so the pulp should not be electively removed; revascularization will allow root formation and maturation to continue, and reduce the risk of subsequent root fracture.[1,19] However, there is a risk that infection present on the root surface or on the apical surface of the pulp at the time of replantation may initiate, or perpetuate, inflammatory resorption, which can rapidly destroy the thin wall of the immature root. If this or any other positive sign of infection does occur, the pulp space should be cleaned and disinfected, and root canal treatment undertaken (see below). Otherwise, regular clinical and radiological reviews should be undertaken at approximately 1, 2, 3, 6 months and 1 year; the patient should be asked to return immediately should any problems develop.

With mature teeth the chances of pulp revascularization are so low that the necrotic pulp should be extirpated through a conventional access cavity prior to removal of the splint. The cleaned and shaped root canal is, initially, filled with a dressing of calcium hydroxide prior to root canal filling with gutta-percha. There appears to be no benefit in leaving calcium hydroxide in the tooth for a prolonged period.[51,52] In addition, calcium hydroxide should not be inserted within one week of injury, to allow periodontal healing to take place at the apex.

ROOT CANAL TREATMENT OF IMMATURE TEETH

The teeth most commonly injured are the incisors. The apices of these teeth are not normally closed until about the age of 13 years; although in a two-dimensional radiograph they may appear closed much earlier than this. It is necessary to produce an apical barrier against which a root filling can be packed. This has, traditionally, been achieved by disinfection of the root canal space and repeated dressing with calcium hydroxide until a biological barrier was achieved. This had the disadvantages of prolonged treatment for a usually anxious child, risk of root fracture due to dentine desiccation with prolonged contact with calcium hydroxide and risk of reinfection due to loss or leakage of temporary fillings.[52,53] More recently, MTA has been used with success to produce an immediate hard matrix barrier.[33,35,36,53–59] It is necessary first to disinfect the canal. Some operators then dress with calcium hydroxide for one week or slightly longer,[56] while others rely on irrigants to disinfect the canal and immediately place a plug of MTA at the apex.[57] When set, this acts as a mechanical barrier; hard tissue will eventually form against the MTA.[35,60] The elimination of infection from the root canal space prior to filling is essential; the canal must be clean and dry. Sometimes a radiolucent area may not resolve immediately. If it persists, this may indicate either a long-standing infection outside the tooth which requires surgery, or an undetected, possibly vertical, root fracture. A small radiolucency may also remain representing scar tissue.

Local anaesthesia is given so that a rubber dam clamp can be placed securely on the tooth and in case the pulp is still partially vital. Palatal local anaesthesia may also be needed, both for clamp application and if vital tissue is encountered. If the tooth is partially erupted

or very crowded a split dam technique may be used, with a caulking agent (OraSeal, Ultradent Products, South Jordan, UT, USA). Occasionally, in the early stages of treatment, if the child is exceptionally anxious, local anaesthesia and a clamp may be avoided and an alternative rubber dam used (Dry Dam, Directa AB, Upplands Väsby, Sweden). However, access may be very limited for endodontics and leakage more difficult to control. It is essential to appreciate that avoiding local anaesthesia and then the child experiencing pain because of residual vital pulp may make future treatment very difficult if not impossible; therefore, there is no substitute for adequate anaesthesia and proper tooth isolation for successful endodontics. The access cavity on the palatal surface of the crown should be sufficiently large, and sufficiently incisally placed, to allow adequate access to the wide root canal; care must be taken to remove all remnants of pulp tissue from the pulp horns, or discolouration of the crown may ensue. Since both sodium hypochlorite and calcium hydroxide dissolve organic matter it is not strictly necessary to have straight-line access to the whole root canal at the expense of tooth tissue conservation. Indeed, to attempt this would often be to weaken the neck of the tooth excessively. The cervical constriction apical to the cingulum should be reduced.[61] Instrumentation should be carried out to 1–2 mm short of the radiographic apex, unless necrotic tissue is encountered at this level, when instruments should be taken further. The length of the root canal is estimated by taking a radiograph with a file of known length in place. If the canal is very wide it may be helpful to wedge the file in place with a pledget of cotton wool.

Excessive filing of the root canal walls must be avoided as the canal walls are already thin; instead the pulp space should be cleaned by copious irrigation with sodium hypochlorite. The irrigation needle should be pre-measured, and the irrigant delivered with gentle pressure using the forefinger to depress the plunger of the syringe, to prevent forcing sodium hypochlorite through the apex. After thorough cleaning, a stiff paste of calcium hydroxide, if used, is packed into the canal with root canal pluggers.[62] Calcium hydroxide is alkaline and has an antimicrobial effect, and thus allows healing to take place. The quality of the calcium hydroxide filling may be checked radiologically before closure of the access cavity with an effective temporary filling (e.g. IRM, Dentsply). The tooth should be reviewed and if symptom-free, the calcium hydroxide is removed, the canal irrigated and dried. MTA can then be inserted into the apical 3–4 mm using pre-measured root canal pluggers (Fig 12.11). Some operators use ultrasound, transmitted by holding an ultrasonic tip in contact with the root canal plugger, to better condense the MTA.[63] A check radiograph is taken and revision undertaken if necessary. If the MTA is short of the apex it may be moistened and advanced a little further with pluggers. As the material takes 3–4 hours to set, if necessary, it can readily

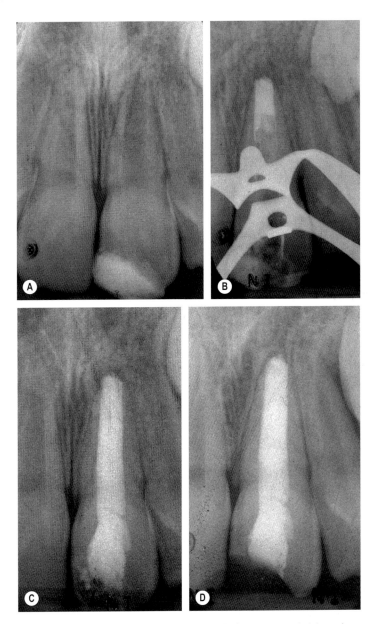

Figure 12.11 (A) The maxillary left central incisor has become non-vital after a traumatic injury; the root canal is wider than that of the right central incisor, signifying that the tooth has been non-vital for some time. (B) The root canal has been disinfected and the apical 4 mm filled with MTA. (C) The canal was then back-filled with gutta-percha and the neck of the tooth filled with etched and bonded composite resin. (D) One year later, healing has taken place.

Table 12.1 Advantages of MTA over calcium hydroxide for managing the immature tooth with an open apex

- Reduced number of treatment appointments.
- Less demanding on both clinical and patient time.
- Less stressful for the patient in terms of overall treatment duration.
- Equal or more favourable treatment outcome.
- Reduced risk of root fracture.
- Reduced risk of reinfection due to loss of temporary filling.
- Greater cost of material more than offset by reduced treatment time.

be removed at this stage using root canal files and thoroughly washing with sterile water.

When correct placement is confirmed, it is allowed to set; a moist cotton pellet may be temporarily inserted into the canal and the access cavity sealed. At a subsequent visit, the canal may be back-filled with gutta-percha (Obtura III Max, Obtura Spartan, Earth City, MO, USA) (Fig 12.11). Alternatively, this may be done immediately after placing the MTA but there is a high risk of disturbing the unset MTA plug. Many operators now fill the whole canal with MTA if there is no contraindication rather than back-filling with gutta-percha. If the apex is wide open, it may be helpful to pack a little sterile resorbable material at the apex to limit extrusion of the MTA (Surgicel, Johnson and Johnson Medical Ltd.). MTA is extremely 'tissue friendly' and extrusion of a little of the material does not seem to adversely affect the outcome. This technique can be demanding as it is difficult to pack the material correctly at the apex; magnification and good lighting are essential so an operating microscope is invaluable. It is recommended that this treatment should be undertaken by a specialist. Adequate time must be allowed, as revision of the filling at a subsequent visit is very challenging. Some authorities cite cost as a contraindication to the use of MTA; however, the clinical time saved due to the reduced number of treatment appointments more than offsets the cost of the material (Table 12.1) Some specialist groups still include the calcium hydroxide method in their guidelines on account of the availability and lower cost of calcium hydroxide, but the opinion is emerging that the MTA is preferable and superior.

Avoidance of Cervical Root Fracture

Non-vital immature teeth have thin roots with weak dentine walls, and are especially at risk of root fracture

at the neck of the tooth[12] (Fig. 12.12). The neck of the tooth may be reinforced using etched and bonded composite resin, allowing space, if indicated, for a post.[64,65] If little coronal tissue remains, a fibre post may be cemented into the root canal. Compared to metal posts, fibre posts have the advantage of some flexibility; if it fails, it is more likely to become decemented rather than cause a root fracture.[66]

Surgical Treatment of Immature Teeth

If attempts to eliminate infection from the periapical tissues are, ultimately, unsuccessful, then a surgical approach may be indicated. In an apprehensive child, sedation or general anaesthesia may be necessary and appropriate consent should be obtained. Surgery may, for example, be necessary to look for a longitudinal root fracture; if present, the tooth would need to be extracted. If apical surgery is to be undertaken, the root canal is normally filled first, and the root canal filling cut back during surgery to allow placement of a root-end filling of MTA. Further details on endodontic surgery are covered in Chapter 10.

Revascularization Treatment of Immature Teeth

A recent development in treatment of these teeth is to clean the root canal and dress with a triple antibiotic paste of ciprofloxacin, metronidazole and minocycline. Care should be taken to avoid discolouration resulting from the use of minocycline.[67] When the canal is considered clean and disinfected, bleeding is induced at the apex and MTA is placed, about 3 mm apical to the cervical constriction, over the subsequent blood clot. This method has been shown to enable continued root growth and thickening of the walls of the root, which is, obviously, a tremendous advantage as it overcomes the problems of a non-vital immature tooth with very thin walls being prone to fracture. The tissue within the pulp space may not be normal pulp, but derived from cells of surrounding tissue. A number of case series have been published showing success with this treatment, which appears very promising.[10,67–75]

Regenerative Treatment of Immature Teeth

This requires stem or progenitor cells, a scaffold to provide a micro-environment for cell growth and differentiation,

Apical to the part of the root which had formed by the time of transplantation, the root should grow and mature normally.[79] Should the pulp become necrotic, root canal treatment is complicated and is best referred to a specialist for management.

COMPLICATIONS

External inflammatory root resorption

This may occur if infection develops in the pulp space and there is damage to the adjacent cementum; this is common in the more severe luxation injuries.[49,50] Microorganisms and their toxins may track along the dentinal tubules to the surface of the root, where the resultant inflammatory reaction attracts osteoclasts, which may destroy a large part of the root within a few weeks (Fig. 12.13). Inflammatory resorption is diagnosed radiologically as a localized area of tooth resorption with a radiolucent area in the adjacent bone. This may occur particularly rapidly in immature teeth, which have thin roots and wide dentinal tubules. It is, therefore, very important to take frequent radiographs and to disinfect the pulp space promptly if this type of resorption is seen. This will halt the resorption and the periodontal structures should heal.[80]

The root canal must be thoroughly cleaned with sodium hypochlorite to kill microorganisms. Calcium hydroxide is then inserted and will create an unsuitable environment for the continued survival of microorganisms in the pulp space or dentinal tubules; it also raises the pH, which discourages osteoclastic activity.[80] When the infection is controlled, the root canal can be filled. Should the coronal seal subsequently fail, microorganisms may re-enter the root canal and potentially stimulate further resorption.

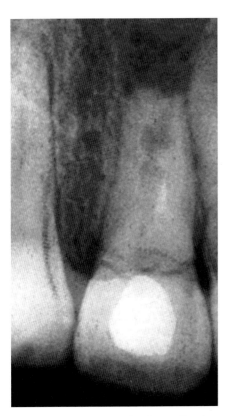

Figure 12.12 The maxillary central incisor suffered a cervical root fracture during long term calcium hydroxide treatment and before root canal treatment was completed.

and a signalling mechanism. This technique is under development and not as yet at the stage of being used clinically; however, it appears promising for the future.[68,76,77,78]

AUTO-TRANSPLANTATION OF AN IMMATURE PREMOLAR INTO THE INCISOR SPACE

This may be undertaken in a patient who requires extraction of premolars as a part of orthodontic treatment. It has a high success rate but relies on careful case selection and meticulous surgical technique. The premolar must be immature, preferably with the root length nearly complete and the apex open. Great care must be taken not to damage the cementum at the neck of the tooth as this may cause cervical resorption. The desired outcome is that the pulp of the transplanted tooth should revascularize, and remain vital. This is followed by pulp canal obliteration.

Cervical external inflammatory root resorption

Sometimes, a late complication of trauma, particularly luxation, is inflammatory resorption close to the neck of the tooth (Fig. 12.14). This may occur in vital as well as root filled teeth and is often unrelated to the pulpal status, as infection has entered from the damaged root surface.[50,81] The resorption spreads around the root canal rather than into it. Cervical resorption may be difficult to differentiate radiologically from internal resorption. However, if two views are taken at different horizontal angles, the lesion in cervical resorption will be seen to change position; it should be possible to distinguish the outline of the root canal superimposed upon it. Root canal treatment,

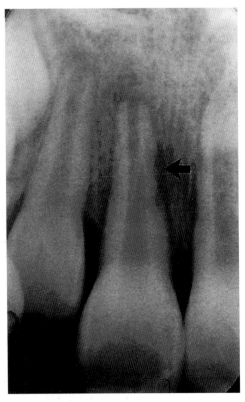

Figure 12.13 The maxillary right central incisor displays external inflammatory root resorption on the mesial aspect (arrowed); there is a radiolucency of the bone adjacent to that in the tooth. The pulp of the tooth became necrotic as a consequence of a luxation injury.

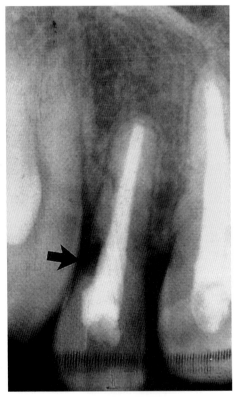

Figure 12.14 Cervical external inflammatory resorption (arrowed) has occurred on the distal surface of the maxillary right lateral incisor approximately three years after trauma. If surgical access is good, the defect may be repaired, or the tooth may need to be extracted as in this example.

or retreatment, is not the appropriate method of dealing with the problem. Where the condition is limited and surgical access is good, surgical repair of the defect may be undertaken. In the case of a vital tooth, only if it is considered that surgical repair will expose the pulp, should root canal treatment be undertaken. If the condition is extensive or surgical access is poor, extraction is usually indicated. CBCT scanning is a very valuable method of assessing the nature and exact location of the resorption.[13,14] It has been suggested that cervical resorption may be associated with bleaching of non-vital teeth.[55] However, this procedure should not cause damage if the dentine tubules of the root are protected and if sodium perborate and water rather than hydrogen peroxide are used.[82,83]

External replacement root resorption

This may occur when there is damage to the periodontal structures as in severe luxation injuries and especially with

avulsions if the periodontal ligament is allowed to dry out.[49,50] Replacement resorption can be detected at follow-up appointments; the tooth lacks mobility and when approximately 20% of the surface is affected gives a ringing note to percussion testing.[84] The condition can often only be observed on radiographs much later when the root has a moth-eaten appearance (Fig. 12.15). Because the cementum barrier is damaged in replacement resorption, the body treats the tooth as bone, and the tooth is gradually resorbed during physiological bone turnover and replaced by bone. In a healthy tooth, the cementum resists osteoclastic activity. Being a physiological process, replacement resorption cannot be treated; therefore, carrying out root canal treatment is of no benefit. The tooth will ultimately be lost, but the time taken is variable and depends on the rate of bone turnover. In some young patients it can progress rapidly, and during the growth phase the ankylosed tooth will inhibit local alveolar bone growth and so appear to sink into the jaw (infraposition) as the surrounding alveolar bone grows.[85,86] Early diagnosis and

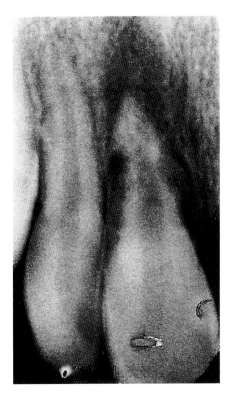

Figure 12.15 The maxillary right central incisor displays replacement resorption on the mesial and distal root surfaces; there is a moth-eaten appearance. The tooth had been replanted 2 hours after avulsion 1 year previously.

treatment planning is, therefore, important. Extraction of an ankylosed tooth in a growing patient is best avoided, unless the space is to be closed, as alveolar atrophy will follow. Before or during the growth spurt, if there is no infection present, the crown and any root filling may be removed and the root retained to preserve alveolar bone.[85-87] If growth is nearly complete it may be appropriate to restore the incisal edge to improve its appearance. In older patients the tooth can be left until symptoms arise from later infection.

Barrier formation coronal to the apex

If vital tissue remains at the apex, and a material such as calcium hydroxide is placed short of the apex, a calcific barrier may form coronal to the apex. This may be desirable if the apical portion remains vital. However, if subsequent infection occurs, treatment will be required. If the barrier is near the apex, apical surgery may be the treatment of choice. If it is more coronal, it may be necessary to instrument through the barrier. In this case it is very

important to have excellent access and vision to avoid perforation. This treatment is best referred to a specialist.

Previous injury

Sometimes a patient presents with a new injury to an already traumatized tooth and the history of the presenting injury may fail to correlate with the findings of the clinical and radiological examinations and special tests. The patient should be questioned specifically about a previous injury.

Root canal retreatment

If a patient presents with signs or symptoms related to a root filled immature tooth and there are technical deficiencies in the previous treatment, root canal retreatment is indicated; it is, generally, more successful than surgery, which is often complicated by a short root with thin walls. Root canal retreatment is covered in Chapter 14. If the technical quality of the previous treatment is already very good, the possibility of recent root fracture must be considered.

Tooth discolouration

Since non-vital teeth tend to discolour, especially if necrotic pulp is allowed to remain within the pulp horns, many patients request to have their teeth bleached. This may be carried out, under rubber dam; root filling is removed to the cervical level and the canal entrance sealed with, for example, glass ionomer cement. Smear layer from the access cavity is removed using an etching agent and a thick paste of sodium perborate and water inserted. A temporary dressing is placed over this and the patient recalled after 1 week. At this visit, the colour improvement is assessed and the treatment may be repeated if required. When the desired lightening is achieved, the access cavity is then restored with composite resin. Care must be taken that the root filling is removed to the cervical constriction but not further beyond, to reduce the risk of cervical external resorption, which has been reported following bleaching.[88] Alternatively, instead of bleaching, a veneer or crown may be necessary.

ORTHODONTIC TREATMENT

Orthodontists are very concerned about causing resorption of root filled, previously traumatized teeth during tooth movement. However, there is no scientific evidence to show that these teeth are more at risk than vital ones.[89,90] It is essential that root canal treatment has been carried out properly prior to orthodontic movement and that infection has been eliminated; where there is any concern about the technical quality of the root canal filling, the root canal treatment should be redone first. There is no hard evidence to support the clinical practice of dressing teeth with calcium hydroxide and delaying placement of the permanent root filling until the completion of orthodontic treatment. This practice incurs increased risk of microleakage or loss of the temporary restoration and the canal becoming reinfected. It also causes additional inconvenience and stress to the patient, as well as risking further complications like root fracture if the tooth is repeatedly opened to replace the calcium hydroxide.[52,91]

LEARNING OUTCOMES

After reading this chapter the reader should be able to:

- understand the importance of correct diagnosis and treatment planning in cases of trauma
- treat simple traumatic injuries
- recognise the significance of and be familiar with methods of preserving pulpal vitality in immature teeth
- appreciate that elimination of infection from the root canal system is critical to achieving a favourable treatment outcome
- discuss modern, and the shortcomings of older, endodontic techniques for treating non-vital immature teeth
- know when it is appropriate to refer a complex case
- describe the common complications following dental trauma and their management.

REFERENCES

1. Andreasen JO, Andreasen FM, Andersson L. Textbook and Color Atlas of Traumatic Injuries to the Teeth, 4th edn. Copenhagen: Blackwell Munksgaard; 2007.

2. Flores MT, Andersson L, Andreasen JO, et al. Guidelines for the management of traumatic dental injuries. I. Fractures and luxations of permanent teeth. II. Avulsion of permanent teeth. III. Primary teeth. Dental Traumatology 2007;23:66–71, 130–136, 196–202.

3. Kinirons MJ. UK National Clinical Guidelines in Paediatric Dentistry. Treatment of traumatically intruded permanent incisor teeth in children. International Journal of Paediatric Dentistry 1998;8:165–168.

4. Kopel HM, Johnson R. Examination and neurologic assessment of children with oro-facial trauma. Endodontics and Dental Traumatology 1985;1:155–159.

5. National Institute for Health and Clinical Excellence. Prophylaxis against infective endocarditis: NICE guidelines. Online. Available: <http://www.nice.org.uk/nicemedia/pdf/CG64NICEguidance.pdf>; 2008.

6. Jacobsen I. Criteria for diagnosis of pulp necrosis in traumatized permanent incisors. Scandinavian Journal of Dental Research 1980;88:306–312.

7. Odor TM, Pitt Ford TR, McDonald F. Use of laser Doppler flowmetry for pulp testing – preliminary findings. International Endodontic Journal 1998;31:189–220 (Abstract).

8. Gazelius B, Olgart L, Edwall B. Restored vitality in luxated teeth assessed by laser Doppler flowmeter. Endodontics and Dental Traumatology 1988;4:265–268.

9. Lee JY, Yanpiset K, Sigurdsson A, Vann WF Jr. Laser Doppler flowmetry for monitoring traumatized teeth. Dental Traumatology 2001;5:231–235.

10. Banchs F, Trope M. Revascularization of immature permanent teeth with apical periodontitis: new treatment protocol? Journal of Endodontics 2004;30:196–200.

11. Andreasen FM, Vestergaard Pedersen B. Prognosis of luxated permanent teeth – the development of pulp necrosis. Endodontics and Dental Traumatology 1985;1:207–220.

12. Cohenca N, Simon JH, Roges R, et al. Clinical indications for digital imaging in dento-alveolar trauma. Part 1: traumatic injuries. Dental Traumatoogy 2007;23:95–104 Review.

13. Cohenca N, Simon JH, Mathur A, Malfaz JM. Clinical indications for digital imaging in dento-alveolar trauma. Part 2: root resorption. Dental Traumatology 2007;23:105–113.

14. Patel S, Dawood A, Ford TP, Whaites E. The potential applications of cone beam computed tomography in the management of endodontic problems. International Endodontic Journal 2007;4:818–830.

15. Roberts JA, Drage NA, Davies J, Thomas DW. Effective dose from cone beam CT examinations in dentistry. British Journal of Radiology 2009;82:35–40.

16. White SC. Cone-beam imaging in dentistry. Health Physiology 2008;95:628–637.

17. Andreasen FM, Andreasen JO. Diagnosis of luxation injuries: the importance of standardized clinical, radiographic and photographic techniques in clinical investigations. Endodontics and

Dental Traumatology 1985;1:160–169.

18. Heide S, Kerekes K. Delayed partial pulpotomy in permanent incisors of monkeys. International Endodontic Journal 1986;19:78–89.

19. Cvek M. Prognosis of luxated non-vital maxillary incisors treated with calcium hydroxide and filled with gutta-percha. A retrospective clinical study. Endodontics and Dental Traumatology 1992;8:45–55.

20. Andreasen JO, Ravn JJ. The effect of traumatic injuries to primary teeth on their permanent successors. II. A clinical and radiographic follow-up study of 213 teeth. Scandinavian Journal of Dental Research 1973;7:284–294.

21. Holan G, Eidelman E, Fuks AB. Long-term evaluation of pulpotomy in primary molars using mineral trioxide aggregate or formocresol. Pediatric Dentistry 2005;27:129–136.

22. Andreasen JO, Andreasen FM, Bakland L, Flores MT. Traumatic Dental Injuries. A Manual. 2nd edn, Copenhagen: Blackwell Munksgaard; 2003

23. Stalhane I, Hedegard B. Traumatized permanent teeth in children aged 7–15 years. Part II. Swedish Dental Journal 1975;68:157–169.

24. Ravn JJ. Follow-up study of permanent incisors with enamel-dentin fractures after acute trauma. Scandinavian Journal of Dental Research 1981;89:355–365.

25. Maguire A, Murray JJ, Al-Majed I. A retrospective study of treatment provided in the primary and secondary care services for children attending a dental hospital following complicated crown fracture in the permanent dentition. International Journal of Paediatric Dentistry 2000;10:182–190.

26. Robertson A, Andreasen FM, Andreasen JO, Noren JG. Long-term prognosis of crown-fractured permanent incisors. The effect of stage of root development and associated luxation injury. International Journal of Paediatric Dentistry 2000;10:191–199.

27. Cvek M. A clinical report on partial pulpotomy and capping with calcium hydroxide in permanent incisors with complicated crown fracture. Journal of Endodontics 1978;4:232–237.

28. Heide S, Mjör I. Pulp reactions to experimental exposures in young permanent monkey teeth. International Endodontic Journal 1983;16:11–19.

29. Fuks AB, Cosack A, Klein H, Eidelman E. Partial pulpotomy as a treatment alternative for exposed pulps in crown-fractured permanent incisors. Endodontics and Dental Traumatology 1987;3:100–102.

30. Granath LE, Hagman G. Experimental pulpotomy in human bicuspids with reference to cutting technique. Acta Odontologica Scandinavica 1971;29:155–163.

31. Nair PN, Duncan HF, Pitt Ford TR, Luder HU. Histological, ultrastructural and quantitative investigations on the response of healthy human pulps to experimental capping with mineral trioxide aggregate: a randomized controlled trial. International Endodontic Journal 2008;41:128–150.

32. Cvek M, Lundberg M. Histological appearance of pulps after exposure by a crown fracture, partial pulpotomy, and clinical diagnosis of healing. Journal of Endodontics 1983;9:8–11.

33. Min KS, Park HJ, Lee SK, et al. Effect of mineral trioxide aggregate on dentin bridge formation and expression of dentin sialoprotein and hemeoxygenase-1 in human dental pulp. Journal of Endodontics 2008;34:666–670.

34. Pitt Ford T, Torabinejad M, Abedi H, et al. Using mineral trioxide aggregate as a pulp-capping material. Journal of the American Dental Association 1996;127:1491–1494.

35. Shabahang S, Torabinejad M. Treatment of teeth with open apices using mineral trioxide aggregate. Practical Periodontics and Aesthetic Dentistry 2000;12:315–320.

36. Torabinejad M, Chivian N. Clinical applications of mineral trioxide aggregate. Journal of Endodontics 1999;25:197–205.

37. Cvek M, Mejàre I, Andreasen JO. Healing and prognosis of teeth with intra-alveolar fractures involving the cervical part of the root. Dental Traumatology 2002;18:57–65.

38. Andreasen JO, Andreasen FM, Mejàre I, Cvek M. Healing of 400 intra-alveolar root fractures. 1. Effect of pre-injury and injury factors such as sex, age, stage of root development, fracture type, location of fracture and severity of dislocation. Dental Traumatology 2004;20:192-202. 2. Effect of treatment factors such as treatment delay, repositioning, splinting type and period and antibiotics. Dental Traumatology 2004;20:203-211.

39. Welbury RR, Kinirons MJ, Day P, et al. Outcomes of root fractured permanent incisors. Paediatric Dentistry 2002;24:98–102.

40. Andreasen FM. Pulpal healing after luxation injuries and root fracture in the permanent dentition. Endodontics and Dental Traumatology 1989;5:111–131.

41. Zachrisson BU, Jacobsen I. Long-term prognosis of 66 permanent anterior teeth with root fracture. Scandinavian Journal of Dental Research 1975;83:345–354.

42. Jacobsen I, Kerekes K. Long-term prognosis of traumatized permanent anterior teeth showing calcifying processes in the pulp cavity. Scandinavian Journal of Dental Research 1977;85:588–598.

43. Jacobsen I, Kerekes K. Diagnosis and treatment of pulp necrosis in permanent anterior teeth with root fracture. Scandinavian Journal of Dental Research 1980;88:370–376.

44. Andreasen JO. Etiology and pathogenesis of traumatic dental injuries. A clinical study of 1298 cases. Scandinavian Journal of Dental Research 1970;78:329–342.

45. Olgart L, Gazelius B, Lindh-Strömberg U. Laser Doppler flowmetry in assessing vitality in luxated permanent teeth. International Endodontic Journal 1988;21:300–306.

46. Andreasen FM, Zhijie Y, Thomsen BL, Andersen PK. Occurrence of pulp canal obliteration after luxation injuries in the permanent dentition. Endodontics and Dental Traumatology 1987;3:103–115.

47. Andreasen FM. Transient apical breakdown and its relation to color and sensibility changes after luxation injuries to teeth. Endodontics and Dental Traumatology 1986;2:9–19.

48. Boyd DH, Kinirons MJ, Gregg TA. A prospective study of factors affecting survival of replanted permanent incisors in children. International Journal of Paediatric Dentistry 2000;10:200–205.

49. Kinirons MJ, Boyd DH, Gregg TA. Inflammatory and replacement resorption in reimplanted permanent incisor teeth: a study of the characteristics of 84 teeth. Endodontics and Dental Traumatology 1999;15:269–272.

50. Tronstad L. Root resorption – etiology, terminology and clinical manifestations. Endodontics and Dental Traumatology 1988;4:241–252.

51. Dumsha T, Hovland EJ. Evaluation of long-term calcium hydroxide treatment in avulsed teeth – an in vivo study. International Endodontic Journal 1995;28: 7–11.

52. Andreasen JO, Munksgaard EC, Bakland LK. Comparison of fracture resistance in root canals of immature sheep teeth after filling with calcium hydroxide or MTA. Dental Traumatology 2006;22:154–156.

53. El-Maligny OA, Avery DR. Comparison of apexification with mineral trioxide aggregate and calcium hydroxide. Pediatric Dentistry 2006;28:248–253.

54. Hatibovi -Kofman S, Raimundo L, Zheng L, et al. Fracture resistance and histological findings of immature teeth treated with mineral trioxide aggregate. Dental Traumatology 2008;24:272–276.

55. Holden DT, Schwartz SA, Kirkpatrick TC, Schindler WG. Clinical outcomes of artificial root-end barriers with mineral trioxide aggregate in teeth with immature apices. Journal of Endodontics 2008;34:812–817.

56. Pace R, Giuliani V, Pini Prato L, et al. Apical plug technique using mineral trioxide aggregate: results from a case series. International Endodontic Journal 2007;40:478–484.

57. Simon S, Rilliard F, Berdal A, Machtou P. The use of mineral trioxide aggregate in one visit apexification treatment: a prospective study. International Endodontic Journal 2007;40:186–197.

58. Steinig TH, Regan JD, Gutmann JL. The use and predictable placement of Mineral Trioxide Aggregate in one-visit apexification cases. Australian Endodontic Journal 2003;29:34–42.

59. Witherspoon DE, Small JC, Regan JD, Nunn M. Retrospective analysis of open apex teeth obturated with mineral trioxide aggregate. Journal of Endodontics 2008;34: 1171–1176.

60. Koh ET, Torabinejad M, Pitt Ford TR, et al. Mineral trioxide aggregate stimulates a biological response in human osteoblasts. Journal of Biomedical Materials Research 1997;37:432–439.

61. Barnett F. The role of endodontics in the treatment of luxated permanent teeth. Dental Traumatology 2002;18:47–56.

62. Metzger Z, Solomonov M, Mass E. Calcium hydroxide retention in wide root canals with flaring apices. Dental Traumatology 2001;17:86–92.

63. Yeung P, Liewehr FR, Moon PC. A quantitative comparison of the fill density of MTA produced by two placement techniques. Journal of Endodontics 2006;32:456–469.

64. Katebzadeh N, Dalton BC, Trope M. Strengthening immature teeth during and after apexification. Journal of Endodontics 1998;24:256–259.

65. Trope M, Maltz DO, Tronstad L. Resistance to fracture of restored endodontically treated teeth. Dental Traumatology 1985;1:108–111.

66. Mannocci F, Cavalli G, Gagliani M. Fibre Posts. In: Adhesive Restoration of Endodontically Treated Teeth. London: Quintessence; 2008. p. 59–73.

67. Reynolds K, Johnson JD, Cohenca N. Pulp revascularization of necrotic bilateral bicuspids using a modified novel technique to eliminate potential coronal discolouration: a case report. International Endodontic Journal 2009;42:84–92.

68. Hargreaves KM, Giesler T, Henry M, Wang Y. Regeneration potential of the young permanent tooth: what does the future hold? Journal of Endodontics 2008;34(7 Suppl): S51–56.

69. Jung IY, Lee SJ, Hargreaves KM. Biologically based treatment of immature permanent teeth with pulpal necrosis: a case series. Journal of Endodontics 2008;34:876–887.

70. Shah N, Logani A, Bhaskar U, Aggarwal V. Efficacy of revascularization to induce apexification/apexogenesis in infected, non-vital, immature teeth: a pilot clinical study. Journal of Endodontics 2008;34:919–925.

71. Thibodeau B, Teixeira F, Yamauchi M, et al. Pulp revascularization of immature dog teeth with apical periodontitis. Journal of Endodontics 2007;33:680–689.

72. King M, Cvek M, Mejàre I. Rate and predictability of pulp revascularisation in therapeutically reimplanted permanent incisors. Endodontics and Dental Traumatology 1986;2:83–89.

73. Ritter AL, Ritter AV, Murrah V, et al. Pulp revascularization of replanted immature dog teeth after treatment with minocycline and doxycycline assessed by laser doppler flowmetry, radiography, and histology. Dental Traumatology 2004;20:75–84.

74. Skoglund A, Tronstad L, Wallenius K. A microangiographic study of vascular changes in replanted and autotransplanted teeth of young dogs. Oral Surgery Oral Medicine Oral Pathology 1978;45: 17–28.

75. Windley W, Teixeira F, Levin L, et al. Disinfection of immature teeth with a triple antibiotic paste. Endodontics and Dental Traumatology 2005;31:439–443.

76. Cordeiro MM, Dong Z, Kaneko T, et al. Dental pulp tissue engineering with stem cells from exfoliated deciduous teeth. Journal of Endodontics 2008;34:962–969.

77. Murray PE, Garcia-Godoy F, Hargreaves KM. Regenerative endodontics: a review of current status and a call for action. Journal of Endodontics 2007;33:377–390.

78. Nakashima M, Akamine A. The application of tissue engineering to regeneration of pulp and dentin in endodontics. Journal of Endodontics 2005;31:711–718.

79. Andreasen JO, Håkansson L. Atlas of Replantation and Transplantation of Teeth. Philadelphia, USA: Saunders; 1992.

80. Hammarström LE, Blomlöf LB, Feiglin B, Lindskog SF. Effect of calcium hydroxide treatment on periodontal repair and root resorption. Endodontics and Dental Traumatology 1986;2:184–189.

81. Patel S, Kanagasingam S, Pitt Ford T. External cervical resorption: a review. Journal of Endodontics 2009;35:616–625.

82. Rotstein I, Mor C, Friedman S. Prognosis of intracoronal bleaching with sodium perborate preparation in vitro: 1-year study. Journal of Endodontics 1993;19:10–12.

83. Rotstein I, Zalkind M, Mor C, et al. In vitro efficacy of sodium perborate preparations used for intracoronal bleaching of discolored non-vital teeth. Endodontics and Dental Traumatology 1991;7:177–180.

84. Andreasen JO, Kristerson L. The effects of limited drying or removal of the periodontal ligament. Periodontal healing after replantation of mature permanent incisors in monkeys. Acta Odontologica Scandinavica 1981;39:1–13.

85. Andersson L, Malmgren B. The problem of dentoalveolar ankylosis and subsequent replacement resorption in the growing patient. Australian Endodontic Journal 1999;25:57–61.

86. Malmgren B, Malmgren O. Rate of infraposition of reimplanted ankylosed incisors related to age and growth in children and adolescents. Dental Traumatology 2002;18:28–36.

87. Cohenca N, Stabholz A. Decoronation – a conservative method to treat ankylosed teeth for preservation of alveolar ridge prior to permanent prosthetic reconstruction: literature review and case presentation. Dental Traumatology 2007;23:87–94.

88. Cvek M, Lindvall AM. External root resorption following bleaching of pulpless teeth with oxygen peroxide. Endodontics and Dental Traumatology 1985;1:56–60.

89. Levander E, Malmgren O. Evaluation of the risk of root resorption during orthodontic treatment: a study of upper incisors. European Journal of Orthodontics 1988;10:30–38.

90. Spurrier SW, Hall SH, Joondeph DR, et al. A comparison of apical root resorption during orthodontic treatment in endodontically treated and vital teeth. American Journal of Orthodontics and Dentofacial Orthopedics 1990;97:130–134.

91. Drysdale C, Gibbs SL, Pitt Ford TR. Orthodontic management of root filled teeth. British Journal of Orthodontics 1996;23:255–260.

Chapter | **13** |

Marginal periodontitis and the dental pulp

I. Rotstein, J.H. Simon

SUMMARY

Endodontic-periodontal diseases often present challenges to the clinician in their diagnosis, treatment and prognosis assessment. Aetiological factors such as microorganisms, as well as contributing factors such as trauma, root resorption, perforation and dental malformation play a role in the development and progression of such diseases. Treatment and prognosis of endodontic-periodontal diseases vary and are dependent on the aetiology, pathogenesis and correct recognition of each specific condition. Therefore, understanding the interrelationship between endodontic and periodontal diseases will enhance the clinician's ability to establish correct diagnosis, assess the prognosis of the teeth involved and select a treatment plan based on biological and clinical evidence.

ANATOMICAL CONSIDERATIONS

The dental pulp and the periodontium are intimately related and connected via exposed dentinal tubules, lateral or accessory canals, and the apical foramen.[1-14] Exposed dentinal tubules in areas devoid of cementum may serve as viable communication pathways between the dental pulp and periodontal ligament. Exposure of dentinal tubules may occur due to developmental defects, disease and following periodontal or surgical procedures. Radicular dentinal tubules extend from the pulp to the cementodentinal junction (CDJ). They run a relatively straight course and range in size from 1 to 3 μm in diameter.[13] The diameter of the tubules decreases with age or as a response to chronic low grade stimuli causing apposition of highly mineralized peritubular dentine. The number of dentinal tubules varies from approximately 8000 mm^{-2} at the CDJ to 57 000 mm^{-2} at the pulpal end. In the cervical area of the root the number of dentinal tubules is about 15 000 mm^{-2}.[13]

© 2009 Elsevier Ltd, Inc, BV
DOI: 10.1016/B978-0-7020-3156-4.00016-4

When the cementum and enamel do not meet at the cemento-enamel junction (CEJ) these tubules remain exposed thereby creating pathways of communication between the pulp and the periodontal ligament. Patients experiencing cervical dentine hypersensitivity are an example of such a phenomenon. Fluid and irritants may flow through patent dentinal tubules. In the absence of an intact enamel or cementum layer, the pulp can become exposed to the oral environment via the gingival sulcus or periodontal pocket. Experimental studies demonstrated that soluble material from bacterial plaque applied to exposed dentine can cause pulpal inflammation indicating that dentinal tubules may provide ready access between the periodontium and the pulp.[15]

Scanning electron microscopic studies have demonstrated that dentine exposure at the CEJ occurred in about 18% of teeth in general and in 25% of anterior teeth in particular.[16] In addition, the same tooth may have different CEJ characteristics presenting dentine exposure on one surface while the other surfaces are covered with cementum.[17] This area is susceptible to the progression of endodontic pathogens, as well as to the effect of root scaling and planing on cementum integrity, trauma, and bleaching-induced pathosis.[18,19,20] Other areas of dentinal communication may be through developmental grooves both palato-gingival and apical.[21] The base of these grooves is often not covered by cementum and accessory canals are often present.

Lateral and accessory canals can be present anywhere along the length of the root. Their incidence and location have been well documented in both animal and human teeth using a variety of methods. These included dye perfusion, injection of impression materials, microradiography, light microscopy and scanning electron microscopy.[2,4,6,8,10,14,22] It is estimated that 30–40% of all teeth have other smaller canal systems and the majority of them are found in the apical third of the root. It was reported that 17% of teeth presented multiple canal systems in the apical third of the root, about 9% in the middle third, and less than 2% in the coronal third.[4] However, it seems that the incidence of periodontal disease associated with these types of canals is relatively low. A study of 1000 human teeth with extensive periodontal disease found only 2% of such canals associated with the involved periodontal pocket.[8]

Other canal systems in the furcation of molars may also be a direct pathway of communication between the pulp and the periodontium.[6,10] The incidence of accessory canals may vary from 23% to 76%.[2,4,23] These accessory canals contain connective tissue and blood vessels that connect the circulatory system of the pulp to that of the periodontium. However, not all these canals extend the full length from the pulp chamber to the floor of the furcation.[23] It was reported that pulpal inflammation may cause inflammatory reaction in the interradicular periodontal tissues.[24] The presence of these patent smaller canals is a potential pathway for the spread of microorganisms and their toxic byproducts from the pulp to the periodontal ligament and vice-versa, resulting in an inflammatory process in the involved tissues.

The apical foramen is the principal route of communication between the pulp and periodontium. Microbial and inflammatory byproducts may exit readily through the apical foramen to cause periapical pathosis. The apex is also a potential portal of entry of inflammatory byproducts from deep periodontal pockets into the pulp. Pulp inflammation or pulp necrosis extends into the periapical tissues causing a local inflammatory response often associated with bone and root resorption.[24] Endodontic therapy aims to eliminate the intraradicular aetiological factors thereby leading to healing of the affected periapical tissues.

EFFECT OF INFLAMED PULP ON THE PERIODONTIUM

When the pulp becomes inflamed, it elicits an inflammatory response in the periodontal ligament at the apical foramen and/or adjacent to smaller openings of the root canal system.[25] Inflammatory byproducts of pulpal origin may permeate through the apex, smaller canals in the apical third of the root canal system or exposed dentinal tubules and trigger an inflammatory vascular response in the periodontium.[26–33] Among those are living pathogens such as certain bacteria strains including spirochetes, fungi and viruses,[26,27,29,33–38] as well as non-living pathogens.[37,39,40,41,42] Many of these are pathogens similarly encountered in periodontal inflammatory disease. In certain cases, pulpal disease will stimulate epithelial growth affecting the integrity of the periapical tissues.[43,44]

In an experimental study, defects of different sizes were created on root surfaces of extracted lateral incisors with open or mature apices. The canals were either infected or filled with calcium hydroxide and then replanted. It was observed that intrapulpal infection promoted marginal epithelial downgrowth on the denuded dentine surface after 20 weeks.[45] The effects of endodontic pathogens on marginal periodontal wound healing on dentinal surfaces surrounded by healthy periodontal ligament have been assessed.[46] It was found that in infected teeth the defect was covered by 20% more epithelium and the non-infected had 10% more connective tissue covering. It appears that the pathogens in a necrotic canal can stimulate epithelial downgrowth along denuded dentine surfaces with marginal communication.

The effect of endodontic infection on periodontal probing depth and the presence of furcation involvement in mandibular molars have also been investigated.[47] In 100 patients with molars with periapical lesions on both roots, the periodontal probing depth was significantly greater than around teeth without periapical lesions. It was suggested that root canal inflammation in molars involved with marginal periodontitis may potentiate periodontitis progression by pathogens spreading through accessory canals and dentinal tubules causing more attachment loss in the furcation.

Periodontal pathogens in pulp and periodontal diseases affecting the same tooth were studied by means of 16S RNA gene directed polymerase chain reaction samples from 31 teeth.[48] Specific polymerase chain reaction methods were used to detect *Actinobacillus actinomycetemcomitans*, *Bacteroides forsythicus*, *Eikenella corrodens*, *Fusobacterium nucleatum*, *Porphyromonas gingivalis* *Prevotella intermedia* and *Treponena denticola*. The pathogens were found in all endodontic samples. In chronic apical periodontitis and chronic marginal periodontitis the same pathogens were found. It was concluded that periodontal pathogens often accompany endodontic infections and support the concept that endodontic-periodontal interrelationships are a critical pathway for both diseases. In addition, foreign bodies and materials may also pass into the periapical tissues. Extrinsic foreign bodies, including foreign lipids, cellulose granulomas and iatrogenic materials, can cause a direct inflammatory response.

EFFECT OF MARGINAL PERIODONTITIS ON THE PULP

The effect of periodontal inflammation on the pulp is controversial and conflicting studies abound.[3,5,12,24,49,51,52,53,55,57,58] It has been suggested that marginal periodontitis has no effect on the pulp, at least, until it involves the apex.[3] On the other hand, several studies suggested that the effect of periodontal disease on the pulp is degenerative in nature including an increase in calcifications, fibrosis and collagen resorption, as well as a direct inflammatory effect.[9,11] It appears that the pulp is usually not severely affected by periodontal disease until recession has opened an accessory canal to the oral environment. At that stage, pathogens leaking from the oral cavity through the accessory canal into the pulp may cause a chronic inflammatory reaction followed by pulpal necrosis. However, as long as the accessory canals are protected by sound cementum, necrosis usually does not occur. Additionally, if the mircovasculature of the apical foramen remains intact the pulp will maintain its vitality.[9] With regard to the root apex, once the apical vasculature is compromised, the pulp will lose its vitality. This is shown in teeth with primary periodontal lesions with secondary endodontic involvement (see later). The effect of periodontal therapy on the pulp is similar during scaling, curettage or periodontal surgery if accessory canals are opened to the oral environment. In such cases, pathogenic invasion and secondary inflammation and necrosis of the pulp can occur.

CLASSIFICATION

There are many ways of classifying the so-called endodontic-periodontal (endo-perio) lesions.[24,52,59,60,61] For differential diagnostic and treatment purposes they are best classified as endodontic, periodontal or combined diseases.[62,63] They include:

1. primary endodontic lesion
2. primary periodontal lesion
3. combined lesions.

The combined lesions include:

1. primary endodontic lesion with secondary periodontal involvement
2. primary periodontal lesion with secondary endodontic involvement
3. true combined lesions.

This classification is based on the theoretical pathways explaining how these lesions are formed.[61] By understanding the pathogenesis, the clinician can then suggest an appropriate course of treatment and better assess the prognosis.

Primary endodontic lesion

An acute exacerbation of a chronic periapical lesion on a tooth with a necrotic pulp may drain coronally through the periodontal ligament into the gingival sulcus (Fig. 13.1A). This condition may mimic a periodontal abscess. However, it is only periodontal in that it passes through the periodontal ligament space (Figs 13.2–13.5). In reality, it is a sinus tract resulting from pulpal disease. Therefore, it is essential that a gutta-percha cone is inserted into the sinus tract and one or more radiographs taken to track the origin of the lesion. When the sinus tract is probed, it is usually narrow and lacks width. A similar situation occurs where drainage from the apex of a molar tooth extends coronally into the furcation area (Fig. 13.6). Direct extension of inflammation from the pulp may also occur into the furcation area of a non-vital tooth when a lateral or accessory canal is present (Fig. 13.7). Primary endodontic lesions usually heal following root canal treatment; the sinus tract extending into the gingival sulcus or furcation disappears at an early stage (usually within a few weeks) once the consequences of the necrotic pulp has been treated. It is important to recognize that an attempt to provide periodontal therapy for this condition will result in failure since if the necrotic pulp has not been diagnosed and treated.

Primary periodontal lesion

These lesions (Fig. 13.1C) are caused by marginal periodontitis, which progresses apically along the root surface

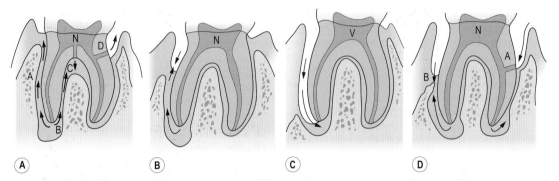

Figure 13.1 Classification of endodontic-periodontal lesions. (A) Primary endodontic lesions: pathway extending from apex to gingival sulcus via periodontium (A); apex to furcation (B); lateral canal to furcation (C); lateral canal to pocket (D). (B) Primary endodontic lesion with secondary periodontal involvement. (C) Primary periodontal lesion extending to the apex. (D) Primary periodontal lesion with secondary endodontic involvement via a lateral canal (A). Combined lesion from coalescence of separate lesions (B). N = Necrotic pulp. V = Vital pulp.

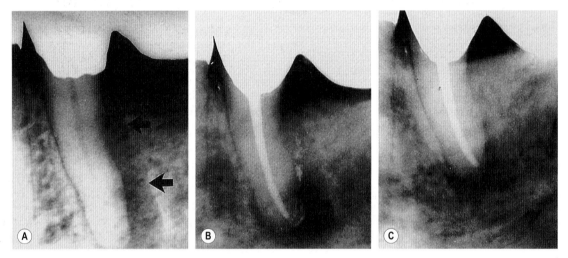

Figure 13.2 Primary endodontic lesion. Mandibular premolar with a radiolucency along the distal surface of the root. (A) Pretreatment, the lesion (arrowed) drained through the gingival sulcus. (B) Immediately after treatment, root canal sealer can be observed in the sinus tract. (C) Six months later, there is evidence of healing and bone filling.

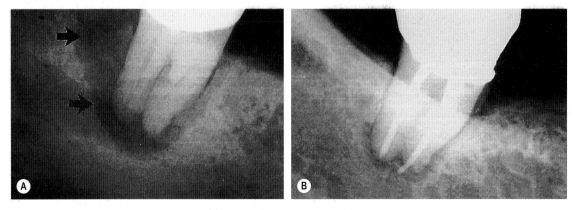

Figure 13.3 (A) Mandibular molar with a narrow probable distal pocket and large radiolucency (arrowed). (B) Marked healing apparent at one-year recall confirming that the original 'pocket' was of endodontic origin.

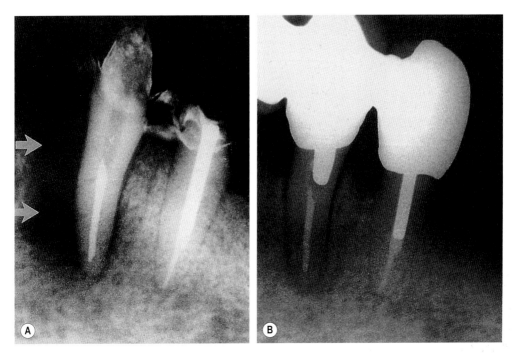

Figure 13.4 Success following treatment of a primary endodontic lesion. (A) Immediate post-treatment radiograph of a mandibular canine showing mesial radiolucency (arrowed). (B) Radiograph at 15 months showing healing.

until the apical region is reached. In such conditions, pulp sensitivity testing will reveal a clinically normal pulpal response (Figs 13.8 & 13.9). In addition, a probable pocket that has width is anticipated, possibly becoming progressively shallower as the probe is moved laterally; there is also an accumulation of plaque and frequently calculus. The prognosis in this condition depends wholly upon the stage of the marginal periodontitis and the efficacy of periodontal therapy. The clinician must also be aware of the radiographic appearance of marginal periodontitis associated with developmental radicular anomalies (see later).

Combined lesions

Primary endodontic lesion with secondary periodontal involvement

If, after a period of time, a suppurating primary endodontic lesion remains untreated, it may become secondarily involved with marginal periodontal breakdown (Fig. 13.1B). Biofilm forms at the gingival margin of the sinus tract and leads to marginal periodontitis. When plaque or calculus is encountered upon probing, the treatment and prognosis of the tooth are altered; the tooth now requires both endodontic and periodontal treatments. If the endodontic therapy is adequate, the prognosis depends on the severity of the marginal periodontal damage and the efficacy of periodontal therapy. With endodontic therapy alone, only part of the lesion will heal to the level of the secondary periodontal lesion.

Primary endodontic lesions with secondary periodontal involvement may also occur as a result of root perforation during root canal treatment, or where pins or posts have been misplaced during coronal restoration (Fig. 13.10). Symptoms may be acute, with periodontal abscess formation associated with pain, swelling, exudation of pus, pocket formation and tooth mobility. A more chronic response may sometimes occur without pain, and involves the sudden appearance of a pocket with bleeding on probing or exudation of pus. When the root perforation is situated close to the alveolar crest, it may be feasible to raise a flap and repair the defect with an appropriate filling material and subsequently reposition the flap apically to expose the repaired perforation. In deeper perforations, or in the roof of the furcation, immediate internal repair of the perforation has a better prognosis than management of an infected one. Many materials have been used for this purpose. Today, Mineral Trioxide Aggregate is most widely used.[64,65]

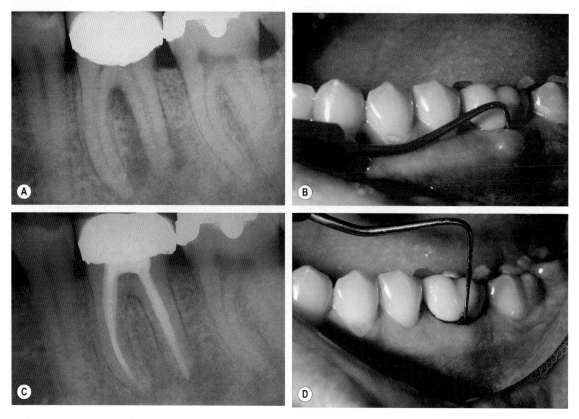

Figure 13.5 Mandibular molar with apical lesion extending into furcation. (A) Preoperative radiograph showing furcal and distal radiolucency. (B) Clinical photograph of gingival swelling and a periodontal probe in the furcation. (C) A 1-year recall radiograph showing furcal and distal radiolucencies healing. (D) Clinical photograph showing minimal pocket depth on the buccal. Healing occurred following root canal treatment alone.

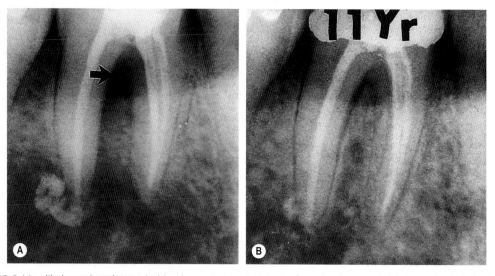

Figure 13.6 Mandibular molar where apical involvement extends into the furcation (arrowed). (A) Immediately following root canal treatment, excess sealer is present at the apex of the distal root. (B) Radiograph 11 years later showing apical and furcation healing.

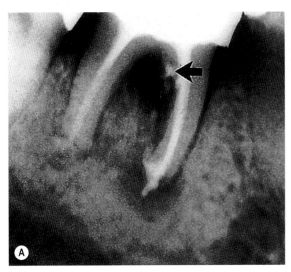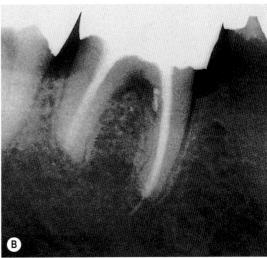

Figure 13.7 Primary endodontic lesion with a lateral canal demonstrated in the furcation. (A) Post-treatment radiograph demonstrating filling material passing through openings into the furcation (arrowed). (B) After 18 months, complete healing of the lesions at the apex and adjacent to the lateral canal is demonstrated.

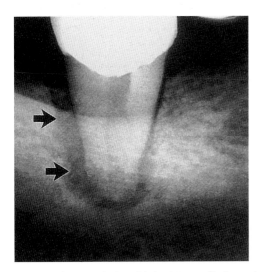

Figure 13.8 Primary periodontal lesion. A mandibular molar presented with a probable distal pocket (arrowed). Pulp testing was positive indicating a lesion of periodontal origin; the tooth was extracted.

Root fractures may also present as primary endodontic lesions with secondary periodontal involvement. These typically occur on root-treated teeth (Fig. 13.11), often with post crowns in situ. The signs may range from a local deepening of a periodontal pocket to more acute periodontal abscess formation. In addition, root fractures have become an increasing problem with molar teeth that have been treated by root resection. In a study of 100 patients, a total of 38 teeth failed during the 10-year period of observation, and 47% of the failures were due to root fractures, with the vast majority being in mandibular molar teeth.[54,56]

Primary periodontal lesion with secondary endodontic involvement

The apical progression of a periodontal pocket can continue until the apex is reached. As a result, the pulp may become necrotic due to irritants permeating via a lateral canal or the apical foramen (Fig. 13.1D). In single rooted tooth the prognosis is usually poor, which is the opposite of that for the primary endodontic lesion. In molar teeth not all the roots may suffer the same loss of supporting tissues to the apex, in which case the possibility of root resection should be considered.

The treatment of marginal periodontitis can also lead to secondary endodontic involvement. Lateral or accessory canals and dentinal tubules can be opened to the oral environment by curettage, scaling or surgical flap procedures (Figs 13.12 & 13.13). In addition, it is possible for a blood vessel within a lateral canal to be severed by a curette during treatment. Also, pulp changes resulting from marginal periodontitis were observed when the main apical foramen was involved.[9] Provided the blood supply through the apex is intact, the pulp has a strong capacity for survival (Fig. 13.10).

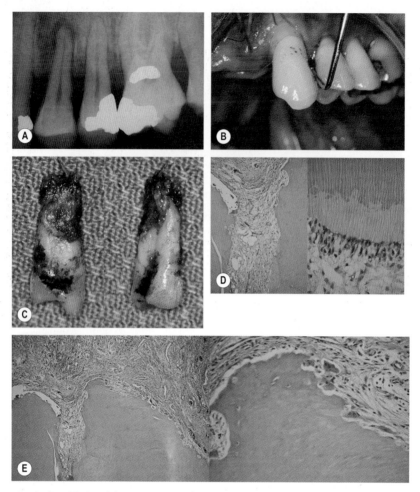

Figure 13.9 Primary periodontal lesion. (A) Preoperative radiograph of maxillary first premolar with a periapical lesion but no obvious endodontic aetiology. (B) Clinical photograph with periodontal probe in place. The pulp will respond normally to pulp sensitivity testing. (C) Two views of the extracted tooth. Note mesial anatomical groove along the root. (D) Micrographs showing vital pulp in the tooth. (E) Micrographs showing inflammatory resorption and periodontitis.

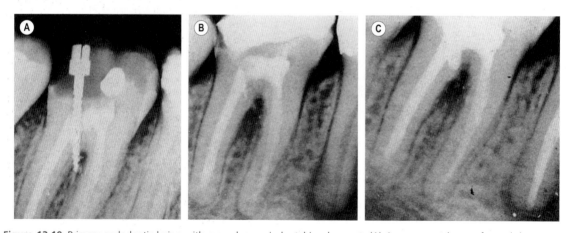

Figure 13.10 Primary endodontic lesion with secondary periodontal involvement. (A) A screw post has perforated the furcation area of a mandibular second molar. (B) After 6 months, furcation bone loss is evident. (C) The perforation has been treated from within the tooth and the pocket has been curetted. Some new bone has formed in the furcation and clinically, no pocket can be probed.

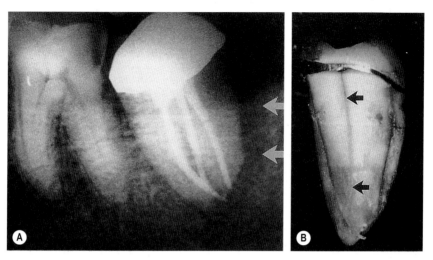

Figure 13.11 Longitudinal fracture. (A) A distal pocket (arrowed) probable to the apex on a mandibular left second molar persisted following root canal treatment, necessitating extraction. (B) Following extraction, a longitudinal fracture on the distal root surface (arrowed) was evident extending the length of the tooth. Fused roots prevented 'anatomical redesigning'.

There is a correlation between cultivable microorganisms from the root canals of human caries-free teeth with advanced periodontitis and those from associated periodontal pockets.[66,67] The microorganisms from the periodontal pocket are a possible source for root canal infection. Support for this concept has come from research in which cultured samples obtained from the pulp tissue and radicular dentine of periodontally involved human teeth showed bacterial growth in 87% of the cases.[49,50] It was suggested that the reservoir of bacteria in the dentine and pulp might contribute to the failure of periodontal therapy. A possibility also exists that these teeth will develop pulpal necrosis.

Sometimes there is lack of correlation between marginal periodontitis and pulp involvement.[55] The histological status of the pulps of 100 periodontally involved teeth was similar to the 22 control teeth with a normal periodontium.[56] Despite conflicting opinions from various research studies,[52,58] it seems, from a clinical standpoint, that plaque-associated marginal periodontitis rarely causes significant pathological changes in the pulp, and this remains true until the periodontal pocket reaches the apical foramen.

True combined lesions

These lesions (Fig. 13.1D) occur where an endodontic lesion progressing coronally becomes continuous with a plaque-infected periodontal pocket progressing apically.[61] The degree of attachment loss in this type of lesion is

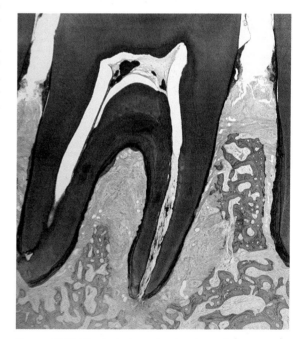

Figure 13.12 Histological examination shows that furcation involvement can be severe in advanced marginal periodontitis. The pulp can become affected through lateral or accessory canals.

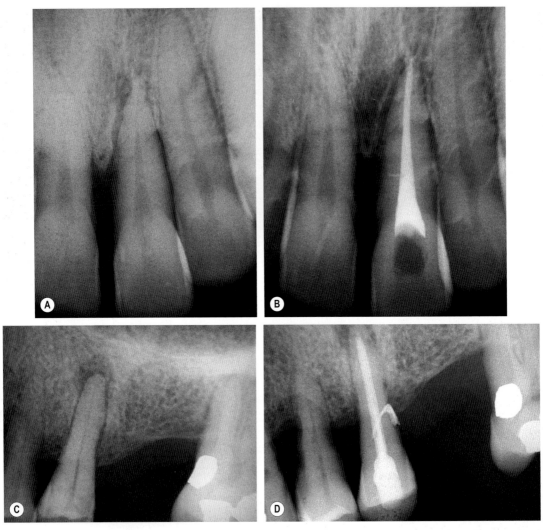

Figure 13.13 Marginal periodontitis with endodontic involvement. (A) Radiograph of an unrestored tooth with generalized periodontitis and a necrotic pulp. (B) After endodontic therapy a communication with the oral environment through a lateral canal has been demonstrated. (C) A similar situation on a premolar with generalized periodontitis and a necrotic pulp. (D) Filling material extruding through a lateral canal suggests how the pulp became necrotic.

invariably large and the prognosis guarded. The prognosis is particularly poor in single rooted teeth, but the situation may be salvaged in molars by sectioning the tooth, if not all the roots are as severely involved. Healing of apical periodontitis may be anticipated following successful endodontic therapy. The periodontal component of this lesion may, or may not, respond to periodontal therapy, depending on the severity of involvement (Fig. 13.14). The radiographic appearance of true combined endodontic-periodontal lesions may be similar to that of a vertically fractured tooth. A fracture that has exposed the

pulp space, with resultant necrosis, may also be labelled a true combined lesion and yet not be amenable to successful treatment. If a sinus tract is present, it may be necessary to raise a flap to determine the aetiology of the lesion (Fig. 13.9).

Diagnosis

The diagnosis of primary endodontic lesion and primary periodontal disease usually present no clinical difficulty. In primary endodontic lesion the pulp is infected and

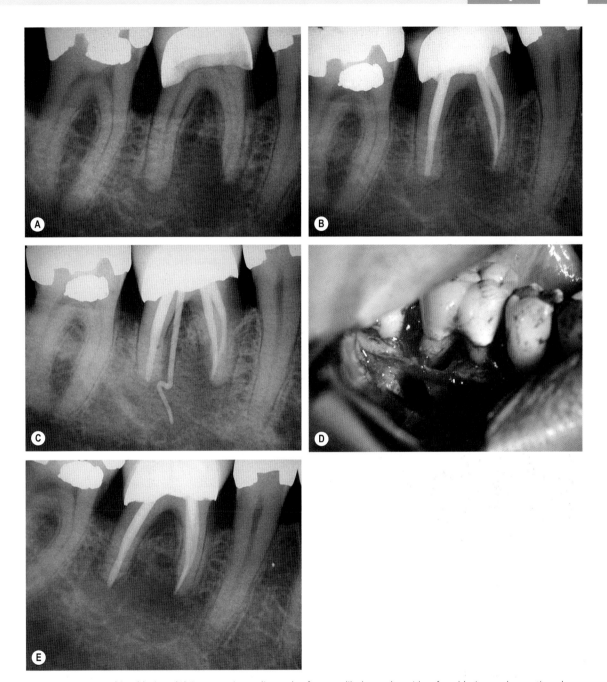

Figure 13.14 A combined lesion. (A) Preoperative radiograph of a mandibular molar with a furcal lesion and necrotic pulp. (B) Endodontic therapy was completed. (C) Recall radiograph with a gutta-percha point in the gingival sulcus. (D) Periodontal surgery and treatment were performed on the cervical and furcal areas. (E) One year after both endodontic and periodontal therapy, the lesions healed.

often non-vital. On the other hand, in a tooth with primary periodontal lesion, the pulp is vital and responsive to sensitivity testing. However, primary endodontic lesions with secondary periodontal involvement, primary periodontal lesions with secondary endodontic involvement, or true combine lesions may be clinically and radiographically very similar. If a lesion is provisionally diagnosed and treated as being primarily due to endodontic disease because of a lack of evidence of marginal periodontitis, and there is soft-tissue healing on clinical probing and bony healing on a recall radiograph, a valid retrospective confirmed diagnosis can then be made. The degree of healing that has taken place following root canal treatment will determine the retrospective classification. In the absence of adequate healing, further periodontal therapy is indicated.

Prognosis

The prognosis depends primarily on the diagnosis of the specific endodontic and/or periodontal disease. The main factors to consider at the time of diagnosis are pulp vitality and type and extent of the periodontal defect. The prognosis and treatment of each type of endodontic-periodontal lesion varies. Primary endodontic lesion should only be treated by endodontic therapy and the prognosis is good. Primary periodontal lesions should only be treated by periodontal therapy. In this case, the prognosis depends on the severity of the periodontal lesion and patient's response. Primary endodontic lesions with secondary periodontal involvement should first be treated with endodontic therapy. The treatment results should be evaluated in 2 to 3 months and only then periodontal therapy should be considered. This sequence of treatment allows sufficient time for initial tissue healing and better assessment of the periodontal condition.[22,68] It also reduces the potential risk of introducing bacteria and their byproducts during the initial healing phase. In this regard, it was suggested that during interim endodontic therapy, aggressive removal of the periodontal ligament and underlying cementum will adversely affect periodontal healing.[1] Areas of the roots that were not aggressively treated showed unremarkable healing.[1] The prognosis of a primary endodontic lesion with secondary periodontal involvement depends primarily on the severity of periodontal involvement, the periodontal therapy and the patient's response.

Primary periodontal lesions with secondary endodontic involvement and true combined endodontic-periodontal lesions require both endodontic and periodontal therapies. It has been demonstrated that intrapulpal infection tends to promote marginal epithelial downgrowth a long a denuded dentin surface.[47] Additionally, experimentally-induced periodontal defects in infected teeth were associated with 20% more epithelium than non-infected teeth.[29] Non-infected teeth showed 10% more connective tissue coverage than infected teeth.[29] The prognosis of primary periodontal lesions with secondary endodontic involvement and true combined lesions depends primarily on the severity of the periodontal disease and periodontal tissues response to treatment.

True combined lesions usually have a more guarded prognosis. In general, assuming the endodontic therapy is adequate, the lesion of endodontic origin will heal. Thus, the prognosis of combined diseases is dependent on the efficacy of periodontal therapy. The prognosis for each classification can be summarized as follows:

Primary endodontic lesion

Treatment: root canal treatment.
Prognosis: excellent.

Primary periodontal lesion

Treatment: periodontal therapy (scaling, curettage, surgery).
Prognosis: dependent on efficacy of periodontal therapy and patient's response.

Combined lesions

Treatment: endodontic and periodontal therapy.
Prognosis: dependent on periodontal therapy and patient's response. The lesion caused by endodontic disease will heal therefore prognosis is dependent on periodontal therapy.

COMPLICATIONS DUE TO RADICULAR ANOMALIES

A particular group of teeth that fails to respond well to treatment is associated with an invagination or a longitudinal developmental radicular groove. Such conditions can lead to untreatable localized marginal periodontitis (Fig. 13.15). These grooves usually begin in the central fossa of maxillary central or lateral incisors over the cingulum, and continuing apically down the root for varying distances. Such a groove is apparently the result of an attempt of the tooth germ to form another root. This fissure-like channel may provide a nidus for biofilm formation and infection, and an avenue for the progression of marginal periodontitis.

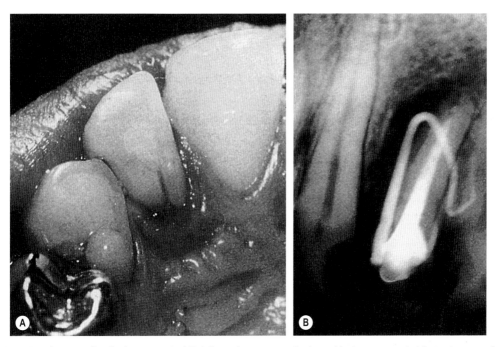

Figure 13.15 Developmental radicular anomaly. (A) A lingual groove on the lateral incisor was probable to the apex. (B) Root canal treatment did not improve the situation and the defect remained probable to a gutta-percha point.

From the time the tooth develops with this anomalous root defect, the potential for isolated marginal periodontitis exists. As long as the epithelial attachment remains intact, the periodontium remains healthy. However, once the integrity of the attachment is breached and the groove becomes inflamed, a self-sustaining infrabony pocket can be formed along its entire length. Radiographically an area of bone destruction follows the course of the groove.

Diagnosis

The correct clinical diagnosis of this condition at an early stage is important. The patient may have symptoms of a periodontal abscess or a variety of endodontic presentations. If the condition is purely periodontal, it can be diagnosed by visual detection following the groove to the gingival sulcus and by probing the depth of the pocket. This pocket is usually tubular in form and localized to this one site, as opposed to a more generalized periodontal condition. The tooth is usually responsive to pulp sensitivity testing. Bone destruction that follows the groove longitudinally may be apparent radiographically. If this entity is also associated with pulp infection, the patient may

present clinically with any endodontic symptoms, and pulp sensitivity testing will be abnormal.

Prognosis

The prognosis for endodontic therapy is guarded, depending on the apical extent of the groove. The clinician must look for the groove because it may have been altered by a previous restoration on the palatal surface. The use of an operating microscope can be advantageous due to enhanced magnification and illumination. The appearance of a teardrop-shaped area on the radiograph should also arouse suspicion. The developmental groove may actually be visible on the radiograph; if so, it will appear as a dark longitudinal line. This condition must be differentiated from a longitudinal fracture, which may give a similar radiographic appearance.

Treatment

In essence, since this lesion is a self-sustaining infrabony pocket, scaling and root planing alone may be inadequate. Although the acute nature of the problem may be alleviated initially, the reason for the inflammation must be eradicated by cutting out the groove and surgical management of the tissues. This can be combined with placement of a biocompatible material in an attempt to improve success.[69] Teeth with large developmental grooves with advance lesions need to be extracted if not treatable and implant treatment should be considered.

ALTERNATIVES TO IMPLANTS

Anatomical redesigning

To assist periodontal therapy and in certain endodontic situations, anatomical redesigning may become necessary. Such redesigning may include root amputation, resection and bicuspidization. It provides a periodontally maintainable environment for the remaining root(s). The reported survival rate is approximately 68%.[70] Generally, such cases should be referred to a specialist to assess prognosis and enhance survival rate. Often, the natural tooth can be retained. However, if the prognosis appears poor, early extraction is advisable to avoid compromising future implant treatment.

Root amputation is the removal of one or more roots from a multirooted tooth, leaving the majority of the crown and any existing coronal restoration intact. Tooth resection involves the removal of one or more roots of a tooth along with their coronal part(s); it is sometimes referred to as hemisection. Bicuspidization is the separation of a multirooted tooth by a vertical cut through the furcation.

Indications for root amputation or tooth resection:

- Advanced marginal periodontitis. The pattern of alveolar bone loss in marginal periodontitis may affect the different roots of a molar tooth unequally. If left untreated, the adjacent healthier root support could eventually become involved by direct extension of the periodontal lesion resulting in poorer prognosis. Removal of the offending root(s) allows the well-supported part of the tooth to be retained as a functional unit with healthy tissues and a normal radiographic appearance.
- Close root proximity. The distobuccal root of the maxillary first molar and the mesiobuccal root of the second molar often tend to flare towards each other. Marginal periodontitis in these sites may lead to angular bone loss, which is difficult to treat leaving the patient with a plaque control management problem. Selective root removal will allow the re-establishment of a proper embrasure area.
- Furcation involvement.
- Extensive radicular caries.
- Root resorption.
- Root fracture or perforation.
- Inability to perform root canal treatment due to calcification or other canal obstructions.

Indications for bicuspidization are:

- Gross perforation in the furcation. However, the length of the remaining roots must be favourable.
- Close root proximity. This prevents periodontal therapy or home maintenance by the patient, which can be improved by root separation.

Contraindications for anatomical redesigning are:

- Poor patient motivation and plaque control. This is particularly important if there has been inadequate improvement following initial periodontal therapy.
- Unfavourable bony support. This relates to all remaining roots of the involved tooth, particularly if it is an abutment for a fixed prosthesis.
- Fused roots. These prevent root removal. A special clinical situation with a more favourable prognosis exists when there is only apical fusion and adequate interradicular bone, allowing for surgical root removal.
- Short thin roots.
- A long root trunk. The furcation area is situated so far apically that considerable supporting bone would need to be sacrificed.
- Surrounding anatomy. This may preclude the formation of a functional band of attached gingiva around the remaining roots.
- Non-negotiable canals. The canals are sclerosed or blocked and root-end surgery is not feasible.
- Non-restorable tooth.

Root amputation

This form of treatment relates primarily to maxillary molar teeth. The root most commonly removed by amputation is the distobuccal of the first molar. Prior to root removal, whenever possible, following root canal treatment the pulp chamber should be sealed with a permanent restorative material extending into the coronal part of the root to be resected (Fig. 13.16). Coronal reshaping and buccolingual narrowing to reduce the occlusal table should also be performed to redirect occlusal forces to the remaining solid roots.

The need for root removal may become apparent during diagnosis and treatment planning instead of treating roots with extensive periodontal breakdown. Root canal treatment is completed and a permanent restorative material placed in the pulp chamber and coronal part of the root to be amputated so that the root end is already sealed when the root is removed. The patient's plaque control needs to reach a satisfactory level and the inflammatory phase resolved before root amputation. A full-thickness mucoperiosteal flap is reflected to expose the furcation area. The furcation is carefully explored with a periodontal probe to ensure that the furcation has not been exposed

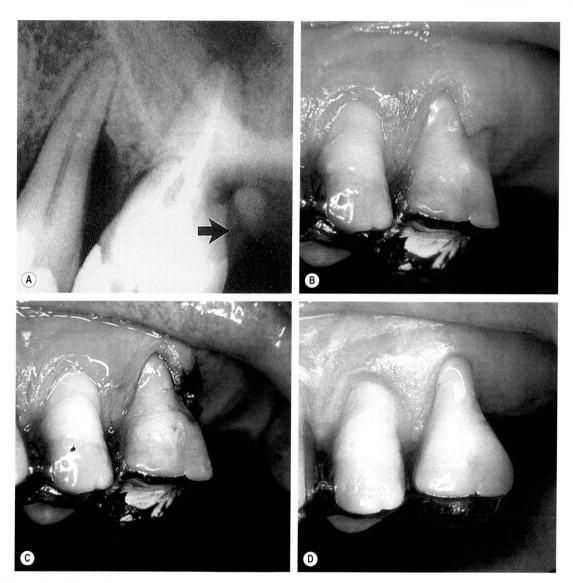

Figure 13.16 (A) Marginal periodontal involvement of the distobuccal root (arrowed) of the maxillary first molar required its amputation. (B) Before amputation. (C) After amputation. (D) The remaining tooth after polishing and smoothening.

on all three surfaces. If so, tooth resection would be required, leaving one root in situ, or otherwise, the tooth would need to be extracted. The cut in the root is made with a long thin bur, long enough to reach from one side of the root to the other. Care must be taken to maintain the correct angulation of the bur, so as not to damage the remaining root(s) or the crown. The bur is held at a 45° angle to the tooth at the level of the furcation. Removal of some of the buccal cortical plate of bone may be required so that the separated root can be gently elevated out of its socket, without undue pressure being

applied to the adjacent tooth or bone. Once the root has been removed, the area of the stump is reshaped with burs, so that it blends imperceptibly into the remaining tooth structure. Enough clearance should also be left between the undersurface of the crown and the gingival tissue to allow for adequate plaque control. The tooth surface is finished with fine burs and then polished. The periodontal condition is re-evaluated at about 3 months after root removal. If the mucogingival and osseous deformities still remain definitive periodontal surgery should be carried out.

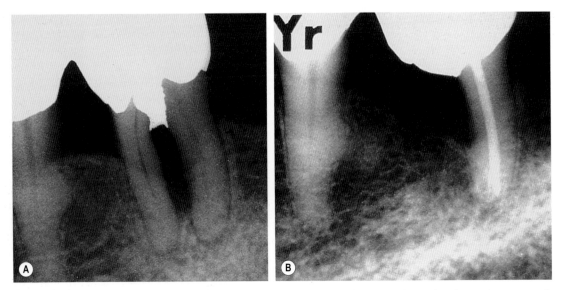

Figure 13.17 (A) A perforation with periodontal breakdown in the furcation of a mandibular molar; the tooth was part of a 4-unit splint. The mesial root was amputated and the coronal restoration recontoured and reduced buccolingually. (B) Recall at 13 years demonstrated long-term stability.

An alternative treatment modality allows for root amputation to be carried out at the time of periodontal surgery; this has the advantage of combining both stages into only one surgical procedure. The disadvantage is that bony healing has yet to occur, and the extent to which this will progress cannot always be predicted; this may also result in more radical reshaping at the site, than might otherwise be required. In this approach, a cavity is cut over the pulp stump with a suitable bur and an appropriate dressing placed over the exposed pulp. Definitive root canal treatment is carried out at a later stage and after the periodontal dressings have been removed.[21]

There may be situations where it is reasonable to amputate the root of a mandibular molar. If such a tooth presents with a periodontally-involved mesial root and it is part of a multiunit bridge or splinted crowns, amputation should be considered. The buccolingual dimension of the occlusal aspect of the tooth and pontics should be reduced to minimize and redirect the occlusal forces if possible (Fig. 13.17). Another situation where an amputation could be considered is when the periodontally involved root of a crowned tooth is adjacent to another crowned tooth. They could be firmly splinted to each other to avoid longitudinal fracture of the remaining root (Fig. 13.18); broad interproximal contact without splinting is not sufficient. Maxillary molars do not normally present such a problem because of the support provided by the two remaining roots. The remaining coronal portion of the amputated root should be contoured to allow for maintenance of periodontal health. The canal at the amputation site should be prepared and filled with a suit-

able restorative material to prevent the accumulation of plaque and development of caries. It is best to place the filling internally prior to root removal. If this is not feasible, the filling should be placed into the resected root end during surgical procedure.

Tooth resection

Tooth resection is often the treatment of choice where there is deep furcation involvement. It is also the treatment of choice where teeth are to be included in a fixed prosthesis.[59] It is advantageous to complete the initial crown preparation first; this will then serve as a guide when entering the furcation. Full-thickness mucoperiosteal flaps are reflected and the tooth is sectioned using a long tapered fissure bur. In maxillary molars, depending on the degree of furcation involvement, it may be possible to retain two roots, provided the furcation is not opened between them, such as mesial and palatal, or distal and palatal, or the two buccal roots. If the furcation is opened mesially, buccally and distally, then only the best supported root is retained. Sometimes this can only be determined after sectioning all three roots and assessing them individually.[6] The bur is positioned in the long axis of the tooth at the most coronal level of the involved furcation. Initial cuts are made in the crown in the direction of the adjacent furcation. The same step is then followed from the adjacent furcation towards the initial cut. The bur is then alternated between the two cuts until they are joined. Mandibular molars are sectioned buccolingually into two halves.

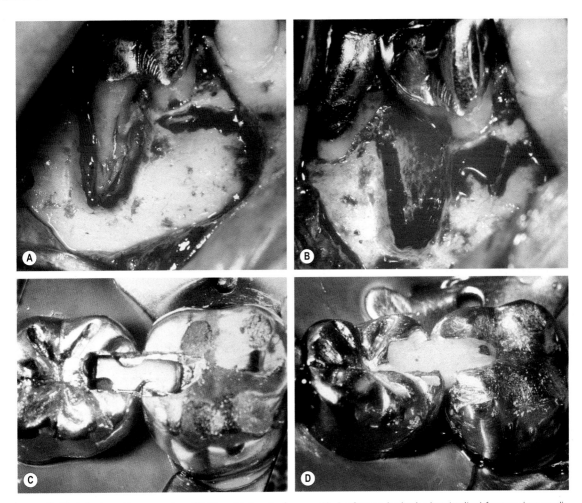

Figure 13.18 Splinting of lower molars. (A) The distal root of a mandibular first molar had a longitudinal fracture (arrowed) necessitating removal. (B) Following amputation of the root and contouring of the remaining structure. (C) An occlusal preparation was made for a metal splint. (D) A restorative filling material has been used to keep the splint in place.

As a general rule it is important to make the cut at the expense of the part that is to be removed (Fig. 13.19A). This minimizes the risk of overcutting the retained section. When sectioning has been completed, the involved part of the tooth is extracted with forceps. In finishing the preparation it is important to remove the overhang of the crown that may be left at the roof of the furcation and to blend the cut surface into the retained portion of the tooth. This should be checked radiographically. When the vertical cut to the furcation ends in close proximity to, or at the level of bone, it is necessary to remove approximately 1 mm of the bone with a sharp scalpel in order to expose some intact cementum beyond the cut surface (Fig. 13.19B). It is not advisable to end the restoration within the cut, leaving raw-cut dentine exposed because of the risk of subsequent development of marginal caries (Fig. 13.20). The biological width of the periodontium must be maintained. This will facilitate the preparation for the restoration that follows (Fig. 13.21). There may be situations where it is necessary to consider occlusal factors, as in amputation, and reduce the size of the occlusal table. Root fracture is a common cause of failure of root resected teeth.[56]

Bicuspidization

This procedure is used on roots of a multirooted tooth, primarily mandibular molars (Fig. 13.22). An adequate length and width of the root and clinical crown are primary considerations in case selection and treatment decision-making. The cut should be directed vertically to the middle of the furcation. It is necessary to expose the margin of the cut surface to facilitate crown preparation later. When there is close root proximity, it is necessary

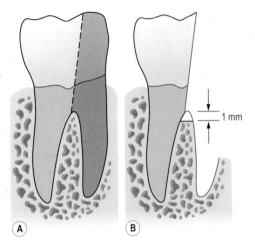

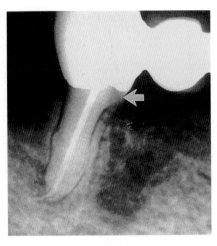

Figure 13.19 Resection. (A) The cut should be made at the expense of the part to be removed. (B) The restoration should not leave the raw cut exposed; 1 mm of the bone should be removed to facilitate preparation.

Figure 13.20 The lack of the 1mm space in bone led the restoration to end on the raw-cut dentine, with the long-term adverse consequence of marginal caries (arrowed).

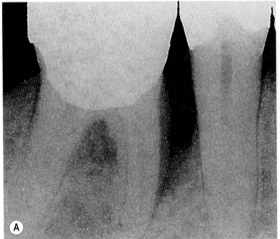

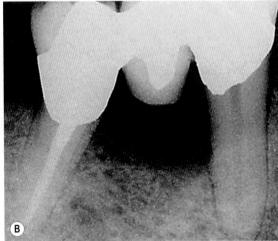

Figure 13.21 (A) Angular bone loss extending close to the apex of the mesial root of the mandibular first molar. The widely displayed roots made hemisection suitable. (B) The mesial root was removed. The distal root underwent root canal treatment and surgery and was used as a bridge abutment.

to separate the roots orthodontically (Fig. 13.23). Both roots are then restored as single units to simulate two premolars.

LEARNING OUTCOMES

After studying this chapter, the reader should know and understand the:

- anatomical structures involved in endodontic-periodontal diseases
- effect of pulpal inflammation on the periodontium
- effect of marginal periodontitis on the dental pulp
- classification of endodontic-periodontal diseases
- treatment modalities for endodontic-periodontal diseases, prognosis and complications.

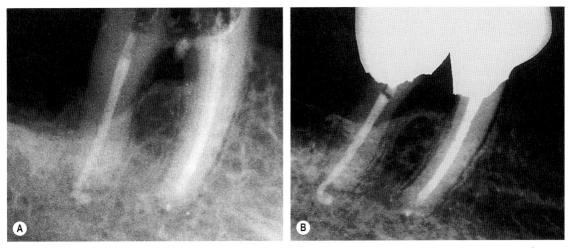

Figure 13.22 (A) Perforation into the furcation of a lower molar necessitated bicuspidization. (B) Recall examination after six years showing enlarged furcation space permitting effective oral hygiene.

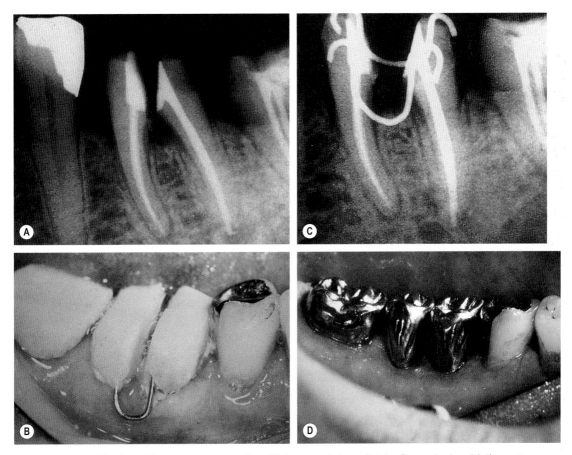

Figure 13.23 Bicuspidization achieved by root separation. (A) Radiograph immediately after sectioning. (B) The roots were separated orthodontically. (C) Radiograph after separation. (D) The separate crowns were cemented.

REFERENCES

1. Blomlöf LB, Lindskog S, Hammarstrom L. Influence of pulpal treatments on cell and tissue reactions in the marginal periodontium. Journal of Periodontology 1988;59:577–583.

2. Burch JG, Hulen S. A study of the presence of accessory foramina and the topography of molar furcations. Oral Surgery, Oral Medicine, Oral Pathology 1974;38: 451–455.

3. Czarnecki RT, Schilder H. A histological evaluation of the human pulp in teeth with varying degrees of periodontal disease. Journal of Endodontics 1979;5: 242–253.

4. De Deus QD. Frequency, location and direction of the lateral, secondary and accessory canals. Journal of Endodontics 1975;1: 361–366.

5. Dongari A, Lambrianidis T. Periodontally derived pulpal lesions. Endodontics and Dental Traumatology 1988;4:49–54.

6. Gutmann JL. Prevalence, location, and patency of accessory canals in the furcation region of permanent molars. Journal of Periodontology 1978;49:21–26.

7. Jansson L, Ehnevid H, Lindskog S, Blomlof L. The influence of endodontic infection on progression of marginal bone loss in periodontitis. Journal of Clinical Periodontology 1995;22:729–734.

8. Kirkham DB. The location and incidence of accessory pulpal canals in periodontal pockets. Journal of the American Dental Association 1975;91:353–356.

9. Langeland K, Rodrigues H, Dowden W. Periodontal disease, bacteria, and pulpal histopathology. Oral Surgery, Oral Medicine, Oral Pathology 1994; 37:257–270.

10. Lowman JV, Burke RS, Pelleu GB. Patent accessory canals: incidence in molar furcation region. Oral Surgery, Oral Medicine, Oral Pathology 1973;36:580–584.

11. Mandi FA. Histological study of the pulp changes caused by periodontal disease. Journal of the British Endodontic Society 1972;6: 80–82.

12. Mazur B, Massler M. Influence of periodontal disease on the dental pulp. Oral Surgery, Oral Medicine, Oral Pathology 1964;17:592–603.

13. Mjör IA, Nordahl I. The density and branching of dentinal tubules in human teeth. Archives of Oral Biology 1996;41:401–412.

14. Rubach WC, Mitchell DF. Periodontal disease, accessory canals and pulp pathosis. Journal of Periodontology 1965;36: 34–38.

15. Bergenholtz G, Lindhe J. Effect of soluble plaque factors on inflammatory reactions in the dental pulp. Scandinavian Journal of Dental Research 1975;83: 153–158.

16. Muller CJ, Van Wyk CW. The amelo-cemental junction. Journal of the Dental Association of South Africa 1984;39:799–803.

17. Schroeder HE, Scherle WF. Cemento-enamel junction-revisited. Journal of Periodontal Research 1988;23:53–59.

18. Ehnevid H, Jansson L, Lindskog S, et al. Endodontic pathogens: propagation of infection through patent dentinal tubules in traumatized monkey teeth. Endodontics and Dental Traumatology 1995;11:229–234.

19. Rotstein I, Friedman S, Mor C, et al. Histological characterization of bleaching-induced external root resorption in dogs. Journal of Endodontics 1991;17:436–441.

20. Rotstein I, Torek Y, Misgav R. Effect of cementum defects on radicular penetration of 30% H_2O_2 during intracoronal bleaching. Journal of Endodontics 1991;17:230–233.

21. Simon JHS, Dogan H, Ceresa LM, Silver GK. The apical radicular groove: its potential clinical significance. Journal of Endodontics 2000;26:295–298.

22. Paul BF, Hutter JW. The endodontic-periodontal continuum revisited: new insights into etiology, diagnosis and treatment. Journal of the American Dental Association 1997;128:1541–1548.

23. Goldberg F, Massone EJ, Soares I, Bittencourt AZ. Accessory orifices: anatomical relationship between the pulp chamber floor and the furcation. Journal of Endodontics 1987;13:176–181.

24. Seltzer S, Bender IB, Ziontz M. The inter-relationship of pulp and periodontal disease. Oral Surgery, Oral Medicine, Oral Pathology 1963;16:1474–1490.

25. Seltzer S, Bender IB, Nazimov H, Sinai I. Pulpitis-induced interradicular periodontal changes in experimental animals. Journal of Periodontology 1967;38: 124–129.

26. Baumgartner JC, Falkler WA. Bacteria in the apical 5 mm of infected root canals. Journal of Endodontics 1991;17:380–383.

27. Dahle UR, Tronstad L, Olsen I. Characterization of new periodontal and endodontic isolates of spirochetes. European Journal of Oral Sciences 1996;104: 41–47.

28. Haapasalo M, Ranta H, Ranta K, Shah H. Black-pigmented Bacteroides spp. in human apical periodontitis. Infection and Immunity 1986;53:149–153.

29. Jansson L, Ehnevid H, Blomlof L, et al. Endodontic pathogens in periodontal disease augmentation. Journal of Clinical Periodontology 1995;22:598–602.

30. Sundqvist G. Associations between microbial species in dental root canal infections. Oral Microbiology and Immunology 1992;7:257–262.

31. Sundqvist G, Johansson E, Sjogren U. Prevalence of black-pigmented Bacteroides species in root canal infections. Journal of Endodontics 1989;15:13–19.

32. Thilo BE, Baehni P, Holz J. Dark-field observation of the bacterial distribution in root canals following pulp necrosis. Journal of Endodontics 1986;12:202–205.

33. Trope M, Tronstad L, Rosenberg ES, Listgarten M. Darkfield microscopy as a diagnostic aid in

differentiating exudates from endodontic and periodontal abscesses. Journal of Endodontics 1988;14:35–38.

34. Baumgartner JC. Microbiologic aspects of endodontic infections. Journal of the California Dental Association 2004;32:459–468.

35. Egan MW, Spratt DA, Ng YL, et al. Prevalence of yeasts in saliva and root canals of teeth associated with apical periodontitis. International Endodontic Journal 2002;35: 321–329.

36. Jung IY, Choi BK, Kum KY, et al. Molecular epidemiology and association of putative pathogens in root canal infection. Journal of Endodontics 2000;26: 599–604.

37. Nair PNR. Pathogenesis of apical periodontitis and the causes of endodontic failures. Critical Reviews in Oral Biology and Medicine 2004;15:348–381.

38. Siqueira JF Jr, Sen BH. Fungi in endodontic infections. Oral Surgery, Oral Medicine, Oral Pathology Oral Radiology and Endodontics 2004;97:632–641.

39. El-Labban NG. Electron microscopic investigation of hyaline bodies in odontogenic cysts. Journal of Oral Pathology 1979;8:81–93.

40. Nair PNR. Cholesterol as an aetiological agent in endodontic failures- a review. Australian Endodontic Journal 1999;25:19–26.

41. Silver GK, Simon JHS. Charcot-Leyden crystals within a periapical lesion. Journal of Endodontics 2000;26:679–681.

42. Tagger E, Tagger M, Sarnat H. Russell bodies in the pulp of a primary tooth. Oral Surgery, Oral Medicine, Oral Pathology Oral Radiology and Endodontics 2000;90:365–368.

43. Nair PNR, Pajarola G, Schroeder HE. Types and incidence of human periapical lesions obtained with extracted teeth. Oral Surgery, Oral Medicine, Oral Pathology 1996;8:93–101.

44. Simon JHS. Incidence of periapical cysts in relation to the root canal. Journal of Endodontics 1980;6:845–848.

45. Blomlof L, Lengheden A, Lindskog S. Endodontic infection and calcium hydroxide–treatment. Effects on periodontal healing in mature and immature replanted monkey teeth. Journal of Clinical Periodontology 1992;19:652–658.

46. Jansson LE, Ehnevid H, Lindskog SF, Blomlof LB. Radiographic attachment in periodontitis-prone teeth with endodontic infection. Journal of Periodontology 1993;64:947–953.

47. Jansson L, Ehnevid H. The influence of endodontic infection on periodontal status in mandibular molars. Journal of Periodontology 1998;69: 1392–1396.

48. Rupf S, Kannengiesser S, Merte K, et al. Comparison of profiles of key periodontal pathogens in periodontium and endodontium. Endodontics and Dental Traumatology 2000;16:269–275.

49. Adriaens PA, Deboever JA, Loesche WJ. Bacterial invasion in root cementum and radicular dentin of periodontally diseased teeth in humans. A reservoir of periodontopathic bacteria. Journal of Periodontology 1988;59: 222–230.

50. Adriaens PA, Edwards CA, Deboever JA, Loesche WJ. Ultrastructural observations on bacterial invasion in cementum and radicular dentin of periodontally diseased human teeth. Journal of Periodontology 1988;59:493–503.

51. Bender IB, Seltzer S. The effect of periodontal disease on the pulp. Oral Surgery, Oral Medicine, Oral Pathology 1972;33:458–474.

52. Bergenholtz G, Lindhe J. Effect of experimentally induced marginal periodontitis and periodontal scaling on the dental pulp. Journal of Clinical Periodontology 1978;5:59–73.

53. Gold SI, Moskow BS. Periodontal repair of periapical lesions: the borderland between pulpal and periodontal disease. Journal of Clinical Periodontology 1987;14: 251–256.

54. Ross IF, Thompson RH. A long term study of root retention in the treatment of maxillary molars with

furcation involvement. Journal of Periodontology 1978;49:238–244.

55. Solomon C, Chalfin H, Kellert M, Weseley P. The endodontic-periodontal lesion: a rational approach to treatment. Journal of the American Dental Association 1995;126:473–479.

56. Langer B, Stein SD, Wagenberg B. An evaluation of root resections: a ten-year study. Journal of Periodontology 1981;52: 719–722.

57. Torabinejad M, Kiger RD. A histologic evaluation of dental pulp tissue of a patient with periodontal disease. Oral Surgery, Oral Medicine, Oral Pathology 1985;59:178–200.

58. Wong R, Hirsch RS, Clarke NG. Endodontic effects of root planing in humans. Endodontics and Dental Traumatology 1989;5: 193–196.

59. Abbott P. Endodontic management of combined endodontic-periodontal lesions. Journal of the New Zealand Society of Periodontology 1998;83:15–28.

60. Belk CE, Gutmann JL. Perspectives, controversies and directives on pulpal–periodontal relationships. Journal of the Canadian Dental Association 1990;56:1013–1017.

61. Simon JH, Glick DH, Frank AL. The relationship of endodontic-periodontic lesions. Journal of Periodontology 1972;43:202–208.

62. Rotstein I, Simon JHS. The endo-perio lesion: a critical appraisal of the disease condition. Endodontic Topics 2006;13: 34–56.

63. Rotstein I, Simon JHS. The endodontic-periodontal continuum. In: Ingle JI, Bakland L, Baumgartner JC. Ingle's Endodontics. 6th edn, BC Decker Inc; 2008. p 638–659.

64. Pitt Ford TR, Torabinejad M, McKendry D, et al. Use of mineral trioxide aggregate for repair of furcal perforations. Oral Surgery, Oral Medicine, Oral Pathology, Oral Radiology and Endodontics 1995;79:756–763.

65. Schmitt D, Lee J, Bogen G. Multifaceted use of ProRoot™ MTA root canal repair material. Journal of the American Academy of

Pediatric Dentistry 2001;23: 326–330.

66. Kipioti A, Nakou M, Legakis N, Mitsis F. Microbiological findings of infected root canals and adjacent periodontal pockets in teeth with advanced periodontitis. Oral Surgery, Oral Medicine, Oral Pathology 1984;58:213–220.

67. Kobayashi T, Hayashi A, Yoshikawa R, et al. The microbial flora from root canals and periodontal pockets of nonvital teeth associated with advanced periodontitis. International Endodontic Journal 1990;23:100–106.

68. Chapple I, Lumley P. The periodontal-endodontic interface. Dental Update 1999;26: 331–334.

69. Al-Hezaimi K, Naghshbandi J, Simon JHS, et al. Successful treatment of a radicular groove by intentional replantation and Emdogain therapy. Dental Traumatology 2004;20: 226–228.

70. Buhler H. Evaluation of root-resected teeth. Results after 10 years. Journal of Periodontology 1988;59:805–810.

Chapter | **14** |

Problems with endodontic treatment

P.J.C. Mitchell

SUMMARY

Problems may be encountered when carrying out endodontic treatment. A patient in pain will require emergency treatment. Achieving adequate anaesthesia allows endodontic treatment to be carried out painlessly. However, failure of anaesthesia may occur in acute inflammation; alternative techniques and supplementary anaesthesia may then be required. There may be problems during primary root canal treatment and non-surgical retreatment. These include gaining access to the root canal system, which may entail the removal of natural obstructions, previous restorations, root filling material and broken instruments; there may also be problems with preparation and filling of the root canal system. Complex problems such as instrument removal and perforation repair are often better attempted by specialists. Less complex problems are more easily approached by general dental practitioners. In this chapter, some of the common problems encountered are outlined, the decision-making process explained and the techniques of management described.

EMERGENCY TREATMENT

It is important that a patient who is in pain is rendered comfortable as soon as possible. The practice of treating the patient with antibiotics and analgesics without attempting to make a correct diagnosis and treat effectively the cause of the pain is not to be recommended. Even in an emergency situation, where the cause of the problem appears to be obvious, an accurate diagnosis must be

© 2009 Elsevier Ltd, Inc, BV
DOI: 10.1016/B978-0-7020-3156-4.00017-6

established before any treatment is provided. This can only be achieved by taking a careful history and conducting a thorough clinical examination, followed by appropriate radiographic examination and special tests. If the clinician has no idea precisely the cause of the pain after the initial examination, active treatment should be delayed, as it might be incorrect and may cause the patient harm.[1] This should be explained to the patient, and analgesics prescribed until symptoms change and the diagnosis becomes clearer. The subject of diagnosis is covered in Chapter 3.

Although the following three conditions: acute pulpitis, acute apical periodontitis and acute periapical abscess, cause patients to present as an emergency, it must be remembered that other non-endodontic conditions can cause pain, e.g. food-packing, sinusitis, parafunction, neuropathic pain and temporomandibular joint syndrome. The differential diagnosis of dental pain in general is covered in Chapter 2.

Where the diagnosis is clear, the emergency treatment consists of applying one or more of these basic surgical principles:

- remove the cause of pain
- provide drainage if fluid exudate is present
- prescribe analgesics if required
- adjust the occlusion if indicated.

Acute pulpitis

The causes of pulp injury, its prevention and treatment have been discussed in Chapter 5. The question is often asked: at what stage should palliative treatment cease and be replaced by pulp extirpation? Ideally, the treatment should be related to the state of the pulp, but this can only be determined indirectly. The clinician thus relies on the history given by the patient and a thorough examination. As a rule of thumb, if the pulp of a mature permanent tooth causes severe and prolonged pain even after exciting factors such as thermal stimuli are removed or the patient is woken at night with pain, then it is likely that the pulp has been irreversibly damaged and pulp extirpation is indicated. The pulp may die even when the symptoms are, apparently those of reversible pulpitis. In a survey of cracked teeth, 20% of teeth without spontaneous pain or short-term response to cold eventually became necrotic.[2] Emergency pulpotomy can usually achieve pain relief, if the clinician does not have time to extirpate the entire pulp.[3] It may be difficult to anaesthetize an acutely inflamed pulp and this problem is covered later in this chapter. Antibiotics have no role in treating irreversible pulpitis.[4]

Acute apical periodontitis

This may be defined as acute inflammation of the periodontium. It is often a direct result of irritation through infection of the root canal system,[5] and may be associated with acute pulpitis. A purulent exudate is not present periapically, and treatment consists of removing any pulp remnants from the root canals, irrigation of the canal system with sodium hypochlorite, drying the canals, sealing in an antibacterial dressing such as calcium hydroxide, and closure of the access cavity. The importance of cleaning the root canal system thoroughly cannot be overemphasized, and the use of ultrasonic instruments that have an internal irrigating facility helps considerably. This approach to treatment has been widely adopted by practising endodontists.[6,7]

Care must be taken not to irritate the periapical tissues by extruding infected intracanal material through the apical foramen. Likewise, over-medicating the canal with an irritant drug may cause it to diffuse periapically and cause inflammation or damage to apical tissues; this is covered later in the chapter. An intracanal medicament is only placed as an empty canal can become rapidly recolonized with bacteria.[8] When a medicament is used, there is little evidence to show that the choice of medicament has any influence on postoperative pain.[9,10]

The tooth may be slightly extruded and the occlusion can be relieved by grinding either the tooth itself or, in exceptional circumstances, the opposing tooth. The guiding principle on occlusal reduction should be to do no permanent harm. However, it was suggested that occlusal reduction is more effective when treating teeth with irreversible pulpitis rather than apical periodontitis.[11] Clinically, heavily worn or heavily restored teeth that require root canal treatment may need to be protected against fracture by placement of an orthodontic band; in these cases the occlusion should be adjusted. The importance of preventing a tooth from fracturing by placing a band, to act as a splint cannot be overemphasized.

Acute periapical abscess

This condition may develop as a sequel to acute apical periodontitis or present as an acute phase of chronic apical periodontitis. Accurate diagnosis may sometimes be difficult. It is common for adjacent teeth to be tender to pressure. It is essential to carry out sensitivity testing of the adjacent teeth so that the correct tooth is treated. Radiography may not be helpful as acute lesions do not become radiologically visible until bone, including the cortical plates, has been resorbed. It is often useful to take a bitewing radiograph as well as a periapical radiograph for diagnostic purposes; coronal leakage or caries may be more evident.

Where a soft tissue swelling exists, the diagnosis is generally easier, but it is important to verify the tooth that is related to the swelling. Relief of pain can be obtained speedily by obtaining drainage and adjusting the occlusion of the causative tooth. The practice of prescribing antibiotics without obtaining drainage is incorrect, and unnecessarily prolongs the patient's misery. Opening into the pulp chamber may cause considerable discomfort because of vibration, but this can be minimized by stabilizing the tooth with fingers, and obtaining access with a small round bur in a high-speed turbine handpiece.

Ideally, the tooth should be allowed to drain until the discharge stops and then the canals irrigated gently with sodium hypochlorite, cleaned of debris and prepared fully, dressed and sealed as normal. Such a regime rarely leads to complications.[12] However, this is not always possible either because of lack of time, the tooth is exceedingly tender or there is copious discharge of exudate. In that case, it is permissible to leave the tooth on open drainage for no longer than 24 hours. At the end of this period the patient should be seen again and the root canal system cleaned of debris, irrigated with sodium hypochlorite and instrumented prior to closure. It is important that the root canal is cleaned and sealed as soon as possible so that food does not pack into the canal and invading microorganisms do not cause a further acute flare-up. The practice of leaving the canal open for weeks, if not months, has nothing to commend it[13] and usually leads to periodic 'flare-ups' due to reinfection from the oral cavity by microorganisms that may be more difficult to eliminate. Leaving the access cavity open for a long period may also lead to caries in the pulp chamber and may make subsequent restoration of the tooth very difficult, if not impossible.

If a tooth is symptom-free while on open drainage but flares up as soon as it is sealed, then the thoroughness of debridement must be questioned. This is probably the commonest cause of postoperative flare-up, for no tooth will settle until the root canal system is thoroughly cleaned. The coronal seal must be effective so if the clinical crown contains caries or inadequate restorations, these must be removed. Sometimes because of anatomical difficulties, or the presence of an immovable obstruction in the root canal, it may not be possible to obtain drainage through the canal. In such instances emergency treatment will depend on the presence or absence of swelling. If a swelling is present and fluctuant, incision and drainage, or aspiration through a large bore needle into a syringe are advisable and this generally relieves acute pain. If there is no swelling, supportive antibiotic therapy may be appropriate, followed by non-surgical or surgical endodontic treatment (see Chapter 10) when the acute symptoms have subsided.

Acute flare-up

Following instrumentation of a symptom-free tooth, in the majority of cases, the patient can expect little pain. If the patient has severe pain, or an established periapical lesion prior to treatment, the likelihood of severe postoperative pain is higher.[9,14] The intensity of pain will reduce with time and is substantially helped by prescribing anal-

gesics so that the pain intensity is reduced after 24 to 48 hours. Patients who present with pain and swelling during a flare-up are best managed by prescribing analgesics and antibiotics.[9] If tolerated, ibuprofen prescribed in 600–800 mg doses is one of the most effective non-steriodal anti-inflammatory drugs for acute dental pain.[15] If the patient is unable to tolerate ibuprofen or aspirin, then paracetamol (acetaminophen) is the analgesic of choice. Flare-ups are more likely to occur in teeth with necrotic pulps,[16,17,18] and with atopic patients, for example, those who suffer from allergies.[17] The incidence of flare-ups has been reported to be as low as 2.5% in teeth undergoing root canal treatment;[18] this is a reflection of the high standard of treatment. A much higher incidence of pain could be expected where treatment is inadequate, or infected debris is extruded through the apical foramen. The incidence of extrusion of debris through the apical foramen is lower when the root canal is prepared using a Crown-down approach and with a Balanced-force technique, than with a Step-back approach and a filing technique.[19]

FAILURE OF ANAESTHESIA IN ACUTE INFLAMMATION

Profound analgesia is essential for pulpotomy or vital pulp extirpation, yet there are occasions where, in spite of normally sufficient dosage and satisfactory technique, adequate analgesia is not obtained. Such occasions are distressing for the patient and embarrassing for the dentist. The main reasons for failure are given below and the subject has been reviewed.[20]

The term 'hot tooth' has been used to describe such a situation. The tooth may be excessively stimulated by heat or cold, and may be tender to bite; it may be difficult, if not impossible, to achieve analgesia of sufficient depth despite repeated local anaesthetic injections. The reasons for this failure are not entirely clear although various explanations have been proposed:

- Pulpal inflammation in the affected tooth produces chemical mediators which cause hyperexcitability of the nerve fibres, particularly C-fibres. The local anaesthetic solution is, therefore, unable to block the conduction of all these impulses.[21]
- There is usually increased vascularity of the tissues in the region of the inflamed tooth and hence the local anaesthetic may be more rapidly removed by the bloodstream, shortening its period of duration.[22]
- It has been shown that there is a tendency for inflammation to increase sensory nerve transmission so countering the effects of anaesthetics.[23]
- There is a possible spread of inflammatory mediators along the myelin sheaths of nerves, which restrict the absorption of the local anaesthetic; this is likely to contribute only a small part.[24]

- The pH of inflammatory products in the region of the tooth may be more acidic, thus making the local anaesthetic solution potentially less effective; however, this is considered unlikely.[22]

Alternative anaesthetic techniques

In endodontic practice, the failure to obtain analgesia ultimately is an infrequent occurrence, and when it does occur it is likely to be with a mandibular molar tooth.[25] It must be noted that an acutely inflamed pulp can remain very painful, in spite of what appears to be an otherwise satisfactory inferior dental nerve block injection. In such instances, several alternative techniques are available:

- application of a sedative dressing to the pulp
- intrapulpal anaesthesia
- intraosseous anaesthesia
- sedation.

Application of a sedative dressing to the pulp

Occasionally, the kindest management of the patient is to accept failure of local anaesthesia, dress the tooth to reduce pulpal inflammation and attempt pulpal extirpation on a subsequent occasion. The pulp may be sedated with a zinc oxide–eugenol dressing,[26] or with a corticosteroid-antibiotic dressing.[27,28]

If the pulp has been exposed and is inflamed, it bleeds copiously and should be allowed to do so for 2–3 minutes to wash out inflammatory mediators. The exposure is then covered with a pledget of cotton wool damped with a medicament such as Ledermix (Haupt Pharma GmbH, Wolfratshausen, Germany). The cotton wool is covered by a fortified zinc oxide–eugenol cement. On the subsequent visit, a local anaesthetic should again be given, and when it appears effective the pulp should be extirpated. It is usually possible to achieve effective anaesthesia, when it had not been on the previous occasion.

Intrapulpal anaesthesia

This may be used to supplement existing inadequate anaesthesia. The technique consists of injecting local anaesthetic solution into the pulp. The needle is advanced into the pulp chamber and the solution injected under pressure; initial pain may be reduced by placing topical anaesthetic gel on the exposed pulp prior to injection. Most topical anaesthetic gels contain either benzocaine or lidocaine (lignocaine) at concentrations of 20–30%. Intracanal use of a topical anaesthetic is also helpful when 'hot' vital pulp tissue is encountered apically.

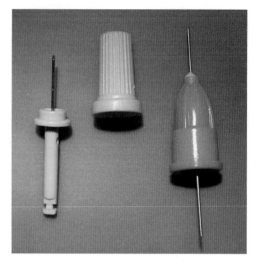

Figure 14.1 Stabident system, consisting of the perforator, perforator cap and injection needle.

Intraosseous anaesthesia

Intraosseous injections of anaesthetic may be delivered either via the periodontal ligament or through the cortical plate. They may be used to supplement existing inadequate anaesthesia.[25] In the case of periodontal ligament injections, special syringes allow small, preset increments of anaesthetic solution to be injected intraosseously through the periodontal ligament. The anaesthetic capsule is inserted into an autoclavable protective sleeve to guard against breakage and a 30-gauge ultra-short needle is used to inject the solution into the ligament. Prior to injection, the gingival sulcus must be disinfected and the soft tissues anaesthetized to reduce discomfort during injection. The primary injection is given on the distal aspect of the tooth, and the needle with the bevel towards the root face is slid into the periodontal ligament space until it is stopped by alveolar bone. The lever is squeezed extremely slowly and about 0.2 ml of anaesthetic solution deposited. The procedure may be repeated on the mesial aspect of the tooth, and in the case of molars on other surfaces.

Intraosseous anaesthetic techniques such as the Stabident system (Fairfax Dental, Miami, FL, USA) use a small disposable 'perforator' to create a hole in the cortical plate of bone through the attached gingiva (Fig 14.1). The soft tissues must be adequately anaesthetized first. Anaesthetic is then delivered into the cancellous bone, within the mandible or maxilla, with a matching needle. Both periodontal ligament injection and injection through the cortical plate produce effective and rapid intraosseous anaesthesia.

These techniques have some disadvantages:

- Infection can be introduced into the tissues unless the soft tissues have been disinfected beforehand.

- The injections are painful unless surface anaesthetic and/or conventional anaesthetic have been administered first.
- Adrenaline (epinephrine) injected intraosseously is rapidly absorbed intravenously. This may result in a noticeable tachycardia. It may, therefore, be wise to use non-adrenaline containing anaesthetics for these injections in patients with cardiac conditions.
- Periodontal ligament injections alter the occlusion of the tooth very slightly by raising it out of its socket, and a careful check of the occlusion of the temporary restoration must be made.
- The anaesthetic is usually only effective for periods of up to 30 minutes.
- It may be difficult to locate the entrance created with the perforator with the injection needle. The X-Tip system (Dentsply, Addlestone, Surrey, UK) overcomes this problem by using a hollow perforator through which the injection needle can be inserted.

Sedation

There are rare and exceptional cases where the use of relative analgesia or intravenous sedation is the only way that a vital pulp can be extirpated, or an abscess drained. Generally, the reasons are not related to the effectiveness of local anaesthesia but to the attitude of the patient. In such instances, before embarking on such a course, the clinician must be satisfied that the patient is fit, the tooth is of sufficient importance to the patient's well-being, and that the patient will accept subsequent treatment without recourse to further intravenous sedation. For further information on sedation the reader is referred elsewhere.[29,30,31,32]

PROBLEMS WITH PREPARATION OF THE ROOT CANAL SYSTEM

Access cavity preparation

The preoperative radiograph must be examined carefully prior to beginning root canal treatment in order to detect the position of the coronal pulp chamber, the position of the canals and the presence of any obstructions that might prevent instrumentation. Access cavity position may vary in teeth that have been 'occlusally realigned' with cast restorations. It is essential to prepare a sufficiently large access cavity so that there are no visual or physical restrictions; the entire roof of the pulp chamber should be removed. If the tooth has been restored with a satisfactory crown, it may be left in place during endodontic treatment. Removal of the crown with a crown and bridge remover (see below) may improve access but hinder rubber dam placement. Use of magnification and axial light will eliminate most access problems when working through a crown. If the crown is technically deficient or secondary caries is present, it should be removed along with any caries, prior to endodontic treatment. Pulp space anatomy and access cavities are covered in Chapter 4.

Problems with primary preparation of the root canal

During primary (non-retreatment) preparation of the root canal, the clinician may encounter various natural problems, which may hinder biomechanical debridement of the entire root canal system. These include intracanal hard tissue formation and acute canal curvature.

Intracanal hard tissue formation

Pulp stones

Pulp stones are not uncommon and may be identified from preoperative radiographs; they normally present little difficulty in removal when ultrasonic instrumentation is utilized. Piezo-electric powered ultrasonic devices are far more efficient for this purpose than magnetostrictive units. The instrument should be worked around the edge of the stone until it becomes loose. It is more difficult, however, to remove a stone from a root canal, particularly if it is attached to the canal wall. In such an instance, if a file can be passed alongside the stone, it may be removed by careful filing.

Tertiary dentine

Tertiary dentine is formed as a sequel to microbiological or physical trauma. Careful examination of the pulp space on the preoperative radiograph will show its size and to what extent it has been filled with tertiary dentine. The depth of the floor of the pulp chamber from the occlusal surface of the tooth should be assessed from the preoperative radiograph; it is essential to have an undistorted image. This should help prevent damage to the floor of the pulp chamber. Tertiary dentine in the original pulp space should be removed carefully with an ultrasonic instrument or a long-shank bur in the slow-speed handpiece. Diamond-coated ultrasonic tips (CPR tips, Sybron Endo, Orange, CA, USA) or periodontal scaling tips (PS tips, EMS, Nyon, Switzerland) are particularly well suited to removing tertiary dentine. They are designed for piezo-electric ultrasonic units and should be used with copious coolant; inadequate cooling may cause burning of the dentine.

Good lighting and magnification is helpful as this dentine is normally very different in colour and texture to primary dentine; it may vary from being porous and yellow in colour to hard, dark and dense. Use of an endodontic explorer (DG16) is highly recommended to help detect the canal orifices. Periodically, the operator should stop and assess whether the cavity is in the correct position. Where the pulp chamber is only partially obliterated, the patent canal orifices are useful landmarks for orientation. If a canal orifice remains elusive, a radiograph should be taken to check that the cavity is not deviating off course in a mesio-distal direction. Once the explorer will stick in the canal orifice, it is usually possible to negotiate the canal with a fine file (e.g. ISO size 06).

Canals that are completely calcified from the pulp chamber to the apical foramen are very rare. Calcification normally begins in the pulp chamber and continues in an apical direction as a result of mild pulpal inflammation.

Sometimes, canals that look completely calcified on a radiograph can be instrumented because a very fine pathway remains within the calcified material. This may not be visible on the radiograph because of inadequate contrast or large film-grain size. For this reason, where endodontic treatment is indicated, an attempt should normally be made to negotiate a fine canal using a small sized file (e.g. ISO size 06), rather than opting for surgery in the first instance (Fig. 14.2). The tertiary dentine which occludes the canal should be removed with an ultrasonic instrument or a long-shank bur in a slow-speed handpiece. Intracanal tertiary dentine is usually much darker than primary dentine, and so magnification and illumination are once again, of great help. Once the canal is patent, preparation is relatively simple. A lubricant with chelating properties such as Slickgel ES (Sybron Endo, Orange, CA, USA) or File-Eze (Ultradent Products, South Jordan, UT, USA) will help to reduce the resistance of a file in a fine canal. It should be made clear that a symptomless tooth with a calcified canal but no periapical radiolucency does not require root canal treatment.[33]

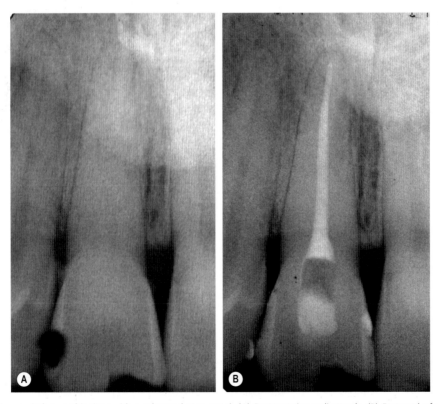

Figure 14.2 A non-vital central incisor with a sclerosed root canal. (A) Preoperative radiograph. (B) Removal of tertiary dentine coronally enabled access to the root canal, which was then cleaned, shaped and filled.

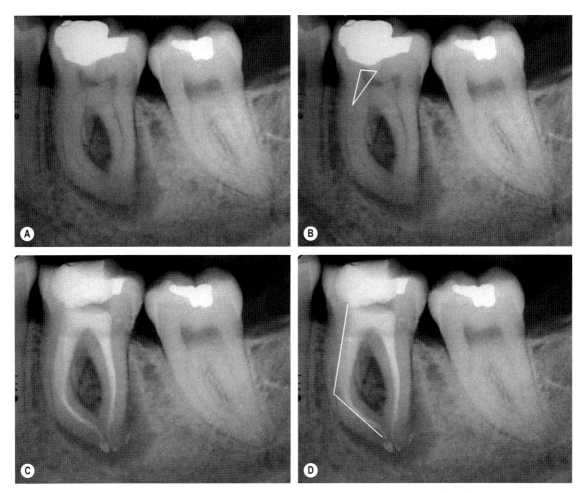

Figure 14.3 (A) A lower first molar with acute canal curvature. (B) Removal of the triangular area during preparation of the coronal part of the canal reduces the overall canal curvature and the stress on instruments. (C) Completed root canal treatment (D) Overall canal curvature has been reduced.

Acute canal curvature

Canals with acute curvature are more demanding to prepare both for the clinician, and on the instruments used. As well as the degree of curvature, the more coronal the position, the harder it is to instrument. Some preparation techniques and the inherent inflexibility of some endodontic instruments tend to straighten the root canal causing procedural errors such as stripping, ledging, zipping and blockages. Canal transportation is less likely when a Crown-down preparation technique is used.[34] If possible, the coronal third of the canal should be opened sufficiently, to allow straight line access to the middle third of the canal (Fig. 14.3). This should not be done at the expense of perforating the canal wall. If the canal is

to be prepared with hand instruments, better results are achieved with a reciprocal technique, such as the Balanced-force technique, rather than with a filing action.[35] The cross-sectional design and material of manufacture of the instrument are of importance in order to ensure maximum flexibility. In general, stainless steel files with a triangular cross-sectional design (e.g. Flexofiles) and nickel-titanium (NiTi) files are most effective.[36,37] Instruments should have a non-cutting tip to reduce the likelihood of ledge formation;[38] they should not be overused but discarded as cyclical fatigue has been shown to be associated with instrument failure.[39] Recapitulation is essential in order to prevent debris build up in the apical portion of the canal and subsequent blockage. Lubricants

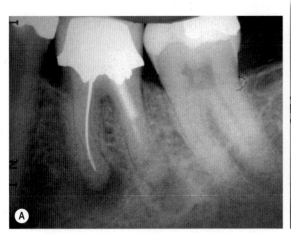
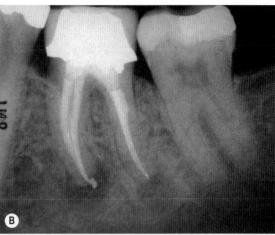

Figure 14.4 A first molar with a silver point and a post requiring root canal retreatment. (A) Preoperative radiograph. (B) The silver point was removed with Steiglitz forceps and the post with ultrasonic instruments. All the canals were prepared and filled with vertical compaction of gutta-percha.

such as Slickgel ES or File-Eze help to increase cutting ability and reduce instrument damage.[40]

Problems with preparation of the previously treated root canal (root canal retreatment)

Iatrogenic obstructions in root canal retreatment include extracoronal restorations, posts, ledges and blocked canals, root filling materials and broken root canal instruments.

Extracoronal restorations

The decision to remove a satisfactory crown prior to root canal treatment may be made to improve access or prevent damage to the crown during access cavity preparation. Improved access may be required for locating additional canals and removing broken root canal instruments. However, removal also risks damage to the crown and underlying tooth structure. There are various devices currently available which may help remove a crown intact. Most rely on the application of a sharp axial force on the crown margin to dislodge the crown. The force may be provided by a sliding weight (e.g. Morrell crown remover, JR Rand, NY, USA), a spring-loaded system (e.g. S-U Crown Butler, Schuler-Dental, Ulm, Germany) or by compressed air (e.g. Kavo crown and bridge remover, Kavo, Biberach/Riss, Germany). In general, cast alloy crowns are easier and more predictable to remove than metal-ceramic crowns, which may fracture. Removal of crown and bridgework intact is, at best an unpredictable process.

Posts

If a post is present and it obstructs root canal retreatment, it should normally, be removed. The method of removal will depend on the type of post present.

Metal posts

Parallel or tapered, passively retained posts may be removed with ultrasonic vibration, a post puller, or a Masserann trepan (Micro-Mega, Besançon, France). Ultrasonic energy may be imparted to the post or its cement lute, via an ultrasonic scaler, in order to aid removal (Fig. 14.4). In general, piezo-electric driven ultrasonic units are more efficient than magnetostrictive units for this purpose; they should be operated at high power with waterspray coolant; lack of adequate cooling will cause heat build-up, which may damage the tooth and the supporting tissues. If cement remains in the bottom of the post hole after post removal, it may be removed with an ultrasonic scaler tip.

Post pullers such as the Gonon (Thomas) post remover (FFDM Pneumat, Bourges Cedex, France) and the Ruddle post remover (SybronEndo, Orange, CA, USA) work by tapping onto the head of the post and extracting it axially using special forceps; the root face is used as an anchorage point. They are efficient at removing both posts that extend above the canal and posts that have fractured within the canal. However, it is inappropriate to try to remove screw posts with axial loading devices as it will lead to root fracture. The Masserann trepan, which is available in different diameters, fits over the post and aims to cut away the cement lute; it works best on parallel-sided posts, and least satisfactorily on oval and tapered cast posts. The Masserann trepan has the potential disadvantage of being destructive as circumferential dentine may be removed with the cement lute.

If a screw post is present, the cement around the head of the post should initially be removed with an ultrasonic instrument. If possible, the type of post should be ascertained and the relevant spanner which was used for placement can be used for removal. Alternatively, the post can be rotated using fine forceps. The tap component of the Ruddle post removal system is designed to screw on to the post end in an anticlockwise direction. This can be utilized with a torque bar, to facilitate the application of force, to unscrew the post.

Posts made from other materials

Post materials such as glass fibre and carbon fibre are designed to be cemented with adhesive luting agents. This method of luting, allied with the fact that these materials are less rigid than metal alloys means that they are unsuitable for removal with ultrasonic instruments or post pullers. Carbon fibre posts can often be split vertically by drilling through with a small Gates-Glidden bur. The remnants within the root canal should then be removed with an ultrasonic file. Some glass-fibre posts may prove impossible to remove and as such, apical surgery may be indicated as per the European Society of Endodontology treatment planning guidelines.[41]

Ledges and blocked canals

Ledges and blockages within canals often occur simultaneously. Inadequate use of irrigant and lack of attention to preparation of a glide path or recapitulation lead to a build-up of debris within the canal. The file, having lost its natural passage to the working length will then create a ledge within the root canal wall. Once created, ledges are very difficult to bypass. If patency to full working length is to be re-established, the canal should first be filled with a lubricant such as Slickgel ES or File-Eze. A small curve is placed in the last 3mm of an ISO size 10 file and the file moved circumferentially around the canal in a watch-winding motion. The file should be of a design with a non-cutting tip, such as a Flexofile. Eventually, the file should encounter 'tight resistance'; the file is now no longer loose in the canal and is engaging the canal beyond the ledge. The file should be worked up and down in a watch-winding action until loose. The next file should pass the ledge more easily, and root canal treatment can then proceed as normal.

Ledging can be avoided in the first instance with generous and frequent irrigation, and if close attention is paid to recapitulation. It was reported that reciprocating or rotary instrumentation techniques tend to produce less canal transportation and apical blockage than filing techniques.[19,42]

Root filling materials

Gutta-percha

Gutta-percha may be removed mechanically, thermomechanically or chemically. If the existing gutta-percha points have been poorly condensed, it is often possible to negotiate a file, e.g. Hedstrom alongside, engage the gutta-percha with a quarter-turn clockwise action and remove it when the file is withdrawn. With well-condensed gutta-percha, the coronal portion should first be removed with Gates-Glidden burs or newer NiTi rotary instruments such as Profile Orifice Shapers (Dentsply). The remaining gutta-percha can then be removed efficiently using rotary NiTi instruments such as Profiles or ProTapers (Dentsply) in the presence of a solvent, e.g. chloroform.[43] Increasing the speed of the instrument to 300–600 rpm may facilitate quicker removal of gutta-percha. Care should be taken to use an instrument with a small tip size so that it does not engage dentine; cutting of dentine at such high speeds is likely to cause instrument separation.

Alternatively, the remaining gutta-percha may be removed with hand files in conjunction with softening agents such as chloroform, methyl chloroform or xylol.[44] Care should be taken not to allow the chloroform to contact the rubber dam as it will be damaged. A file will then pass easily into the mass of gutta-percha, which clings to the file as it is withdrawn. This should be cleaned off before the file is reinserted.

Carrier-based systems

The use of rotary NiTi files in conjunction with chloroform works particularly well for removing carrier-based systems such as Thermafil (Dentsply). The gutta-percha around the coronal portion of the carrier should be removed to a depth of about 4–5 mm. A size 35–40 Flexofile should be carefully 'screwed' in, alongside, to engage the carrier. If the file is then gripped with silver point forceps (e.g. Steiglitz forceps, Henry Schein Minerva Dental, Gillingham, UK) or artery forceps and axial force is applied in a coronal direction, the carrier and remaining gutta-percha can normally be removed in one piece. With chloroform in the canal, any last traces of gutta-percha may be removed with a paper point; this is known as 'wicking'. After all the gutta-percha has been removed, canal preparation proceeds as for initial treatment.

Silver points

Silver points are rarely used as a root filling material today as they do not fill the canal well and corrode easily.[45] They are easy to remove if loosely placed, if the head of the point protrudes into the pulp chamber and it is possible to gain purchase. Corroded silver points or those that are tightly jammed-in are challenging to remove.

If a silver point is embedded in restorative material, great care should be taken not to cause damage when

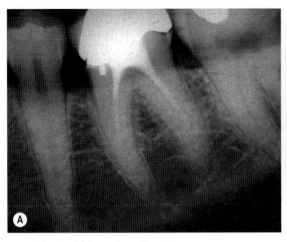
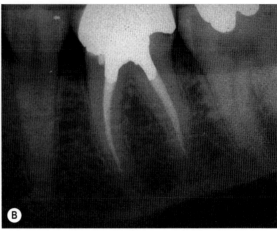

Figure 14.5 Endomethasone root fillings are soft and do not normally create problems for retreatment. (A) Preoperative radiograph of a mandibular molar, the canals were filled with Endomethasone. (B) Postoperative radiograph showing completed root canal retreatment using gutta-percha and placement of an amalgam core in the access cavity.

trying to free the head from the surrounding material; an ultrasonic scaler should be used to remove the last remnants. Once the access cavity is clean, the points may be gripped with either a pair of Steiglitz forceps or a Masserann extractor and removed. Gentle and even pressure should be applied as silver points are very soft and may otherwise break.

If the silver point is entirely within the root canal, removal is more difficult; one or two Hedstrom files may be passed around the point, braided together in order to engage it, facilitating removal. Occasionally, silver points may have been cemented with resin-based sealers such as AH 26 (Dentsply). These silver points may prove very difficult to remove and require long periods of ultrasonic vibration. Unfortunately, because of the softness of the metal, this often causes disintegration of the silver point within the canal. For further information on silver point removal, the reader is referred to a review.[46]

Cement root fillings

Soft pastes such as Endomethasone (Septodont, St. Maur, France) rarely prove difficult to remove (Fig. 14.5); endodontic instruments tend to pass straight through them. Hard setting materials, e.g. AH 26 and SPAD (Quetigny, France), are very difficult to remove; in a straight canal it may be possible to remove such a material with an ultrasonically energized file. Occasionally, voids in the material may allow the passage of a small file. Once the canal is patent, root canal retreatment is relatively straightforward. If a hard-setting paste proves impossible to bypass, surgical retreatment may be indicated.

Broken root canal instruments

The use of rotary NiTi canal preparation systems is now commonplace; research has shown that instrument separation is a small problem and most commonly occurs in the hands of inexperienced practitioners.[47] Management of separated instruments may be considered according to where in the canal the instrument has separated. In essence, the likelihood of removal of the separated instrument depends on whether it can be seen; with good illumination and magnification, this is dependent on whether the instrument has separated in the straight part of the canal or beyond the curve.

Within the straight part of the canal

If an instrument is present in the pulp chamber, it may be possible, provided access is sufficient, to grip and remove it using Steiglitz forceps, a Masserann extractor (Fig. 14.6) or the IRS system (Dentsply). If the instrument is entirely within the canal, removal is more difficult; these cases are best treated by specialists. The most conservative and efficient way of retrieving these instruments is by using ultrasonic instrumentation[48] if the fragment is small, or with a Masserann extractor, or IRS if the fragment is large (Fig 14.7). The instrument should be vibrated using slender ultrasonic tips, e.g. ProUltra titanium tips (Dentsply) or an ultrasonic file. As most separated endodontic files and burs have flutes which are wound in a clockwise direction, the ultrasonic tip should be applied in an anticlockwise direction around the instrument until it is worked loose (Fig. 14.8). In the case of spiral fillers, however, the reverse is true. Care should be taken not to work in a completely dry field as ultrasonic energy can create significant heat

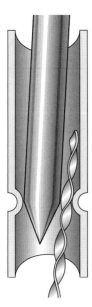

Figure 14.6 Diagram of a Masserann extractor, which contains a tube with a constriction; into this a stylet is inserted to trap the broken instrument against the constriction. The broken instrument is removed when the whole assembly is withdrawn.

build-up, which may, potentially, damage the tooth and periodontium. Sometimes, if removal is impossible, an instrument may be bypassed, in which case preparation should then proceed as normal. In carefully selected cases, there is no evidence that such an action adversely affects the prognosis.[49]

Beyond the curve

If an instrument is not visible because it has separated within the curved part of a canal, removal is unpredictable, but sometimes possible with ultrasonic instrumentation.[50] Great care should be taken however, as significant damage to the root may occur from attempted removal. If it is not possible to remove the instrument, attempts should be made to bypass and incorporate it into the root canal filling. In some cases, it may only be possible to clean, shape and fill the canal to the fractured end of the instrument;[1] in teeth without periapical radiolucencies this does not seem to adversely affect the prognosis.[49]

If removal is unsuccessful, should the patient continue to experience pain, swelling, or a discharging sinus tract after root canal retreatment, then assessment for endodontic surgery is needed. It is worth pointing out that the instrument is very likely to be made from a non-corrodible alloy (e.g. stainless steel or NiTi); therefore, it is not the instrument that causes any continuing inflammation, but the associated infection.

Prevention of instrument fracture

Rotary NiTi instruments appear to break because of cyclic fatigue, i.e. they have been used too many times,[39] or torsional failure.[51] Current United Kingdom guidelines, in line with that issued by the Department of Health (England) advised dentists to ensure that endodontic files and reamers are treated as single use;[52] this should mean that instrument fracture through fatigue is significantly reduced. Torsional failures may still occur with new instruments in canals with abrupt curvature, a great angle of curvature or curvature in the coronal portion of the root canal; this may be mitigated by regular disposal of instruments and greater use of hand files beforehand. Coronal curvatures tend to place greater stress on the thicker sections of a rotary instrument and they are more prone to fatigue.[53] If the tip of a hand file becomes bent at a sharp angle during use, it should not be straightened and reused but discarded. All instruments should be regularly inspected during root canal preparation for signs of distortion. The breaking of an instrument in a root canal is distressing to the operator and may alarm the patient; its retrieval is also very time-consuming. For these reasons, the use of damaged instruments is a false economy.

Hypochlorite accidents

The consequences of unintentional extrusion of sodium hypochlorite into the periapical tissues have been reported in the literature.[54,55,56] Factors that can contribute to this happening include overpreparation of the apical foramen, a pre-existing open apex, poor working length control and not using a dedicated endodontic irrigation needle and syringe. Irrigating syringes should never be jammed into the apical part of canal and irrigation should always be performed relatively passively without excessive hydraulic pressure. It is essential that sodium hypochlorite is not dispensed in such a way that it may be confused with local anaesthetic solution; severe pain, necrosis and swelling will occur if sodium hypochlorite is injected into the soft tissues.[1]

Sodium hypochlorite is a tissue solvent and is highly caustic to soft tissues at therapeutic concentrations. Contact with tissues may cause acute pain, swelling and bruising[54,57] or even paraesthesia.[56] A case of life threatening airway obstruction has also been reported.[58] The treatment of sodium hypochlorite accidents is mostly empirical and includes further irrigation with sterile saline or water,[54] antibiotics[54] and painkillers. Other treatment modalities that have been suggested include local anaesthesia, cold compresses and antihistamines,[59] extraction of the tooth[60] or surgical intervention.[57,58,61]

In general, extrusion of calcium hydroxide does not appear to cause similar problems as extrusion of sodium hypochlorite and healing does not appear to be delayed.[62] The exception to this is when calcium hydroxide is

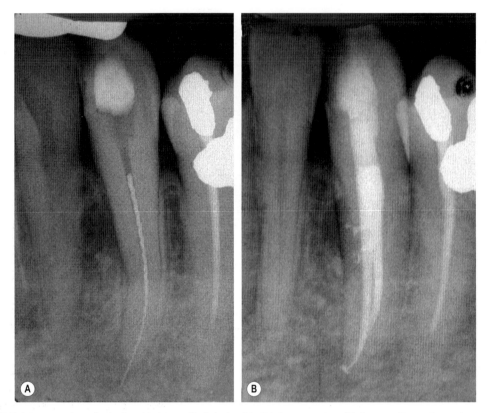

Figure 14.7 A long section of a broken Hedstrom file is lodged in this lower canine. (A) Preoperative radiograph. (B) Postoperative radiograph; the instrument was removed with a Masserann extractor and a second canal was also discovered.

extruded into the inferior alveolar canal; this may cause permanent nerve damage so advice should be sought from a maxillofacial surgeon as soon as possible. One should be very cautious about the use of spiral fillers to place calcium hydroxide in lower premolars and molars for this reason.

PROBLEMS WITH FILLING OF THE ROOT CANAL SYSTEM

Complications during treatment and retreatment can create particular problems in filling the root canal system. Non-iatrogenic problems as a result of inflammatory processes or the death of the pulp in an immature tooth may also pose a challenge.

Non-iatrogenic problems with root canal filling

Chronic inflammatory processes within the pulp may lead to internal hard tissue resorption (internal resorption).

This process ceases following pulpectomy. The root canal shape following preparation, however, is irregular and difficult to fill. Warm gutta-percha filling techniques lend themselves better to this type of problem (Fig. 14.9).

Resorption of dental hard tissue is common in the presence of chronic apical periodontitis;[63] this is known as external inflammatory resorption. In severe cases of external inflammatory resorption, the apical constriction may be lost. This leads to difficulty in creating a sufficiently robust 'end-point' at the apex that will prevent extrusion of root filling material. Over-filling and a poor apical seal are likely to occur. Traditionally, the problem may be overcome by employing a root-end closure technique such as that used in immature teeth but Mineral Trioxide Aggregate (MTA) is gaining wider acceptance as an apical sealant (see Chapter 12); MTA may be used to fill the canal apically (Fig. 14.10) to avoid the laborious process of inducing apical closure. MTA is biocompatible[64,65] creates a good seal[66] and stimulates hard tissue formation.[67] The MTA should be placed in the canal using a specially-designed carrier such as an MTA gun (Dentsply) and condensed with vertical pluggers such as Machtou pluggers (Dentsply). The MTA can be con-

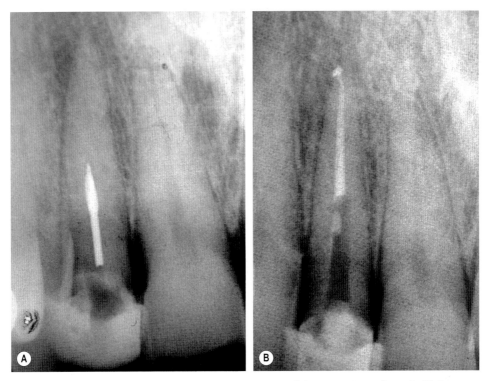

Figure 14.8 A Gates-Glidden drill has broken in this upper lateral incisor. (A) Preoperative radiograph. (B) Postoperative radiograph; the instrument was removed with an ultrasonic file, the root canal treatment completed and post space prepared.

densed further using an ultrasonically-aided file without water spray.[68]

Iatrogenic problems with root canal filling

During root canal retreatment, irregularities within the root canal, such as ledges and elbows are often encountered. An evenly tapered root canal is easiest to fill with most techniques.[69] The use of a warm gutta-percha technique enables three-dimensional filling of irregular canals where cold lateral condensation would not be effective. Dealing with perforations within the root canal system are challenging for the operator. Traditionally, materials such as amalgam and gutta-percha have been used to repair these defects; these materials have been associated with high rates of failure,[70] probably due to microleakage. Modern perforation repair materials such as MTA appear to give good results in the absence of infection.[71,72,73]

In general, coronally-sited perforations should be cleaned well with sodium hypochlorite to disinfect the dentine and sealed as early as possible; this prevents extrusion of infected material through the defect during preparation of the root canal and will reduce interappointment microleakage. Deeper perforations may be created by stripping the inner wall of a curved canal (strip perforations) or injudicious post placement. These are often extremely difficult to manage and should be referred to a specialist. Magnification and good illumination are essential in deep perforation repair. Deeper perforations may have to be repaired at the time of root canal filling.

LEARNING OUTCOMES

After reading this chapter, the reader should:

- recognize some of the problems encountered in endodontic treatment
- understand how these problems may be prevented
- be aware of the techniques designed to deal with these problems
- appreciate how these problems may affect prognosis
- be able to manage the less complex problems
- know when to refer to a specialist.

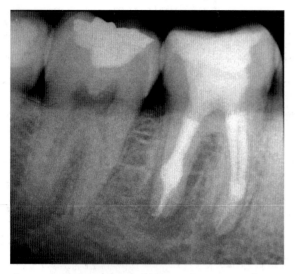

Figure 14.9 A lower molar with internal resorptive defect; this was filled with gutta-percha using warm vertical compaction.

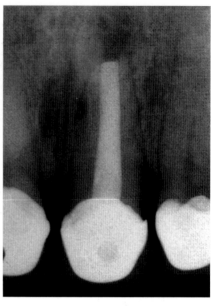

Figure 14.10 An upper central incisor with an immature apex; the root canal has been filled apically with MTA using Machtou pluggers and an ultrasonically-activated file.

REFERENCES

1. Gutmann JL, Dumsha TC, Lovdahl PE. Problem Solving in Endodontics: Prevention, Identification, and Management, 4th edn. St Louis, MO, USA: Elsevier, Mosby; 2005.

2. Krell KV, Rivera EM. A six year evaluation of cracked teeth diagnosed with reversible pulpitis: treatment and prognosis. Journal of Endodontics 2007;33: 1405–1407.

3. Hasselgren G, Reit C. Emergency pulpotomy: pain relieving effect with and without the use of sedative dressings. Journal of Endodontics 1989;15: 254–256.

4. Keenan JV, Farman AG, Fedorowicz Z, Newton T. Antibiotic use for irreversible pulpitis. Cochrane Database of Systematic Reviews 2005, Issue 2. Art. No.: CD004969. DOI: 10.1002/14651858.CD004969. pub2.

5. Hashioka K, Yamasaki M, Nakane A, et al. The relationship between clinical symptoms and anaerobic bacteria from infected root canals. Journal of Endodontics 1992;18:558–561.

6. Dorn SO, Moodnik RM, Feldman MJ, Borden BG. Treatment of the endodontic emergency: a report based on a questionnaire – Part I. Journal of Endodontics 1977;3:94–100.

7. Dorn SO, Moodnik RM, Feldman MJ, Borden BG. Treatment of the endodontic emergency: a report based on a questionnaire – Part II. Journal of Endodontics 1977;3:153–156.

8. Byström A, Sundqvist G. The antibacterial action of sodium hypochlorite and EDTA in 60 cases of endodontic therapy. International Endodontic Journal 1985;18:35–40.

9. Torabinejad M, Cymerman JJ, Frankson M, et al. Effectiveness of various medications on postoperative pain following complete instrumentation. Journal of Endodontics 1994;20:345–354.

10. Trope M. Relationship of intracanal medicaments to endodontic flare-ups. Endodontics and Dental Traumatology 1990;6:226–229.

11. Rosenberg PA, Babick PJ, Schertzer L, Leung A. The effect of occlusal reduction on pain after endodontic instrumentation. Journal of Endodontics 1998;24:492–496.

12. August DS. Managing the abscessed tooth: instrument or close? Journal of Endodontics 1977;3:316–318.

13. Bence R, Meyers RD, Knoff RV. Evaluation of 5000 endodontic treatments: incidence of the opened tooth. Oral Surgery, Oral Pathology, Oral Medicine 1980;49:82–84.

14. Genet JM, Wesselink PR, Thoden van Velzen SK. The incidence of preoperative and postoperative pain in endodontic therapy. International Endodontic Journal 1986;19:221–229.

15. Oxford league table of analgesic efficiency: ⟨www.medicine.ox.ac.uk/ bandolier/booth/painpag/acutrev/ analgesics/leagtab.html⟩.

16. Mor C, Rotstein I, Friedman S. Incidence of interappointment emergency associated with endodontic therapy. Journal of Endodontics 1992;18:509–511.

17. Torabinejad M, Kettering JD, McGraw JC, et al. Factors associated with endodontic interappointment emergencies of teeth with necrotic pulps. Journal of Endodontics 1988;14:261–266.

18. Trope M. Flare-up rate of single-visit endodontics. International Endodontic Journal 1991;24:24–27.

19. Al-Omari MA, Dummer PM. Canal blockage and debris extrusion with eight preparation techniques. Journal of Endodontics 1995;21:154–158.

20. Wong MK, Jacobsen PL. Reasons for local anesthesia failures. Journal of the American Dental Association 1992;123:69–73.

21. Ahlberg KF. Influence of local noxious heat stimulation on sensory nerve activity in the feline dental pulp. Acta Physiologica Scandinavica 1978;103:71–80.

22. Meechan, JG, Robb, ND, Seymour RA. Pain and Anxiety Control for the Conscious Dental Patient. Oxford, UK: Oxford University Press; 1998.

23. Rood JP, Pateromichelakis S. Local anaesthetic failures due to an increase in sensory nerve impulses from inflammatory sensitisation. Journal of Dentistry 1982;10:201–206.

24. Hudson N. Inflammatory conditions. In: Digest Report. Society for the Advancement of Anaesthesia in Dentistry. London, UK; 1960.

25. Cohen HP, Cha BY, Spangberg LSW. Endodontic anesthesia in mandibular molars: a clinical study. Journal of Endodontics 1993;19:370–373.

26. Hume WR. In vitro studies on the local pharmacodynamics, pharmacology and toxicology of eugenol and zinc oxide–eugenol. International Endodontic Journal 1988;21:130–134.

27. Ehrmann EH. The effect of triamcinolone with tetracycline on the dental pulp and apical periodontium. Journal of Prosthetic Dentistry 1965;15:144–152.

28. Schroeder A. Cortisone in dental surgery. International Dental Journal 1962;12:356–373.

29. Roberts GJ. Inhalation sedation (relative analgesia) with oxygen/nitrous oxide gas mixtures: 1. Principles. Dental Update 1990;17:139–146.

30. Roberts GJ. Inhalation sedation (relative analgesia) with oxygen/nitrous oxide gas mixtures: 2. Practical techniques. Dental Update 1990;17:190–196.

31. Scully C, Cawson RA. Medical problems in dentistry, 5th edn. Amsterdam: Elsevier, Churchill Livingstone; 2005.

32. Skelly AM. Sedation in dental practice. Dental Update 1992;19:61–67.

33. Jacobsen I, Kerekes K. Long-term prognosis of traumatized permanent anterior teeth showing calcifying processes in the pulp cavity. Scandinavian Journal of Dental Research 1977;85:588–598.

34. Morgan LF, Montgomery S. An evaluation of the crown-down pressureless technique. Journal of Endodontics 1984;10:491–498.

35. Sepic AO, Pantera EA, Neaverth EJ, Anderson RW. A comparison of Flex-R files and K-type files for enlargement of severely curved molar root canals. Journal of Endodontics 1989;15:240–245.

36. Al-Omari MA, Dummer PM, Newcombe RG, Doller R. Comparison of six files to prepare simulated root canals. 2. International Endodontic Journal 1992;25:67–81.

37. Esposito PT, Cunningham CJ. A comparison of canal preparation with nickel-titanium and stainless steel instruments. Journal of Endodontics 1995;21:173–176.

38. Sabala CL, Roane JB, Southard LZ. Instrumentation of curved canals using a modified tipped instrument: a comparison study. Journal of Endodontics 1988;14:59–64.

39. Haïkel Y, Serfaty R, Bateman G, et al. Dynamic and cyclic fatigue of engine-driven rotary nickel-titanium endodontic instruments. Journal of Endodontics 1999;25:434–440.

40. Yguel-Henry S, Vannesson H, von Stebut J. High precision, simulated cutting efficiency measurement of endodontic root canal instruments: influence of file configuration and lubrication. Journal of Endodontics 1990;16:418–422.

41. European Society of Endodontology. Quality guidelines for endodontic treatment: consensus report of the European Society of Endodontology. International Endodontic Journal 39:921–930. 2006.

42. Pettiette MT, Delano EO, Trope M. Evaluation of success rate of endodontic treatment performed by students with stainless-steel K-files and nickel titanium hand files. Journal of Endodontics 2001;27:124–127.

43. Ferreira JJ, Rhodes JS, Pitt Ford TR. The efficacy of gutta-percha removal using ProFiles. International Endodontic Journal 2001;34:267–274.

44. Wennberg A, Ørstavik D. Evaluation of alternatives to chloroform in endodontic practice. Endodontics and Dental Traumatology 1989;5:234–237.

45. Brady JM, del Rio CE. Corrosion of endodontic silver cones in humans: a scanning electron microscope and X-ray microprobe study. Journal of Endodontics 1975;1:205–210.

46. Hülsmann M. The retrieval of silver cones using different techniques. International Endodontic Journal 1990;23:298–303.

47. Mandel E, Adib-Yazdi M, Benhamou LM, et al. Rotary Ni-Ti Profile systems for preparing curved canals in resin blocks: influence of operator on instrument breakage. International Endodontic Journal 1999;32:436–443.

48. Nagai O, Tagi N, Kayaba Y, et al. Ultrasonic removal of broken instruments in root canals. International Endodontic Journal 1986;19:298–304.

49. Crump MC, Natkin E. Relationship of broken root canal instruments to endodontic case prognosis: a clinical investigation. Journal of the American Dental Association 1970;80:1341–1347.

50. Suter B, Lussi A, Sequeira P. Probability of removing fractured instruments from root canals. International Endodontic Journal 2005;38:112–123.

51. Sattapan B, Nervo GJ, Palamara JE, Messer HH. Defects in rotary nickel-titanium files after clinical use. Journal of Endodontics 2000;26:161–165.

52. Cockcroft, B. Letter from Chief Dental Officer. Department of Health April 2008. ⟨www.library. nhs.uk/SpecialistLibrarySearch/ Download.aspx?resID=260319⟩; 2008.

53. Inan U, Aydin C, Tunca YM. Cyclic fatigue of ProTaper rotary nickel-titanium instruments in artificial canals with 2 different radii of curvature. Oral Surgery Oral Medicine Oral Pathology Oral Radiology and Endodontics 2007;104:837–840.

54. Ehrich DG, Brian Jr JD, Walker WA. Sodium hypochlorite accident: inadvertent injection into the maxillary sinus. Journal of Endodontics 1993;19:180–182.

55. Gursoy UK, Bostanci V, Kosger HH. Palatal mucosa necrosis because of accidental sodium hypochlorite injection instead of anaesthetic solution. International Endodontic Journal 2006;39:157–161.

56. Reeh ES, Messer HH. Long-term paraesthesia following inadvertent forcing of sodium hypochlorite through a perforation in maxillary incisor. Endodontics and Dental Traumatology 1989;5:200–203.

57. Gatot A, Arbelle J, Leiberman A, Yanai-Inbar I. Effects of sodium hypochlorite on soft tissues after its inadvertent injection beyond the root apex. Journal of Endodontics 1991;17:573–574.

58. Bowden JR, Ethunandan M, Brennan PA. Life-threatening airway obstruction secondary to hypochlorite extrusion during root canal treatment. Oral Surgery, Oral Medicine, Oral Pathology, Oral Radiology and Endodontics 2006;101:402–404.

59. Hülsmann M, Hahn W. Complications during root canal irrigation – literature review and case reports. International Endodontic Journal 2000;33:186–193.

60. Neaverth EJ, Swindle R. A serious complication following the inadvertent injection of sodium hypochlorite outside the root canal system. Compendium of Continuing Education in Dentistry 1990;11:474, 476, 478–481.

61. Kavanagh CP, Taylor J. Inadvertant injection of sodium hypochlorite into the maxillary sinus. British Dental Journal 1998;185:336–337.

62. De Moor RJ, De Witt AM. Periapical lesions accidentally filled with calcium hydroxide. International Endodontic Journal 2002;35:946–958.

63. Lomçali G, Sen BH, Cankaya H. Scanning electron microscopic observations of apical root surfaces of teeth with apical periodontitis. Endodontics and Dental Traumatology 1996;12:70–76.

64. Torabinejad M, Hong CU, Pitt Ford TR, Kettering JD. Cytotoxicity of four root end filling materials. Journal of Endodontics 1995;21:489–492.

65. Torabinejad M, Hong CU, Pitt Ford TR, Kariyawasam SP. Tissue reaction to implanted super-EBA and mineral trioxide aggregate in the mandible of guinea pigs: a preliminary report. Journal of Endodontics 1995;c21:569–571.

66. Torabinejad M, Watson TF, Pitt Ford TR. Sealing ability of a mineral trioxide aggregate when used as a root end filling material. Journal of Endodontics 1993;19:591–595.

67. Shabahang S, Torabinejad M, Boyne PP, et al. A comparative study of root-end induction using osteogenic protein-1, calcium hydroxide and mineral trioxide aggregate in dogs. Journal of Endodontics 1999;25:1–5.

68. Lawley GR, Schindler WG, Walker III WA, Kolodrubetz D. Evaluation of ultrasonically placed MTA and fracture resistance with intracanal composite resin in a model of apexification. Journal of Endodontics 2004;30:167–172.

69. Schilder H. Cleaning and shaping the root canal. Dental Clinics of North America 1974;18:269–296.

70. Benenati FW, Roane JB, Biggs JT, Simon JH. Recall evaluation of iatrogenic root perforations repaired with amalgam and gutta-percha. Journal of Endodontics 1986;12:161–166.

71. Lee SJ, Monsef M, Torabinejad M. Sealing ability of a mineral trioxide aggregate for repair of lateral root perforations. Journal of Endodontics 1993;19:541–544.

72. Pitt Ford TR, Torabinejad M, McKendry DJ, et al. Use of mineral trioxide aggregate for repair of furcal perforations. Oral Surgery, Oral Medicine, Oral Pathology, Oral Radiology, Endodontics 1995;79:756–762.

73. Torabinejad M, Chivian N. Clinical applications of mineral trioxide aggregate. Journal of Endodontics 1999;25:197–205.

Chapter | **15** |

Restoration of endodontically treated teeth

F. Mannocci, M. Giovarruscio

SUMMARY

There have been many recent advances in the methods available for restoring endodontically treated teeth. Most are related to adhesive techniques and as a result, composite resin/ceramic materials and non-metallic posts have become popular. These techniques, including the choice of restoration, are discussed in this chapter. However, regardless of the technique or the type of restoration, the survival of endodontically treated teeth may be improved by preserving as much useful tooth structure as possible and ensuring that the stress within the tooth and restoration is kept to a minimum.

INTRODUCTION

The completion of root canal treatment does not signal the end of patient management. The endodontically treated tooth has to be restored to both form and function. In addition, there is now a greater appreciation that coronal leakage may cause failure. Therefore, the quality of the coronal restoration has an influence on treatment outcome. The restoration of endodontically treated teeth has changed considerably in recent years. The availability of adhesive techniques has expanded treatment modalities. Amalgam cores and cast metal posts are being replaced by adhesive techniques and fibre posts; all-ceramic and composite resin crowns are chosen for better aesthetics. Non-adhesive techniques and restorations are still practised. However, in this chapter, the emphasis will be on adhesive restorations for endodontically treated teeth. Consequently, other restorative techniques have not been covered in any detail. The techniques suggested in this chapter are a matter of preference for the authors.

© 2009 Elsevier Ltd, Inc, BV
DOI: 10.1016/B978-0-7020-3156-4.00018-8

EFFECTS OF ENDODONTIC TREATMENT ON THE TOOTH

The fracture of endodontically treated teeth can have dire consequences[1] and, in some cases, extraction is the only possible option. The loss of tooth substance as a result of endodontic and restorative procedures may be one of the reasons for the increased number of crown/root fractures that was observed in endodontically treated teeth compared to vital teeth with similar restorations.[2] The loss of the marginal ridge/s in particular, has been found to increase cuspal flexure *in vitro*.[3] The physical properties of the remaining dentine may also be altered by the effect of medicaments and irrigants.[4] In addition, there is loss of proprioception when the pulp tissue is removed; non-vital teeth have a higher load perception and can withstand up to twice the amount of loading compared with vital teeth before registering discomfort.[5] Other potential reasons for the increased susceptibility to fracture of endodontically treated teeth include changes in the chemical composition of coronal and root dentine as a result of moisture loss and alterations in collagen alignment.[2] However, apart from perhaps a very small increase in the modulus of elasticity,[6] which could be interpreted to be consistent with making the tooth more brittle, most other research has failed to show any change in the inherent physical properties of dentine.[7]

In a recent study on the impact of endodontic treatment on tooth rigidity,[8] access cavity and post space preparations resulted in a significant reduction in root rigidity. In a micro-computed tomography study on extracted premolar teeth, the amount of hard tooth tissue structure lost due to caries removal, access cavity preparation, root canal preparation and post (fibre and cast) space preparation were investigated.[9] Access cavity and post space preparation caused the greatest loss of hard tooth tissue; the loss of coronal tooth structure caused by cast post space preparation was greater than that caused by fibre post preparation.[9] From the available evidence, mostly related to premolar teeth, the loss of tooth structure is the most significant factor in the weakening of endodontically treated teeth. Since adhesive restorative techniques do not require the creation of macromechanical retention, there is, consequently, a reduction in hard tooth structure loss.

SURVIVAL OF THE ENDODONTICALLY TREATED TOOTH

The failure rate of endodontically treated teeth restored with metal-ceramic crowns were reported to be significantly higher than that of vital teeth.[10] However, a recent systematic review[11] showed that endodontically treated teeth restored with crowns have a higher long-term survival rate (81 ± 12% after 10 years) compared with teeth without crown coverage (63 ± 15% after 10 years). Interestingly, in the first 3 years, the survival rate of teeth without crown coverage was found to be satisfactory (84 ± 9%) but there was a significant decrease in survival rate after this period.[11] These results are in agreement with those of two randomized clinical trials on endodontically treated premolars restored without crown coverage.[12,13] Teeth restored with fibre posts and direct composite resin were found to be more effective than amalgam in preventing root fractures but less effective in preventing secondary caries.[13] Therefore, an adequate assessment of the tooth prognosis is essential[14] (see Chapter 3). It was shown that endodontically treated teeth are more often extracted as a result of restorative rather than endodontic failures. It is generally acknowledged that such failures are the result of mistakes made in the treatment planning phase.[15]

TIMING THE RESTORATIVE PROCEDURE

Some patients are willing to go to almost any length to try and hold on to a tooth, even if the prognosis is acknowledged to be guarded. Others may be unmotivated to embark on any complex treatment, or may wish only to invest in options they consider entirely predictable. Therefore, it is essential that endodontic treatment is part of an overall strategic patient management plan. It would be better to consider extraction and construction of a fixed prosthesis supported by a tooth or implant if the restorability is questionable (see Chapter 3). Although finance should never dictate treatment planning, in reality it remains a factor to consider when decision-making. In certain circumstances, after considering the costs of the endodontic treatment and restoration, and reviewed in the light of the prognosis for the tooth, extraction and replacement may be preferable to preservation. If tooth retention is desired, often a combination of endodontic, periodontal and restorative treatment may be necessary to rescue a tooth (Figs. 15.1 & 15.2).

However, once the decision to root treat and restore has been taken, the next decision will be how long to wait after root canal treatment before placing the final restoration. There is no set answer but the following factors should be considered:

- pre-existing endodontic status
- quality of the root canal filling
- position of the tooth in the mouth
- type of restoration planned.

Following completion of root canal treatment, if the result is technically satisfactory and the tooth is symptom-free, it would be reasonable to proceed immediately to placement of the final restoration, especially when dealing with a previously vital, uninfected tooth. Although previously vital, if the tooth is tender to biting or lateral pressure after satisfactory completion of root canal treatment, it should be put on probation for 2 to 3 weeks. Hopefully, at the end of this period, the tooth is more comfortable and the final restoration can then proceed. If not, then an extended period of monitoring or a review of the possible causes for continuing symptoms including the need for retreatment should be considered.

If there was apical periodontitis prior to treatment but the periapical radiolucency is less than 2 mm in diameter and the root filling is satisfactory, then if symptom-free, the tooth should be treated in the same way as for vital teeth and restored without delay. In contrast, if the periapical radiolucency is greater than 2 mm in diameter, the root filling is technical satisfactory and the tooth is symptom-free, a short probationary period may be necessary. Regardless of whether a tooth is vital or non-vital, if the quality of the root filling is unsatisfactory, root canal retreatment should be considered prior to placement of the final restoration. Similarly, in cases where the prognosis is in doubt for whatever reason, it is prudent to delay the final restoration until there is clinical evidence, and in some cases, radiological evidence, of healing. If the decision is taken to wait for evidence of healing, it is imperative that the remaining tooth structure is protected by an adequate interim restoration, which also prevents coronal leakage. If adequate cusp coverage is difficult to achieve with interim plastic restorations, the placement of an orthodontic band is indicated to prevent tooth/root fracture.

RESTORATION CHOICE

The choice of restoration for an endodontically treated tooth is dependent on the amount of coronal tooth tissue left. In fact, this single most important factor will dictate the retention of the restoration and the fracture susceptibility of the tooth. Most randomized clinical trials on the restoration of endodontically treated teeth are focused on posterior teeth. The data on the survival of anterior teeth are only available from studies in which both anterior and posterior teeth have been included.[16,17] The suggestion from existing literature is there is a relationship between the fracture resistance of endodontically treated teeth and the residual amount of tooth structure. Hence, the life expectancy of endodontically treated teeth may not necessarily be increased by the choice of restoration but rather by the amount of tooth structure preserved. Anterior and posterior endodontically treated teeth present differing restorative demands. Anterior teeth may be less prone to fracture but compared with posterior teeth, aesthetics is a major consideration.

Anterior teeth

Composite resin restoration

In anterior teeth where there has been little previous restoration, a combination of composite resin placed over a base of glass ionomer cement may suffice. Composite resin is the most appropriate material for restoring the access cavity given its physical properties, high quality surface finish and the good seal achieved with bonding. Where an eugenol-containing root canal sealer has been used, care should be taken to ensure that the root canal filling is removed to the level of the cervical neck of the tooth if potential discoloration of the dentine is to be avoided. If the tooth is discoloured, bleaching techniques may be used, particularly, if the discolouration is mild (Fig.15.3). Internal and external bleaching techniques may be applied.

Ceramic or composite resin veneers

If the coronal tooth tissue loss is less than one-third, the palatal aspect of the tooth is to be preserved but it is impossible to obtain a good aesthetic result using a direct restoration, then a ceramic or composite resin veneer may be placed. Veneers normally cover the entire labial surface of the tooth including the incisal edge and through to the proximal contacts (Fig.15.4). Ceramic or composite resin veneers are seldom recommended for endodontically treated anterior teeth as it is not easy to incorporate the access cavity within such restorations.

Metal-ceramic crowns

Amongst non-adhesive techniques, metal-ceramic crowns have become the most commonly prescribed indirect restoration for endodontically treated anterior teeth. A reduction of the labial surface of approximately 1.8–2 mm is necessary. The extent of tooth reduction may compromise the strength of the remaining tooth tissue; so caution should be exercised before prescribing such a restoration. Far from preserving residual tooth structure, it may actually promote its loss. In general, crowning of anterior teeth is indicated if the amount of tooth structure left is not sufficient for a direct restoration and for aesthetic reasons.

Gold-porcelain infusion crowns

They offer two main advantages. The labial tooth reduction required (1–1.2 mm) is less extensive compared with that for a metal-ceramic crown; this is of potential benefit in terms of strength and tooth preservation. In addition, the colour of the underlying gold allows for a

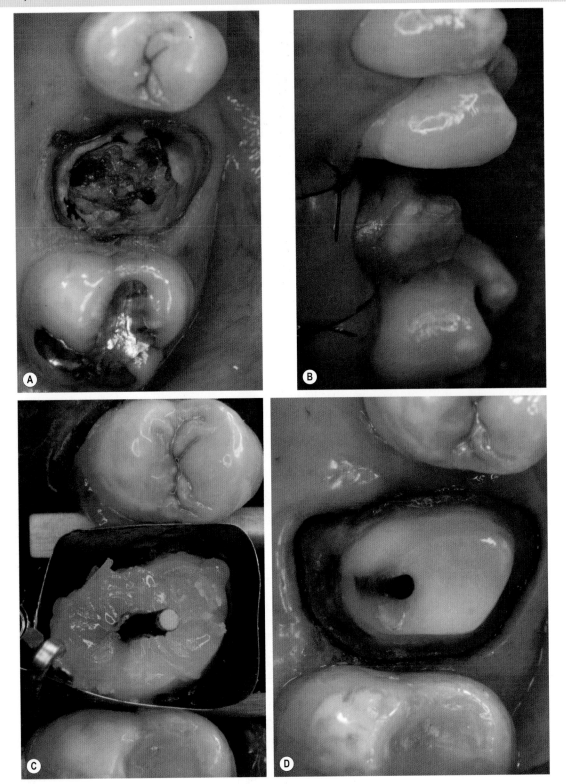

Figure 15.1 A badly broken down maxillary first molar (A) requiring crown lengthening (B) before being restored with a fibre post and composite core (C, D) followed by a metal-ceramic crown (E-G). From Mannocci et al 2008[14] with permission of Quintessence Publishing Co. Ltd.

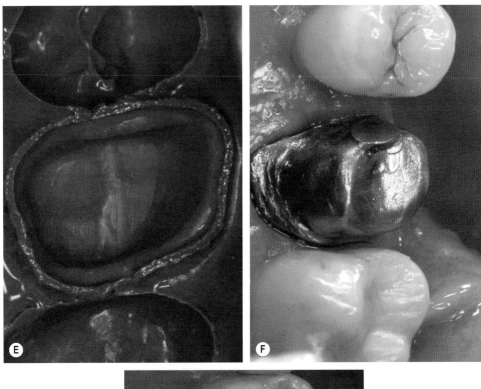

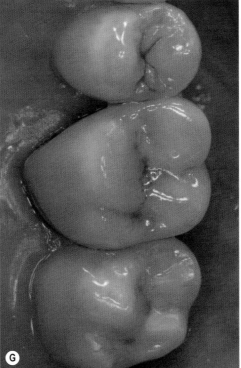

Figure 15.1, cont'd.

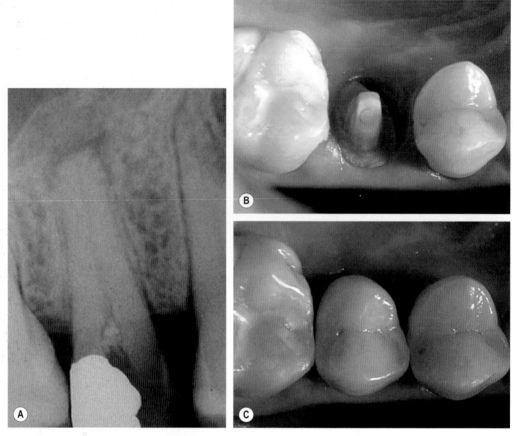

Figure 15.2 A broken down maxillary second premolar (A). Following root canal treatment and crown lengthening, the tooth was restored using a fibre post and composite core (B) followed by a metal-ceramic crown (C).

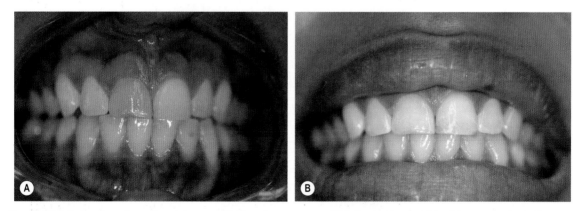

Figure 15.3 A discoloured maxillary right central incisor due to trauma (A) following internal bleaching, an aesthetically improved result was obtained (B) without the need for a cosmetic restoration. Reproduced courtesy of R Moazzez.

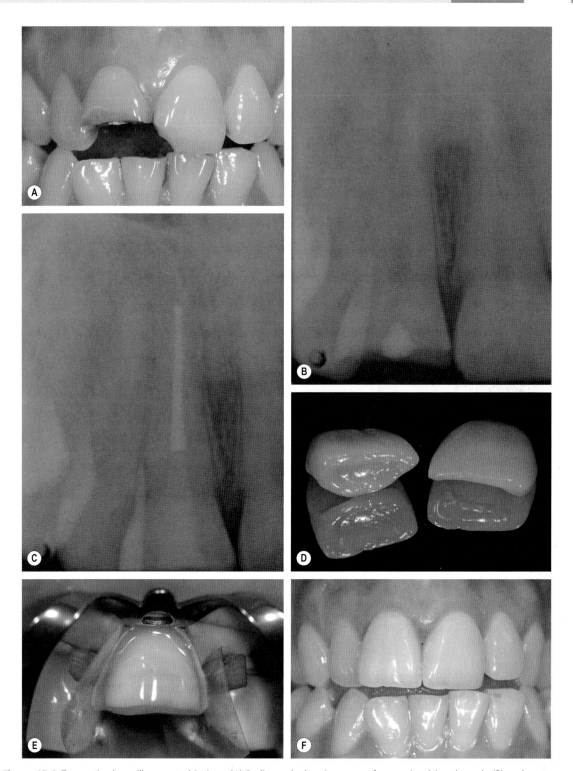

Figure 15.4 Traumatized maxillary central incisors (A) Radiograph showing crown fracture involving the pulp (B) and root canal treatment was needed (C). Ceramic veneers were then made for both teeth (D). These were cemented with composite resin under rubber dam isolation (E). An excellent aesthetic result was achieved (F) and the supragingival margins ensure good periodontal health.

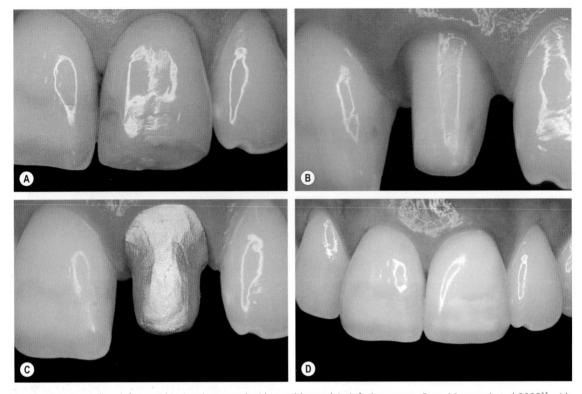

Figure 15.5 A maxillary left central incisor is restored with a gold-porcelain infusion crown. From Mannocci et al 2008[14] with permission of Quintessence Publishing Co. Ltd.

better aesthetic result, especially at the cervical area (Fig.15.5).

All-ceramic crowns

All ceramic crowns are more fragile than metal-ceramic crowns. However, the advantages of all-ceramic crowns are:

- labial tooth reduction required is, again, less than that for metal-ceramic crowns;
- absence of a metallic substructure allows a better aesthetic result, especially in areas close to the soft tissues.

Endodontically treated teeth are often discromic and therefore, opaque ceramic cores are indicated. As abutments for bridges, all ceramic crowns are only indicated for three-unit bridges in cases of high aesthetic requirement; in such cases, a zirconium construction is indicated.

Resin crowns

Resin crowns require less tooth tissue reduction (typically 0.8–1 mm) and the aesthetics is good. However, they are just as expensive as metal-ceramic and all-ceramic crowns, and yet they are not as durable. They may be considered as interim rather than final restorations.

Posterior teeth

Amalgam restoration

A conventional amalgam restoration, including interproximal extension but no cuspal coverage is largely contraindicated because of the high risk of cuspal or root fracture.[18] Amalgam restorations providing a minimum of 2 mm of cuspal coverage was regarded as particularly suitable for mandibular molars but aesthetic concerns have diminished its popularity. In a study on the long-term survival of extensive amalgam restorations that involve the rebuilding of cusps and the provision of auxiliary retention, it was reported that clinical survival was independent of retention method, operator, tooth type and the extent of the restoration;[19] the cumulative survival rate was 88% at 100 months. In maxillary molars, the coverage of the functional palatal cusp is mandatory; the coverage of the buccal cusps may not be necessary if there is no contact in lateral movements. However, in mandibular molars, all the cusps should be covered and protected.

Amalgam restorations are also used as core build-ups prior to crowning of posterior teeth; there are no clinical studies on the performance of amalgam as a core material. The amalgam is packed into the pulp chamber, and if necessary, the root canal space to provide intraradicular retention. If the pulp chamber is less than 4 mm deep, a metal post is necessary to help retain the amalgam core. For intraradicular retention, a minimum of 3 mm of amalgam should be packed into the root canal space.

Composite resin restoration

In general, composite resin restorations cannot be regarded as definitive restorations in posterior teeth except in cases where there has been very limited loss of tooth structure; for example, small interproximal boxes and little or no cuspal overlay (Fig.15.6). There is no consensus on the minimum thickness of composite resin required to protect cusps from fracture. Coverage of all cusps with less than 2.5 mm thickness of composite resin has been suggested. In most cases, the loss of tooth structure caused by proximal caries and the resultant large and deep access cavity makes the placement, shaping and finishing of a direct composite resin restoration difficult to perform. The problem may be compounded if cuspal coverage has to be provided. In such cases, a direct composite filling may result in a poor reconstruction of the coronal anatomy and deficient contact points will not be capable of preventing food impaction. Composite resin restorations are also used as core build-ups prior to provision of crowns. They may be used in conjunction with posts if radicular retention is required.

Gold onlays

Gold onlays may be an excellent option for the restoration of endodontically treated teeth but they have, largely, been abandoned because of poor aesthetics. They have the advantage of allowing for the preservation of sound tooth structure. The impression procedure is relatively simple because the margins are supragingival and periodontal health is easy to maintain. Gold onlays are still appropriate in cases where aesthetics if not a major concern. If this type of restoration is planned, coverage of all cusps is advisable.

Gold crowns

Like gold onlays, this type of restoration is still appropriate in teeth where aesthetics is not of paramount importance such as the maxillary second molar (Fig.15.7), or where there is limited interocclusal space and as bridge abutments. Gold crowns permit the preservation of a greater amount of sound tooth structure compared to metal-ceramic crowns as tooth reduction required is comparatively less.

Composite resin and ceramic onlays/crowns

Such restorations are contraindicated in teeth that are meant as bridge abutments. An initial direct, self-curing composite resin core build-up is generally indicated; the colour should be a shade different from that of dentine, in order to differentiate the composite from the dentine. This core will serve as a guide in designing a cavity for optimal material thickness. Posts are not normally used for retention of the core. The onlay preparation is similar to that used for vital teeth. A minimum thickness of 1.5–2 mm is required for the composite resin or ceramic material. The margins are normally a 90° shoulder finish, and the internal line angles of the cavity are rounded. Proximal boxes should only be extended above the contact points and internal walls should be divergent. Coverage of all the cusps with a thickness of no more than 2.5–3 mm is usually recommended. Glass ionomer cement or flowable composite resin may be placed over the root filling and in the pulp chamber in order to achieve the required thicknesses and internal form of the cavity preparation. Ceramic onlay/crowns are normally cemented with adhesive resins.

All ceramic crowns are not really suitable in posterior teeth because of the risk of fracture; although they are sometimes used in premolars for aesthetic reasons. There is no clear evidence to favour ceramic or composite resin onlays/crowns, but composite resin onlays/crowns are, in general, less expensive and easier to repair (Fig.15.8).

Metal-ceramic crowns

Cuspal coverage is required where tooth structure loss is more than that associated with an access cavity. Metal-ceramic crowns are most extensively used for restoring posterior teeth (Fig.15.1) and as bridge abutments. Unfortunately, a disadvantage is that heavy tooth reduction is necessary to create sufficient room for provision of metal-ceramic crowns.

POSTS

Indications for posts

In the restoration of endodontically treated teeth, the placement of a post is generally suggested if the amount of residual tooth structure is not sufficient to support a core made of a plastic material (amalgam or composite). Composite resin as a core material has been tested extensively in clinical trials. In a controlled clinical study of up to 17 years[17] and another after 5 to 10 years,[20] teeth restored with crowns and composite resin cores performed

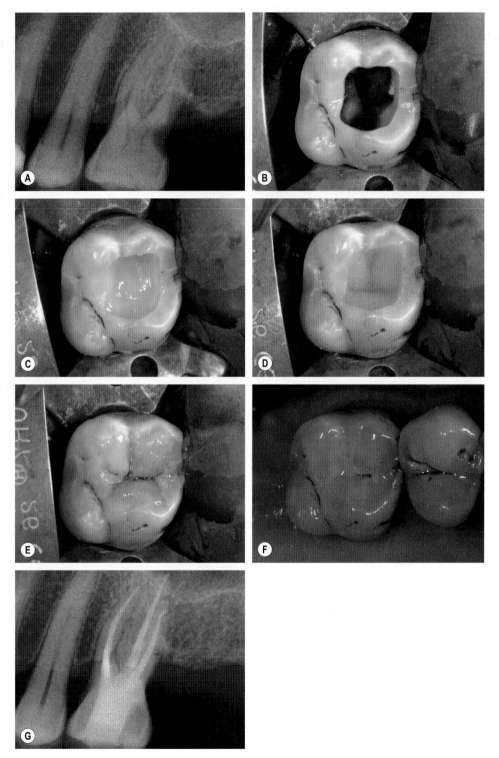

Figure 15.6 A maxillary first molar with distal root caries penetrating into the pulp chamber (A). The tooth was restored with two separate composite resin fillings after completion of the root canal treatment (B-F); this restoration will form an ideal core should a crown be needed in the future. Radiograph following completion of endodontic and restorative treatment (G).

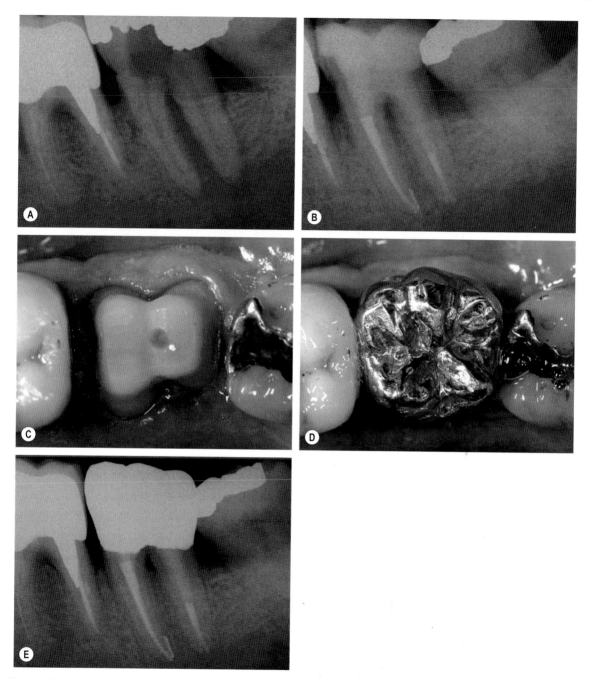

Figure 15.7 A mandibular second molar with a significant interradicular endodontic lesion (A). Following completion of root canal treatment, the tooth was restored with a fibre post and composite resin (B, C), and a gold crown placed (D). The review radiograph after 2 years shows evidence of healing (E).

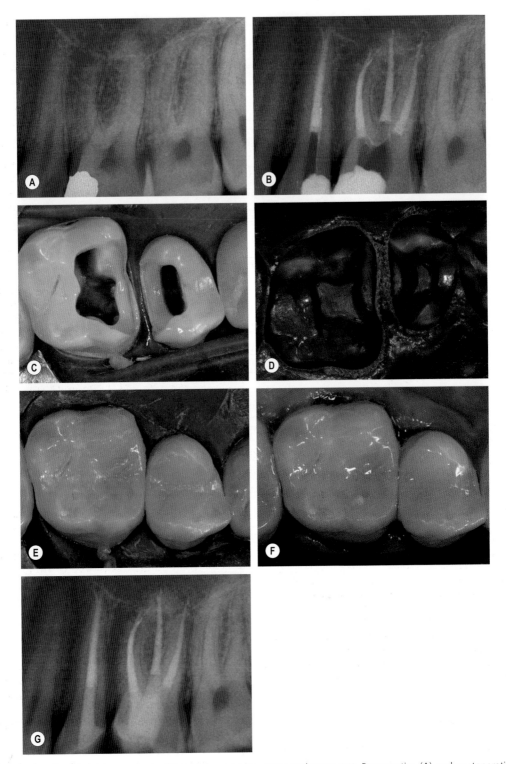

Figure 15.8 Maxillary second premolar and first molar requiring root canal treatment. Preoperative (A) and postoperative radiographs (B). Since there is still a considerable amount of residual tooth structure left (C), both teeth were restored with composite onlays (D-F). Radiograph after completion of endodontic and restorative treatment (G); the composite resin onlays are radiolucent, hence not obvious radiologically.

similarly to those restored with prefabricated metal and cast posts.

The idea that the placement of a post does not reinforce a tooth is indeed very popular and remains debatable. However, this concept was challenged in two recent studies; a 2-year[21] and a 3-year[22] randomized clinical trials on endodontically treated premolars restored with crowns and fibre posts reported the increased probability of survival. In other words, there were more teeth not restored with a fibre post lost due to crown or root fractures.

Clearly there are many clinical cases in which the use of a post is not indicated. The classical example being the restoration of a mandibular molar with a ceramic or composite onlay where there is a wide and deep pulp chamber, and a considerable amount of tooth structure left (Fig. 15.6). In these cases, the preparation of a post space will not only result in a significant loss of tooth structure, but also an increased risk of root perforation.

There is a recent systematic review of the literature[23] on root canal posts for the restoration of root filled teeth. Only one randomized clinical trial was found comparing fibre and cast posts, providing evidence of a longer survival rate for fibre post restored teeth, but the evidence was regarded as weak. In a micro-computed tomography study on the restoration of teeth with three residual coronal walls, the modification of the post space for a fibre post into that required for a cast post of the same size and shape more than doubled the loss of hard tooth tissue.[9]

A recent literature review[24] on clinical studies of fibre posts reported that fibre-reinforced composite posts outperform metal posts in the restoration of endodontically treated teeth; however, the evidence cannot be considered as conclusive. The placement of a fibre-reinforced composite post would seem to protect against failure, especially under conditions of extensive coronal destruction; the most common type of failure with fibre-reinforced composite posts is debonding.[24]

The number of variables involved in designing clinical studies on the restoration of endodontically treated teeth does not allow for its application to all teeth. For example, both the above mentioned clinical studies were carried out on premolar teeth, and clearly the clinical context may be very different, for instance, with anterior teeth or with molars. The available evidence do not rule out the use of cast posts; however, since the use of cast posts may result in a significantly greater loss of tooth structure compared to fibre posts,[9] their use should be limited to those cases in which no additional dentine has to be removed to allow for their cementation.

Length of posts

The rules regarding the length, diameter and root/post ratio are based on laboratory studies[25] or anecdotal evidence. The length of the post classically assumed to be ideal is when it reaches two-thirds the length of the root. Unfortunately, most roots have curvatures that begin far more coronally; therefore, this rule cannot be applied in many cases (Fig.15.9). However, in a finite element analysis, it was shown that the extension of posts to the apical third of the root allows for ideal stress distribution to the alveolar bone.[26] It was also shown that the tensile strength of the dentine in the apical third of the root is far higher than that of the coronal third.[27] In conclusion, a post that is longer than the clinical crown of the tooth is advisable to limit the chance of decementation and root fracture. Longer posts will ensure an even better distribution of stresses; however, particularly in long roots, posts that reach, for example, three-quarters of the length of the canal may be extremely difficult or impossible to remove if non-surgical retreatment be necessary; in such cases, apical surgery is the only option left to address endodontic failure.

Post length cannot be considered in isolation without reviewing the length of the root canal filling that must remain if the apical seal is to be preserved.[28] There does not appear to be a satisfactory answer to this question. The minimum acceptable length of root filling is 5 mm[29] but it is based on the use of traditional root canal sealers and luting cement for posts. With more modern materials, a minimum of 4 mm of root filling should be acceptable to ensure the preservation of an adequate apical seal. If this is not possible, it is a restorative dilemma deciding on whether to compromise the length of root canal filling or the length of the post. If the length of root canal filling falls below 3 mm, the relative frequency of periapical lesions increases significantly.[30]

Diameter of posts

In most cases, if the canal is adequately shaped during root canal treatment, the enlargement that is necessary to obtain a correct post space preparation is minimal; again, it is impossible to define rules that are valid for all root types. In order to avoid root perforations or the excessive removal and weakening of root structure, post space preparation is best carried out by the clinician that root treated the tooth, who is best placed to appreciate the inherent root morphology of the tooth concerned.

The ferrule effect

A ferrule effect may be defined as the envelopment of the tooth structure by a crown. The ability to obtain a ferrule effect is regarded as pivotal to the success of any extracoronal restoration, irrelevant of the core that has been placed. Evidence in favour of this concept are limited to laboratory studies.[31] The ideal extent of a ferrule remains contentious, with the complete envelopment of at least 2.0 mm of coronal tooth tissue regarded as optimal.[31] This should

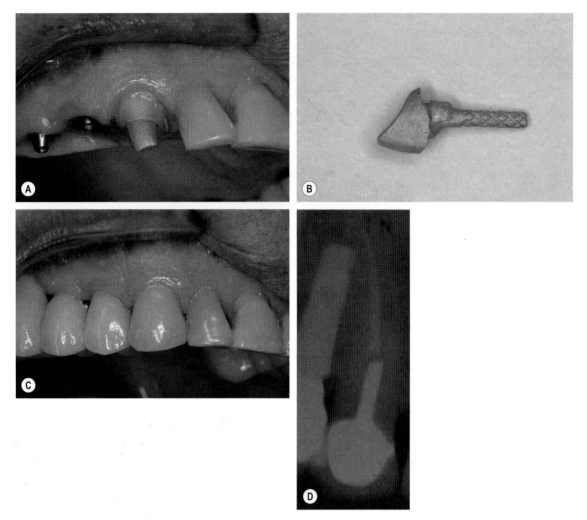

Figure 15.9 A maxillary right canine that looks easy to restore with a cast post and core (A, B) followed by a metal-ceramic crown (C). However, the canal curvature in the coronal third is such that an ideal length of post cannot be achieved (D). Reproduced courtesy of L Howe.

provide adequate resistance to the lateral forces imparted on the restored tooth. Ideally, this ferrule should be continuous around the entire circumference of the tooth.

A recent randomized clinical trial[21] found that in premolar teeth with almost complete loss of coronal tooth structure restored with fibre posts and composite, the presence of a ferrule did not improve tooth survival. Therefore, any ferrule should be considered in the context of the individual case, with respect to the occlusion and the quality and nature of the post and core in that particular case. Adhesive techniques may allow thinner sections of coronal tissue to be preserved in a way which is not possible with traditional methods.

Ideal properties of post/cores

The ideal properties of post/cores include:

- adequate compressive strength
- strong enough to prevent flexion of the core during parafunctional movement
- resistance to leakage of oral fluids at the core/tooth interface
- ease of manipulation
- ability to bond to the remaining tooth structure
- thermal coefficient of expansion and contraction similar to tooth tissue

- minimal potential for water absorption and inhibition of dental caries.

Although not ideal, composite resins have the majority of these properties and are the material of choice as both post and core materials. As a core build-up material composite resin may be bonded to the remaining tooth structure using dentine adhesives.

Properties of fibre posts

Studies have shown that the mechanical properties of carbon, glass and quartz fibre posts are substantially similar; for this reason, the more aesthetic glass and quartz fibre posts have now replaced carbon fibre posts.[32] The modulus of elasticity of fibre posts is generally lower than that of metal posts but, nonetheless, it is three to four times higher than that of dentine.[32] The main difference, in terms of mechanical properties between fibre and metal posts is the loss of flexural strength that affects fibre posts that are exposed to cyclic loading in a wet environment or thermocycled.[32] As a result of this, the mode of failure of fibre post restored teeth is unlikely to be root fracture but normally, decementation that may or may not be associated with the development of caries at the interface between the tooth and the restoration.

The adhesion of the fibre posts to the composite core is mainly micromechanical. The irregularities on the surface of the post provide the retention for the bonding resin. It was reported that silanization of fibre posts may increase the retention of the composite cores[33] but these results have not been confirmed by others.[34]

Clinical and technical aspects of fibre post restorations

Tooth isolation

As with all clinical procedures that involve adhesive dentistry, the use of the rubber dam is preferred.

Removal of the gutta-percha and canal enlargement

This is easily carried out using Gates-Glidden or Largo drills (Fig.15.10A). Heated instruments such as System B (SybronEndo, Orange, CA, USA) may also be used to remove gutta-percha root filling. If a drill is used, overenlargement of the canal should be avoided; it is preferable to filling any potential gaps between the post and the canal with composite resin rather than risk root perforation. The need for a bur matching the post is usually not necessary but if desired, it should be used with caution to reduce the risk of root perforation.

Removal of temporary cement and sealer remnants

The removal of temporary cement and any sealer remnants is easily accomplished with the use of ultrasonic tips and preferably aided by magnification with an operating microscope (Fig.15.10B).

Drying of the root canal

The canal needs to be dried before the application of the bonding system. Paper points (Fig.15.10C) or a controlled stream of air from a Stropko irrigator (Vista Dental, Racine, WI, USA) may be used for this purpose. Once the required size of post has been selected, it is advisable to try the post in the root canal (Fig.15.10D).

Bonding systems

Both three-step bonding systems and self-etching primers can be used for the cementation of fibre posts as the bond strength to root dentine achieved with these two types of bonding agents is similar. The primer is applied on both the root dentine and the post. It is advisable to use a self- or dual-curing resin. Microbrushes are needed to ensure a uniform distribution of the bonding agent into the depth of the root canal (Fig.15.10E).

Composite resin cement

Conventional core or dual-cured composite resins are also preferred for the cementation of the post. These materials have mechanical properties closer to that of dentine. Light-cured composite resins are too thick to be inserted properly into the root canal whereas flowable composite and composite resin cements have a much lower modulus of elasticity and may, therefore, be the weakest part of the restoration.

Insertion of composite resin

In order to minimize void formation within the composite resin in the canal, it should be injected using a syringe with a special tip specifically designed for this purpose. The composite resin is injected into the canal starting from the bottom of the post space until it is completely filled. Ultrasound transmitted via a tip placed in contact with the syringe may help ensure a more uniform distribution of the composite resin into the root canal (Fig.15.10F).

Insertion of the post

The post is simply inserted into the root canal. There is no need to place composite resin onto the post itself.

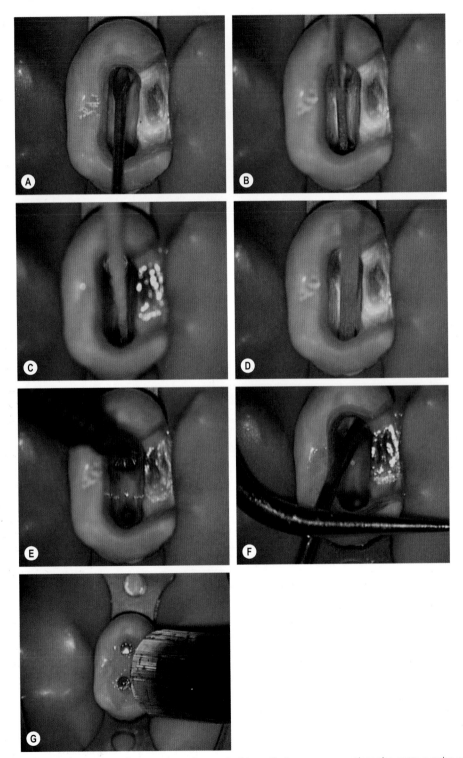

Figure 15.10 Fibre post placement and composite resin core build-up. Post space preparation; the gutta-percha root filling is removed with a Gates-Glidden drill (A). Sealer and temporary cement remnants are removed with an ultrasonic tip with magnification (B). The root canals are dried with paper points (C) and the chosen fibre post is tried in the root canal (D). The primer is placed into the root canal using microbrushes (E); a specially-designed tip is used to introduce the composite resin into the root canal and with the help of ultrasound (F). The core is made with light-cured composite resin (G).

Composite resin core build-up

The composite resin core is created immediately using the same self-curing material. A light-cured composite resin may also be used to complete the core build-up (Fig.15.10G). Following which, crown preparation can be carried out at the same visit.

LEARNING OUTCOMES

Following completion of this chapter, the reader should be able to discuss the:

- effects of endodontic treatment on teeth
- factors influencing the survival of endodontically treated teeth including the preservation of tooth structure and ensuring the stress within the tooth and restoration is minimized
- timing of the restoration for endodontically treated teeth
- choice of restoration for both anterior and posterior teeth, and the different restorative requirements
- adhesive techniques for the restoration of endodontically treated teeth including fibre post and composite resin cores
- importance of the ferrule effect for the success of any extracoronal restoration.

REFERENCES

1. Eckerbom M, Magnusson T, Martinsson T. Reasons for and incidence of tooth mortality in a Swedish population. Endodontics and Dental Traumatology 1992;8:230–234.
2. Gutmann JL. The dentin-root complex: anatomic and biologic considerations in restoring endodontically treated teeth. Journal of Prosthetic Dentistry 1992;67:458–467.
3. Reeh ES, Messer HH, Douglas WH. Reduction in tooth stiffness as a result of endodontic and restorative procedures. Journal of Endodontics 1989;15:512–516.
4. Grigoratos D, Knowles J, Ng YL, Gulabivala K. Effect of exposing dentine to sodium hypochlorite and calcium hydroxide on its flexural strength and elastic modulus. International Endodontic Journal 2001;34:113–119.
5. Randow K, Glantz PO. On cantilever loading of vital and non vital teeth. Acta Odontologica Scandinavica 1986;44:271–277.
6. Huang TJG, Schilder H, Nathanson D. Effects of moisture content and endodontic treatment on some mechanical properties of human dentin. Journal of Endodontics 1991;18:209–215.
7. Sedgley CM, Messer HH. Are endodontically treated teeth more brittle? Journal of Endodontics 1992;18:332–335.
8. Lang, H, Korkmaz Y, Schneider K, Raab WHM. Impact of endodontic treatments on the rigidity of the root. Journal of Dental Research 2006;85:364–368.
9. Ikram O, Patel S, Sauro S, et al. Micro-computed tomography of tooth tissue volume changes following endodontic procedures and post space preparation. International Endodontic Journal 2009;42:1071–1076.
10. Walton TR. An up to 15-year longitudinal study of 515 metal-ceramic FPDs: Part 1. Outcome. International Journal of Prosthodontics 2002;15:439–445.
11. Stavropoulou A, Koidis P. A systematic review of single crowns on endodontically treated teeth. Journal of Dentistry 2007;35:761–767.
12. Mannocci F, Bertelli E, Sherriff M, et al. Three year clinical comparison of survival of endodontically treated teeth restored with either full cast coverage or direct composite restoration. Journal of Prosthetic Dentistry 2002;88:297–301.
13. Mannocci F, Qualtrough AJ, Worthington H, et al. Randomized clinical comparison of endodontically treated teeth restored with amalgam or with fiber posts and resin composite: five year results. Operative Dentistry 2005;30:9–15.
14. Mannocci F, Gagliani M, Cavalli G. Adhesive restorations of endodontically treated teeth. Berlin: Quintessence; 2008.
15. Salvi GE, Siegrist Guldener BE, Amstad T, et al. Clinical evaluation of root filled teeth restored with or without post-and-core systems in a specialist practice setting. International Endodontic Journal 2007;40:209–215.
16. Creugers NH, Mentink AG, Fokkinga WA, Mentink AG. 5-year follow-up of a prospective clinical study on various core restorations. International Journal of Prosthodontics 2005;18:34–39.
17. Fokkinga WA, Kreulen CM, Bronkhorst EM, Creugers NH. Composite resin core-crown reconstructions: an up to 17-year follow-up of a controlled clinical trial. International Journal of Prosthodontics 2008;21:109–115.
18. Hansen EK, Asmussen E, Christansen NC. In vivo fractures of endodontically treated posterior teeth restored with amalgam. Endodontics and Dental Traumatology 1990;6:49–55.
19. Plasmans PJ, Creugers NH, Mulder J. Long-term survival of extensive amalgam restorations.

Journal of Dental Research 1998;77:453–460.

20. Jung RE, Kalkstein O, Sailer I, et al. A comparison of composite post buildups and cast gold post-and-core buildups for the restoration of nonvital teeth after 5 to 10 years. International Journal of Prosthodontics 2007;20:63–99.

21. Ferrari M, Cagidiaco MC, Grandini S, et al. Post placement affects survival of endodontically treated premolars. Journal of Dental Research 2007;86:729–734.

22. Cagidiaco MC, García-Godoy F, Vichi A, et al. Placement of fiber prefabricated or custom made posts affects the 3-year survival of endodontically treated premolars. American Journal of Dentistry 2008;21:179–184.

23. Bolla M, Muller-Bolla M, Borg C, et al. Root canal posts for the restoration of root filled teeth. Cochrane Database of Systematic Reviews, 1:CD004623; 2007.

24. Cagidiaco MC, Goracci C, Garcia-Godoy F, Ferrari M. Clinical studies of fiber posts: a literature review. International Journal

of Prosthodontics 2008;21: 328–336., 2007.

25. Standlee JP, Caputo M, Hanson EC. Retention of endodontic dowels: effect of cement, dowel length, diameter and design. Journal of Prosthetic Dentistry 1978;39:400–405.

26. Lanza A, Aversa R, Rengo S, et al. 3D FEA of cemented steel, glass and carbon posts in a maxillary incisor. Dental Materials 2005;21:709–715.

27. Mannocci F, Pilecki P, Bertelli E, Watson TF. Density of dentinal tubules affects the tensile strength of root dentin. Dental Materials 2004;20:293–296.

28. DeCleen MJ. The relationship between the root canal filling and post space preparation. International Endodontic Journal 1993;26:53–58.

29. Mattison GD, Delivanis PD, Thacker RW, Hassell KJ. Effect of post preparation on the apical seal. Journal of Prosthetic Dentistry 1984;51:785–789.

30. Kvist T, Rydin E, Reit C. The relative frequency of periapical

lesions in teeth with root canal-retained posts. Journal of Endodontics 1989;15:578–580.

31. Tan PL, Aquilino SA, Gratton DG, et al. In vitro fracture resistance of endodontically treated central incisors with varying ferrule heights and configurations. Journal of Prosthetic Dentistry 2005;93:331–336.

32. Mannocci F, Sherriff M, Watson TF. Three point bending test of fiber posts. Journal of Endodontics 2001;27:758–761.

33. Vano M, Goracci C, Monticelli F, et al. The adhesion between fibre posts and composite resin cores: the evaluation of microtensile bond strength following various surface chemical treatments to posts. International Endodontic Journal 2006;39:31–39.

34. Aksornmuang J, Foxton RM, Nakajima M, Tagami J. Microtensile bond strength of a dual-cure resin core material to glass and quartz fibre posts. Journal of Dentistry 2004;32:443–450.

Index

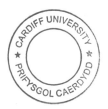